G000036705

Complications of Laparoscopy and Hysteroscopy

Second Edition

Complications of Laparoscopy and Hysteroscopy

Second Edition
Edited by

Randle S. Corfman, PhD, MD
Director
Midwest Center for Reproductive Health, P.A.;
Assistant Clinical Professor of Obstetrics and Gynecology
Department of Obstetrics and Gynecology and Family Practice
University of Minnesota
Minneapolis, Minnesota

Michael P. Diamond, MD
Professor of Obstetrics and Gynecology
Wayne State University School of Medicine;
Director of Reproductive Endocrinology and Infertility
Hutzel Hospital
Detroit, Michigan

Alan H. DeCherney, MD
Professor and Chairman
Department of Obstetrics and Gynecology
UCLA School of Medicine
Los Angeles, California

b
Blackwell
Science

Blackwell Science
Editorial offices:
Commerce Place, 350 Main Street, Malden, Massachusetts
02148, USA
Osney Mead, Oxford OX2 0E1, England
25 John Street, London WC1N 2BL, England
23 Ainslie Place, Edinburgh EH3 6AJ, Scotland
54 University Street, Carlton, Victoria 3053, Australia
Other Editorial offices:
Blackwell Wissenschafts-Verlag GmbH Kurfürstendamm 57,
10707 Berlin, Germany Zehetnergasse 6,
A-1140 Vienna, Austria
Distributors:
USA
  Blackwell Science, Inc.
  Commerce Place
  350 Main Street
  Malden, Massachusetts 02148
  (Telephone orders: 800-215-1000 or 617-388-8250; fax
orders: 617-388-8270)

Canada
  Copp Clark, Ltd.
  2775 Matheson Blvd. East
  Mississauga, Ontario
  Canada, L4W 4P7
  (Telephone orders: 800-263-4374 or 905-238-6074)
Australia
Blackwell Science Pty, Ltd.
54 University Street
Carlton, Victoria 3053
(Telephone orders: 03-9347-0300;
 fax orders: 03-9349-3016)

Outside North America and Australia
Blackwell Science, Ltd.
c/o Marston Book Services, Ltd.
P.O. Box 269
Abingdon
Oxon OX14 4YN
England
(Telephone orders: 44-01235-465500;
fax orders: 44-01235-465555)

The Blackwell Science logo is a trade mark of Blackwell Science
Ltd., registered at the United Kingdom
Trade Marks Registry

Acquisitions: Joy Denomme
Production: Irene Herlihy
Manufacturing: Lisa Flanagan
Typeset by Best-set Typesetter Ltd., Hong Kong
Printed and bound by Braun-Brumfield, Inc.
©1997 by Blackwell Science, Inc.
Printed in the United States of America

97 98 99 00 5 4 3 2 1
All rights reserved. No part of this book may be reproduced in
any form or by any electronic or mechanical means, including
information storage and retrieval systems, without permission
in writing from the publisher, except by a reviewer who may
quote brief passages in a review.

Library of Congress Cataloging-in-Publication Data
Complications of laparoscopy and hysteroscopy / edited by
Randle S. Corfman, Michael P. Diamond, Alan H.
  DeCherney.—2nd ed.
      p. cm.
   Includes bibliographical references and index.
   ISBN 0-86542-507-8
   1. Laparoscopy—Complications.   2. Hysteroscopy—
Complications.
   I. Corfman, Randle S.   II. Diamond, Michael P.   III.
DeCherney, Alan H.
   [DNLM: 1. Genital Diseases, Female—surgery.   2.
Laparoscopy.
   3. Hysteroscopy.   4. Intraoperative Complications—etiol-
ogy.   WP
   660 C737 1997]
   RG107.5.L34C65   1997
   617.5′5059—dc21
   DNLM/DLC
   for Library of Congress   97-15481
                                         CIP

Notice: The indications and dosages of all drugs in this book have been recommended in the medical literature and conform to the practices of the
general community. The medications described do not necessarily have specific approval by the Food and Drug Administration for use in the diseases
and dosages for which they are recommended. The package insert for each
drug should be consulted for use and dosage as approved by the FDA.
Because standards for usage change, it is advisable to keep abreast of revised
recommendations, particularly those concerning new drugs.

Contents

v

List of Contributors

Fred Allgood, CST, SFA
Freelance Surgical First Assistant
Fort Worth, Texas

Salim Bassil, MD
Assistant Clinical Professor
Department of Gynecology
Catholic University of Louvain;
Cliniques Universitaires St. Luc
Brussels, Belgium

Gunther Bastert, MD
Department of Obstetrics and Gynecology
Ruprecht-Karls-University
Heidelberg, Germany

Steven R. Bayer, MD
Assistant Professor
Tufts University School of Medicine;
New England Medical Center
Boston, Massachusetts

Edward M. Beadle, MD, FACOG
Assistant Clinical Professor of Obstetrics
    and Gynecology
University of Minnesota Hospital and Clinics;
Department of Obstetrics and Gynecology
Fairview Hospital
Minneapolis, Minnesota

Charla M. Blacker, MD, FACOG
Assistant Professor of Obstetrics and Gynecology
Wayne State University School of Medicine;
Director, In Vitro Fertilization
Hutzel Hospital
Detroit, Michigan

Philip G. Brooks, MD
Clinical Professor of Obstetrics and Gynecology
UCLA School of Medicine;
Attending Physician
Cedars-Sinai Medical Center
Los Angeles, California

Mary Carter, BS, CST, SFA
Freelance Surgical Assistant
Harris Methodist Hospital
Fort Worth, Texas

Linda M. Chaffkin, MD
Associate Director
Reproductive Endocrinology and Infertility Associates
Hartford, Connecticut

Paula D. M. Chantigian, MD
Obstetrician Gynecologist
Olmstead Medical Group
Rochester, Minnesota

Robert C. Chantigian, MD
Assistant Professor of Anesthesiology
Mayo Medical School;
Consultant in Anesthesiology
Mayo Clinic
Rochester, Minnesota

M. Dwight Chen, MD
Assistant Professor
Department of Obstetrics and Gynecology
University of Minnesota Medical School
Minneapolis, Minnesota

Alan B. Copperman, MD
Department of Obstetrics, Gynecology,
    and Reproductive Science
Mount Sinai School of Medicine
New York, New York

Randle S. Corfman, PhD, MD
Director
Midwest Center for Reproductive Health, P.A.;
Assistant Clinical Professor of Obstetrics and
    Gynecology
Department of Obstetrics and Gynecology and
    Family Practice
University of Minnesota
Minneapolis, Minnesota

Gordon D. Davis, MD
Director of Laser Surgery
Phoenix Integrated Residency Program for
    Obstetrics and Gynecology
McHarry Medical College
Nashville, Tennessee;
St. Joseph's Hospital and Medical Center
Tulane University Charity Hospital of New Orleans
New Orleans, Louisiana

Alan H. DeCherney, MD
Professor and Chairman
Department of Obstetrics and Gynecology
UCLA School of Medicine
Los Angeles, California

Michael P. Diamond, MD
Professor of Obstetrics and Gynecology
Wayne State University School of Medicine;
Director of Reproductive Endocrinology and Infertility
Hutzel Hospital
Detroit, Michigan

Don Dodson, RN, BSN, CRNFA
Certified Registered Nurse First Assistant
Freelance Surgical Assistant
Fort Worth, Texas

Jacques Donnez, MD, PhD
Professor of Gynecology
Catholic University of Louvain;
Head of Department
Cliniques St. Luc
Brussels, Belgium

Lisa D. Erickson, MD
Associate Physician
Abbott Northwestern Hospital
Minneapolis, Minnesota

Jeffrey E. Everett, MD
Department of Surgery
University of Minnesota Hospital and Clinics
Minneapolis, Minnesota

Joseph R. Feste, MD
Clinical Associate Professor
Department of Obstetrics and Gynecology
Baylor College of Medicine;
Clinical Associate Professor
Department of Obstetrics and Gynecology
The University of Texas Health Science Center at
    Houston
Woman's Hospital of Texas
Houston, Texas

Jeffrey M. Fowler, MD
Assistant Professor
Department of Obstetrics and Gynecology
University of Minnesota Hospital and Clinics
Minneapolis, Minnesota

Robert R. Franklin, MD
Clinical Professor
Obstetrics and Gynecology Department
Baylor College of Medicine;
Medical Staff
Columbia Woman's Hospital of Texas
Houston, Texas

William G. Gamble, MD, FACS
Clinical Professor
Department of Surgery
University of Minnesota;
Director, Division of Surgery
Park Nicollet Clinic-Health System Minnesota
Minneapolis, Minnesota

David A. Grainger, MD
Associate Professor of Obstetrics and Gynecology
Director of Reproductive Endocrinology
University of Kansas School of Medicine
Wichita, Kansas

Jamie A. Grifo, MD, PhD
Assistant Professor
The Center for Reproductive Medicine
Department of Obstetrics and Gynecology
Cornell University Medical College
Cornell, New York

George M. Grunert, MD, FACOG, FACS
Instructor
Department of Obstetrics and Gynecology
Baylor College of Medicine;
Director of Assisted Reproductive Technology Program
Woman's Hospital of Texas
Houston, Texas

Muguette Guilbert
CCA
Faculté de Médecine de CAEN
Practicien Hospitalier
Centre Hospitalier
Thonon, France

Gary Holtz, MD (*deceased*)
Clinical Associate Professor
Medical University of South Carolina
Charleston, South Carolina;
Department of Obstetrics and Gynecology
E. Cooper Community Hospital
Mt. Pleasant, South Carolina

Benjamin R. Jacobs, MD
Chairman
Department of Anesthesiology
Paoli Memorial Hospital
Paoli, Pennsylvania

Grace M. Janik, MD, FACOG
Reproductive Endocrinologist

Assistant Clinical Professor
Department of Obstetrics and Gynecology
Medical College of Wisconsin
Director of Columbia IVF
Milwaukee, Wisconsin

D. Alan Johns, MD
Clinical Associate Professor
Department of Obstetrics and Gynecology
University of Texas Southwestern Medical School
Dallas, Texas;
Director GYN Laparoscopy Center
Harris Methodist Fort Worth
Fort Worth, Texas

Piyush N. Joshi, BBS
Professor of Surgery (Urology)
James H. Quillen College of Medicine;
Director, Transplant Program
Johnson City Medical Center
Johnson City, Tennessee

Charles H. Koh, MD, FACOG, FRCOG
Associate Clinical Professor
Department of Obstetrics and Gynecology
Medical College of Wisconsin;
Co-Director
Milwaukee Institute of Minimally Invasive Surgery
    and Reproductive Specialty Center
Milwaukee, Wisconsin

Bertil Larsson, MD, PhD
Associate Professor of Obstetrics and Gynecology
Department of Obstetrics and Gynecology
Karolinska Institutet
Danderyd Hospital
Danderyd, Sweden

Barbara S. Levy, MD
Clinical Assistant Professor Obstetrics and Gynecology
University of Washington School of Medicine
Seattle, Washington

Stephen R. Lincoln, MD
Assistant Professor
Department of Obstetrics and Gynecology
University of Tennessee–Memphis
Memphis, Tennessee

C.Y. Liu, MD, FACOG
Director
Chattanooga Women's Laser Center
Columbia-East Ridge Hospital
Chattanooga, Tennessee

Franklin D. Loffer, MD
Director of Gynecologic Endoscopy
Maricopa Medical Center
Phoenix, Arizona

Anthony A. Luciano, MD
Professor of Obstetrics and Gynecology
University of Connecticut School of Medicine
Farmington. Connecticut;
Director of Reproductive Endocrinology and Fertility
New Britain General Hospital
New Britain, Connecticut

Charles M. March, MD
Professor of Obstetrics and Gynecology
University of Southern California School of Medicine;
Attending Physician
Department of Obstetrics and Gynecology
Southern California University Hospital
Los Angeles, California

Dan C. Martin, MD, FACOG
Clinical Associate Professor
University of Tennessee, Memphis;
Reproductive Surgeon
Baptist Memorial Hospital
Memphis, Tennessee

Peter F. McComb, MB, BS, FRCSC, FACOG
Professor of Obstetrics and Gynecology
University of British Columbia
Vancouver Hospital and Health Sciences Center
Vancouver, British Columbia
Canada

Deborah A. Metzger, MD
Reproductive Medicine Institute
Hartford, Connecticut

Magdy Milad, MD, FACOG
Assistant Professor of Obstetrics and Gynecology
Northwestern University Medical School;
Director of Gynecologic Endoscopy
Northwestern Memorial Hospital
Chicago, Illinois

Robin L. Molsberry, MD
Director
Department of Obstetrics and Gynecology
St. Luke's/Roosevelt Hospital Center
New York, New York

Robert S. Neuwirth, MD
Director of Hysteroscopic Surgery
Babcock Professor of Obstetrics and Gynecology
Columbia College of Physicians and Surgeons
St. Luke's/Roosevelt Hospital Center
New York, New York

Camran Nezhat, MD
Clinical Professor of Gynecology/Obstetrics and Surgery
Stanford University School of Medicine
Stanford, California;
Director
Stanford Endoscopy Center for Training and Technology
Palo Alto, California

Ceana Nezhat, MD
Clinical Assistant Professor of Gynecology and
  Obstetrics
Stanford University School of Medicine
Stanford, California;
Co-Director
Stanford Endoscopy Center for Training and Technology
Palo Alto, California

Farr Nezhat, MD
Clinical Professor of Gynecology and Obstetrics
Stanford University School of Medicine
Stanford, California;
Co-Director
Stanford Endoscopy Center for Training and Technology
Palo Alto, California

Michelle Nisolle, MD, PhD
Clinical Assistant Professor
Department of Gynecology
Cliniques Universitaires St. Luc
Brussels, Belgium

Steven J. Ory, MD
Private Practice
Northwest Center for Reproductive Endocrinology
 and Infertility
Margate/Palm Beach Gardens, Florida

Chau-Su Ou, MD
Assistant Professor of Obstetrics and Gynecology
University of Washington, Seattle;
Attending Physician
Department of Obstetrics and Gynecology
Seattle, Washington

James B. Presthus, MD
Assistant Clinical Professor
Baylor College of Medicine
Houston, Texas;
University of Minnesota Hospital
Methodist Hospital
St. Louis Park, Minnesota

David B. Redwine, MD
Director
Endometriosis Institute of Oregon
Bend, Oregon

Stefan Rimbach, MD
Department of Obstetrics and Gynecology
Ruprecht-Karls-University
Heidelberg, Germany

Scott Roberts, MD, MS
Assistant Professor of Obstetrics and Gynecology
University of Kansas S.M.–Wichita;
Attending, Maternal/Fetal Medicine
Wesley Medical Center
Wichita, Kansas

Jeffrey B. Russell, MD, FACOG
Assistant Professor of Obstetrics and Gynecology
Thomas Jefferson University
Philadelphia, Pennsylvania;
Director
Reproductive Endocrine Division
Department of Obstetrics and Gynecology
The Medical Center of Delaware
Newark, Delaware

Jacques Salvat, MD
CCA
Faculté de Médecine Grenoble
La Tronche, France;
Service Chief
Centre Hospitalier
Thonon, France

Joseph S. Sanfilippo, MD
Professor of Obstetrics and Gynecology
University of Louisville School of Medicine
Louisville, Kentucky

Stephen F. Schiff, MD, FACS
Assistant Clinical Professor of Surgery
Brown University School of Medicine
Providence, Rhode Island

Daniel S. Seidman, MD
Fellow
Department of Gynecology and Obstetrics
Stanford University School of Medicine
Stanford, California

Jeffrey C. Seiler, MD
Private Practice of Gynecology
Columbia New Port Richey Hospital
New Port Richey, Florida

Gerald J. Shirk, MD
Attending Surgeon
St. Luke's Hospital
Cedar Rapids, Iowa

Paul D. Silva, MD
Department of Obstetrics and Gynecology
Gundersen/Lutheran Medical Center
La Crosse, Wisconsin

David G. Silverman, MD
Associate Professor of Anesthesiology
Yale University School of Medicine
New Haven, Connecticut

Mireille Smets, MD
Department of Gynecology
Cliniques Universitaires St. Luc
Brussels, Belgium

Richard M. Soderstrom, MD, FACOG
Clinical Professor of Obstetrics and Gynecology

University of Washington School of Medicine
Seattle, Washington

Christopher Sutton, MA, MB, BCh, FRCOG
Clinical Tutor and Lecturer
Charing Cross and Westminster Medical School
Royal London Medical School
University of London
London, England;
Consultant Gynaecologist
Chelsea and Westminster Hospital
Royal Surrey Hospital
Guildford, Surrey
England

Samuel S. Thatcher, MD, PhD, FACOG
Attending Physician
Center for Applied Reproductive Science
Johnson City Medical Center
Johnson City, Tennessee

John Tripoulas, MD
The Center for Reproductive Medicine
Department of Obstetrics and Gynecology
Cornell University Medical College
Cornell, New York

Togas Tulandi, MD, FRCSC
Professor of Obstetrics and Gynecology
Director
Division of Reproductive Endocrinology
    and Infertility
McGill University
Montreal, Quebec
Canada

Rafael F. Valle, MD, FACOG, FACS
Professor of Obstetrics and Gynecology
Northwestern University Medical School;
Attending Physician
Northwestern Memorial Hospital and
Prentice Women's Hospital and Maternity Center
Chicago, Illinois

Alain Vincent-Genod, MD
CES
Faculté de Médecine Grenoble
La Tronche, France;
Practicien Hospitalier
Centre Hospitalier
Thonon, France

Diethelm Wallwiener, MD
Department of Obstetrics and Gynecology
Ruprecht-Karls-University
Heidelberg, Germany

James M. Wheeler, MD, MPH
Attending Physician
Woman's Hospital of Texas
Houston, Texas

Christina Williams, MD, FRCS
Fellow
Department of Obstetrics and Gynecology
University of British Columbia;
Vancouver Hospital and Health Sciences
    Center
Vancouver, British Columbia
Canada

Preface to Second Edition

A great amount of water has passed under the bridge, so to speak, since the writing of the inaugural edition of *Complications of Laparoscopy and Hysteroscopy*. The text was published at what appears to have been the peak of entry of new techniques and technology to endoscopic surgery. It was with some trepidation that we, as surgeons, approached these new entries in the surgical repertoire, particularly in light of the fact that new skills must be learned and that many, if not most, of the techniques had withstood neither the rigors of prospective studies nor time.

We have since seen a bit of a plateau in terms of new technology as it applies to endoscopic surgery. With this respite has come the opportunity to give scrutiny to the techniques available to the endoscopic surgeon. The second edition provides the reader with a more mature look at the relatively fledgling surgical discipline of endoscopic surgery. We have asked authors to reexamine their topics and to provide updates where updates are due. Finally, we have added new topics to permit greater coverage of the subject at hand.

We thank our colleagues for their willingness to share their vast experience with us. Their intellectual honesty is greatly valued. We also wish to thank the staff at our institutions for their willingness to coordinate the endless details inherent in preparing the manuscripts for this text.

Randle S. Corfman, PhD, MD
Michael P. Diamond, MD
Alan H. DeCherney, MD

Preface to First Edition

Endoscopic surgery, particularly in gynecology, has been around for a good many years. Until relatively recently this mode of access to the abdominal and pelvic milieu has been utilized chiefly as a diagnostic tool. The introduction of laparoscopy, for example, occurred for many of us in the form of a triage prior to proceeding with a laparotomy to surgically correct an abnormality or treat a pathologic process. The vast majority of operative laparoscopic procedures in gynecology, for example, fell into the category of sterilization procedures in the female patient. In both groups of patients a selection bias existed toward those patients with a very low likelihood of suffering from a complication of the procedure, since any "at risk" patient would undergo a laparotomy or minilaparotomy mode of access to the area in question. It may be reasoned, then, that as the complexity of surgery increases so will the number of complications.

Fledgling endoscopic surgeons were inhibited by the lack of instrumentation for performing surgical procedures which were deemed elementary by traditional standards. Further, only one person could see through the endoscope, making it extremely awkward to perform the most simple surgical maneuvers. With the development of the chip video camera a great many barriers fell, not the least of which was the ability of others to assist in the endoscopic surgery. Suddenly it became obvious to a few that a much greater breadth of surgical procedures was possible if specialized instrumentation could be developed. These events led to a wave of "minimally invasive" surgical procedures which rapidly spread to surgical specialties which now include gynecologic, general, thoracic, and urologic surgery.

The rapid developments in technology overwhelmed the ability of academic training programs and postgraduate education systems to adequately train individuals in endoscopic surgery techniques. In many instances, in fact, academic centers viewed endoscopic surgery as a dangerous gimmick with which they wanted no part. This attitude, combined with the tremendous pressure in the private sector to expeditiously add operative endoscopy to the surgeon's repertoire or suffer financial losses, shaped the environment within which the new discipline matured. In an uncharacteristic posture for medicine precious few prospective studies were conducted before widespread application of endoscopic surgical techniques had occurred. Economic pressures continued to mount upon the practicing surgeon.

It was perhaps inevitable that the learning curve would be accompanied by a variety of complications and difficulties in performing endoscopic surgery. Errors in the practice of surgery are inevitable, as is true for medicine in general. These adverse outcomes are further compounded by the lack of emphasis in endoscopic surgery in training programs. It may be argued, in fact, that the greatest evolution in endoscopic surgical techniques occurred in the private sector where emphasis upon publication is not so compelling. A venue for sharing ideas for avoidance, recognition, and treatment of complications during endoscopic surgery has been lacking.

The focus of this book is to provide a venue for many of the most knowledgeable endoscopic surgeons in the world to share their insights and experience in avoiding, recognizing, and dealing with complications of endoscopic surgery. The editors' goal has been to provide surgeons with varying expertise in endoscopic surgery with pearls of wisdom that will contribute to furthering the development of endoscopic surgery, ultimately elevating patient care. It is recognized that some overlap occurs between various chapters. It is our belief that such cross coverage will provide the reader with beneficial contrasts, further broadening the value of the book.

Appreciation is expressed to the many colleagues and mentors to have been willing to openly share their experiences with authors.

Without the skillful help of Camilla Kelley this book could not have been completed.

Victoria Reeders MD and Michael Snider of Blackwell Scientific Publications must be thanked for their endless patience and encouragement.

Finally, we express our appreciation for the encouragement and support freely given by our families through the years.

Randle S. Corfman, PhD, MD,
Michael P. Diamond, MD
Alan H. DeCherney, MD

1 | Assisting with the Management of Endoscopic Complications

Fred Allgood, Mary Carter, and Don Dodson

Assistance is a very special part of any operative procedure, with the assistant being charged with enhancing the performance of the operating surgeon. In endoscopic surgery, however, this role is expanded beyond that of anticipation, exposure, and the other necessary functions that the assistant normally carries out. It is essential that the assistant prevent, if possible, complications due to malfunctioning equipment and efficiently manage them when they occur. In this role, he or she will be able to rapidly inform operating room personnel about any special needs, thereby enabling the surgeon to concentrate on the problem at hand. The best way for assistants to approach laparoscopic complications is by appropriate preparation—that is, by having the necessary equipment on hand and ensuring that it functions properly.

Several areas in which proper preparation can prevent many complications will be addressed in this chapter.

Positioning the patient

Careful positioning of the patient preoperatively will prevent nerve injury, facilitate exposure, and make use of the instruments easier.

Legs and pressure points

Advanced laparoscopic procedures are often of long duration and require access to the abdominal-perineal area. For this reason, a total leg support system is often used (1). The legs are placed into the supports such that no pressure is applied to the knees or calves. The feet should rest comfortably in the support. To prevent a nerve palsy, special attention should be given to the medial and lateral aspects of the knee and ankle. Any areas that appear to have pressure points are then padded, with the bottom of the foot ultimately bearing most of the weight. Care must be given to the lower limbs such that the feet are not in a position to sequester venous supply.

Exposure

The stirrups are placed low in relation to the table. With the thighs in this position, probes and graspers can be moved without causing interference when the surgeon manipulates them (Fig. 1.1). The legs are separated widely enough to allow insertion of instruments for uterine manipulation or for vaginal or rectal identification. The arm on the operative surgeon's side is safely tucked beside the patient. With this positioning, the laser can be moved close to the table without encountering resistance from the laser arm as the surgeon advances it through the operative sleeve.

Particular attention should be given to repositioning the patient undergoing laparoscopically assisted vaginal hysterectomy. During the time that the patient is in a steep Trendelenburg position, she will frequently slide cephalad. When moving the patient caudad, the assistant should ensure that the tucked arm and hand are not compromised. The legs should be adducted slightly before raising to high lithotomy. This positioning requires the efforts of the entire surgical team, with the heightened awareness of potential patient movement potentially preventing any nerve injury.

Instrumentation

The proper tools are essential for performing any job correctly. Operative laparoscopy is no different.

The tools need to be immediately available for use. If a particular instrument is missing, the surgeon should be notified before surgery begins. If a favorite instrument breaks during a procedure, the proper steps should be taken to replace it immediately or suggestions should be given as to an alternative.

Hospitals buy many instruments—but not always the

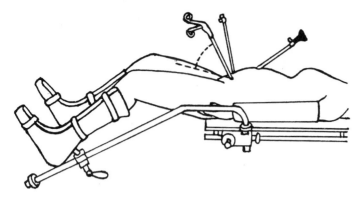

Fig. 1.1 Position of patient with lowered legs to facilitate maneuverability of instruments.

right ones. Different structures (e.g., fimbria, ovary, or ureter) require different types of grasping forceps, for example. Grasping a fimbria with an alligator-type forceps could have disastrous effects. Therefore, all personnel at the operative field should be aware of which instrument is introduced and its intended purpose.

Like forceps, specialized types of scissors are employed in endoscopy. It is essential to become familiar with the different types of scissors and their usage. Because scissors can become dull, several pairs should be included on the sterile field.

Probably the most common element to fail during surgery is the rubber gasket. If the gasket is too large, worn, or cut, the pneumoperitoneum will be lost. In addition, gaskets can be cut by trocars or instruments. When inserting gaskets into the sleeves, caution should be used. Two or three gaskets should be available for each sleeve on the back table; although they may not be needed, it is better to be prepared in case of mishap.

Equipment

The surgeon who performs laparoscopic surgery may be using technology that did not exist just a few years ago. While the equipment itself may be extremely complicated, manufacturers have strived to make operation of the systems as "user-friendly" as possible. Both the surgeon and the assistant should take the time to learn some of the basics of the equipment's operation.

Most components include a video-output and video-input. Troubleshooting these connections is usually as easy as tracing a flow of video-out from the camera controller through the various components.

Light sources

Current versions of light sources represent vast improvements over earlier models. Nevertheless, high-resolution camera and monitor offer little help if the light source does not project the true color of the tissue.

The light generated by today's light sources is extremely hot. Surgical drapes, paper, or linen and the patient can be burned in seconds if the fiber-optic cord is rested on the drapes while the light is on. This mistake can be prevented by not turning on the light source until the scope is in the sleeve.

Monitors

Video monitors should be placed to facilitate easy viewing by the surgical team. If two monitors are employed, the color should be equally balanced on both. The surgeon and the assistant should also view structures that are equal.

It is important to be familiar with faults that can interrupt the monitor picture. Any component that is in the video-out/video-in flow to the monitor can cause a fault in the monitor. If a VCR is not turned on, the monitor will not receive a signal. A video printer can cause the monitor picture to freeze while a picture is captured; pushing the source button on the printer control will revert back to a live picture.

Take the time to understand the video components available in the operating room. Insist that all equipment be uniform and compatible so that all components work in harmony (2). In addition, listen to the nurses and technicians who use the equipment everyday—they are usually the best resources regarding equipment operation.

Insufflators

Several types of insufflators are available. Some include a safety mechanism with a preset value for intraabdominal pressures that, if exceeded, initiates an alarm. Others have a means of establishing high flow rates to rapidly stabilize pneumoperitoneum, especially when evacuation of the carbon dioxide (CO_2) laser plume is in progress. If the team stays alert to the possibility that high intraabdominal pressures could cause significant complications, such a situation can be effectively managed.

When assisting with laparoscopic procedures, it is necessary to focus one's attention on the monitor or on the instruments in use. If the insufflation pressure monitor is not visible, a too low or too high intraabdominal pressure will become apparent by a soft or rigid abdomen, respectively. Pressure problems can have several causes:

Low Abdominal Pressure

Pressure limiting control	Set too low
Tank pressure	Off/empty/low
Insufflator tubing	Attached to unit and sleeve
Gaskets	Torn or improper size
Stopcocks	Open
Anatomical	Open vag cuff or similar problem
Insufflator unit	Malfunction

High Abdominal Pressure

Pressure limiting control	Set too high
Insufflator tubing	Kinked or water present in line
Anatomical	Patient awaking/Valsalva
Insufflator unit	Malfunction

If the pressure is excessively high, then carbon dioxide should be released from the abdomen as quickly as possible. One can suction the excess via a probe already in place or release the Silastic tubing from the side port of the trocar sleeve until the pressure returns to a safe level. Several complications can occur from hyperinsufflation: subcutaneous emphysema in the abdomen, thorax, and neck (3); intraperitoneal emphysema; hypotension (4), pneumothorax (5); and, although rare, gas embolism (6).

Consider the following example. Laparoscopy with laser vaporization of endometrial implants, partial transection of uterosacral ligaments, lysis of omental adhesions with monopolar scissors, and chromopertubation via an Eder catheter was performed on a 23-year-old patient. During the procedure, the patient was placed in a maximum Trendelenburg position. Very high intraabdominal pressures were encountered twice during the procedure. Before the laparoscope was removed, the patient's oxygen saturation decreased from 98% to 60%. Her blood pressure fell rapidly from normal levels to a systolic pressure of 40 mm Hg. Her heart rate decreased from normal to severely bradycardia (30–40 beats/minute). After vigorous resuscitation, her vital signs improved; after 10 minutes, the patient was mildly hypoxic, hypotensive, and mildly bradycardiac (heart rate of 60 beats/minute). Stable vital signs returned within 20 to 30 minutes after the initial onset, and she was extubated. Because of the short duration of the event and her rapid recovery, the cause of the episode was assumed to be a gas embolism (although it was not proven).

Excessive intraabdominal pressures (greater than 20 mm Hg) have also been associated with anesthetic complications. Therefore, careful monitoring of intraabdominal pressures is imperative.

Electrical equipment

For operative laparoscopy, both monopolar and bipolar electrosurgical units should be available along with the proper cords and grounding pads. As is the case in open procedures, the position of the electrode tip should be monitored to prevent thermal injuries. In addition, in laparoscopy the active electrode should always extend fully from the end of the metal sleeve before the current is engaged. A suction-irrigation system can be invaluable in exposing bleeding points. Caution should be taken to ensure that a nonconducting liquid irrigant (such as glycene) is used to prevent accidental thermal injuries. Electrosurgical complications will be covered in more detail in another chapter of this book.

Nothing is more frustrating for the surgeon, assistant, nurses, and technicians than for the surgeon to activate the electrosurgical unit and have nothing happen. The simple cause of the problem is a break in the electrical circuit. The solution can prove somewhat more challenging, however. The easiest strategy is to start at the source and follow the circuit through to the electrodes, checking the following items:

- Is the unit plugged in?
- Is the power on?
- Is the ground pad on and plugged in with no ground alarm?
- Are all settings correct–off standby, proper instrument setting (bipolar, monopolar), and proper power setting?
- Is the foot switch connected if needed?
- Is the power cable connected to the unit and instruments?
- Does the power cable need replacing?
- Is the instrument assembled properly?
- Does the instrument need replacing?

In the event that none of these steps corrects the problem, the electrosurgical unit should be changed and the circuit rechecked.

Safe, proper use of the electrosurgical unit is the responsibility of all personnel in the surgical suite. The assistant should free the surgeon from the frustration of checking the circuit and allow him or her to concentrate on the procedure—thereby making the operating room a much happier place.

Assisting during surgery

Assisting is a very special part of any operative procedure. A good assistant can make a good case go even better. A bad assistant can turn a good case into a disaster.

Do's and don'ts for assistants

Do make suggestions that might help the procedure. The surgeon and the assistant should work as a team. Each team member has his or her task to perform. A surgeon should keep lines of communication with the assistant open, which greatly enhances the ability of the entire team to grow and mature.

Don't try to do the procedure. Two surgeons can make a great team in operative laparoscopy, if they work together. If one is merely waiting for the opportunity to perform the operation his or her way, then the surgeon misses the point. Good operative laparoscopy is a four-handed procedure. Not everyone can be in charge.

Don't let your mind wander back to the mayo stand if you are a scrub nurse functioning as a first assistant. It is hard enough to do just one job—let someone else run the mayo and the back table. In other words, don't let your attention be diverted from the surgical field. If you are trying to assist a surgeon and your attention is drawn away, you break the line of communication. Concentrating on the job at hand is very important.

Do be aware of any changes taking place in the operating room during the procedure or between cases. These changes can consist of personnel entrances and exits, equipment malfunctions, or a shortage of critical supplies. In fact, just about anything that can affect the operating surgeon or the procedure itself can represent a potential problem.

Do arrive early and check the availability of necessary supplies and equipment.

"Freeze, don't move!"

During the actual procedure, the best move for an assistant is sometimes no move at all! Holding something in place can be very difficult. Everyone suffers from a tendency to have the hand follow the eyes—in other words, when you move your head, your hands want to follow. To illustrate this problem, try holding a probe in a certain position, removing the camera, and turning your head to the right and back. Now connect the camera and check the position of your probe. It probably will not be in the same location. Maintaining a stable position can be critical, especially during the use of laser.

To prevent unwanted movement, try to operate in a comfortable position. Develop moves that allow your arms to rest at your sides. Operative laparoscopic procedures can be very long, and you do not need to add to your discomfort.

Conclusion

The more occasions that a team works together, the more smoothly that it will actually work together. If possible, a surgeon should find an assistant and work with him or her on all possible occasions. Through experience, the two will develop a sense of what each other is thinking and anticipate the other's moves. A good assistant can save both the surgeon and the patient time and aggravation.

Laparoscopy is a learned skill; the only way to become proficient is to practice it over and over. The same principles of retraction, tension, and exposure used in open surgery apply in endoscopy. Acquiring the skill to perform these tasks laparoscopically is immensely difficult, however. The assistant should be able to perform the tasks as the surgeon, such as insertion of the Veress needle and trocars, manipulation of structures, suturing, and knot tying and stapling. By possessing the skills, the assistant can enable greater flexibility in the procedure and will know exactly what the surgeon is attempting and the best method to help.

Above all, remember that the surgeon remains in charge of the operation. The assistant can make suggestions, but the ultimate word is that of the surgeon. An assistant should not try to push the surgeon into doing a procedure with which he or she is uncomfortable. An assistant is not present to perform the surgery but to do as the title suggests—*assist.* Everything is easier when you do not have the scissors in your hand.

REFERENCES

1. Rothrock JC. The RN first assistant, 2nd ed. Philadelphia: J.B. Lippincott, 1993:131.
2. Bailey RW, Flowers JL. Complications of laparoscopic surgery. St. Louis: Quality Medical Publishing, 1995:59.
3. Bard PA, Chen L. Subcutaneous emphysema associated with laparoscopy. Anasth Analg 1990;71:101–102.
4. Phillips JM, ed. Endoscopy in gynecology. Downey: American Association of Gynecologic Laparoscopists, 1978.
5. Yacoub OF, Cardona I Jr, Coveler LA, Dodson MG. Carbon dioxide embolism during laparoscopy. Anesthesiology 1982;57:533–535.
6. Shulman D, Aronson HB. Capnography in the early diagnosis of carbon dioxide embolism during laparoscopy. Can Anaesth Soc J 1984;31:455–459.

2 Anesthesia for Laparoscopy

Robert C. Chantigian and Paula D. M. Chantigian

Introduction

Laparoscopic surgery has an excellent safety record with many advantages over conventional laparotomy, including lower morbidity, shorter hospital stays, and less overall expense (1, 2). As a result, its application is expanding from predominately gynecological procedures to general surgical procedures (e.g., cholecystectomies, herniorrhaphies, appendectomies).

Anesthetic considerations unique to laparoscopic surgery relate primarily to the effects of establishing and maintaining a pneumoperitoneum, the effects of the insufflation gas itself, the blind introduction of instruments, and the positioning of the patient. This chapter will briefly address various aspects of the surgical procedure and potential complications as they relate to the anesthetic management of the patient. Some special clinical considerations will also be reviewed.

Surgical procedure

Several aspects of intra-abdominal laparoscopic surgery may affect the delivery of anesthesia.

Insufflation gas

Air, oxygen, nitrous oxide (N_2O) and carbon dioxide (CO_2) have been used to distend the abdominal cavity. Currently, carbon dioxide (the most soluble gas) and nitrous oxide (slightly less soluble) are the most commonly used agents because of their greater solubility in blood, relative availability, and safety. Approximately five times as much carbon dioxide or nitrous oxide is needed to produce symptoms of embolism when compared with air or oxygen (3, 4).

For diagnostic procedures, either carbon dioxide or nitrous oxide is commonly used. For procedures involving electrocautery, 100% carbon dioxide (gray tank*) is the only safe insufflation gas, as air (yellow tank*),

oxygen (green tank*), and nitrous oxide (blue tank*) support combustion (5, 6). A mixture of 14% carbon dioxide and 86% oxygen (gray tank with a green strip at the top of the tank*) should not be used for insufflation when electrocautery is employed, as an intra-abdominal fire may occur (6).

An intra-abdominal fire should be suspected when a flame arises from the tip of the electrocautery unit, the video screen turns orange-red, or the abdominal wall transilluminates. Although this event may last only a few seconds, it could lead to thermal injury. In one case report of an intra-abdominal fire (6), a laparotomy was immediately performed after the fire and the only damage seen was a charred falciform ligament. The surgical procedure was completed, the abdomen was irrigated with saline, and the patient made a normal recovery.

Insufflation volume and rate

Gas is usually introduced into the peritoneal cavity through an insufflation needle (Veress, Tuohy, or Palmer) followed by the placement of one or more trocars. The insertion of the needle or trocar can produce visceral or vascular perforation (7). Manipulation of the needle can cause a profound vasovagal response and/or can tear tissues bound by adhesions. Some clinicians use an open laparoscopic technique to avoid the blind introduction of the insufflation needle and any trocars.

Approximately 2 to 5 liters of gas is necessary to produce the recommended initial intra-abdominal pressures of 12 to 15 mm Hg (1 mm Hg = 1.36 cm H_2O). This gas volume is dependent on the volume of the peritoneal cavity and the muscle tone of the abdominal wall. The initial insufflation rate is approximately 1.0 liter of gas per minute.

All color codes described in this chapter apply to tanks used in the United States. Color codes may vary in other countries.

e the pneumoperitoneum is obtained, gas is
ited as necessary to maintain the desired distention
re. Many insufflation devices permit a high flow
p to 6.0 liters per minute, as well as automatic
ation to maintain a preset pressure.

Intra-abdominal pressure

To adequately visualize the abdominal cavity without
producing marked physiologic abnormalities, the intra-
abdominal distention pressure is usually maintained at
12 to 15 mm Hg. Although some surgeons maintain
slightly higher pressures, few, if any, currently use pressures exceeding 40 mm Hg.

Abdominal wall muscle relaxation allows a larger
volume of gas to be insufflated and provides better visualization of the intra-abdominal contents while maintaining the same intra-abdominal pressure. Under general
anesthesia, muscle relaxants or deep general anesthesia
can be used. With regional anesthesia (spinal or
epidural), anesthetic levels to approximately T_{2-6} will
produce adequate relaxation. Local infiltration anesthesia does not provide abdominal wall relaxation.

Potential complications

Cardiovascular complications

The two most common cardiovascular abnormalities
noted during laparoscopy are alterations in blood
pressure (mean arterial blood pressure = cardiac
output × systemic vascular resistance) and cardiac
arrhythmias. Cardiac output is determined by preload,
contractility, afterload, heart rate, and heart rhythm.

Hypertension may be caused by several factors,
including a light level of general anesthesia and an elevated blood carbon dioxide level (this condition is more
prevalent when carbon dioxide is insufflated). The physiologic effects of the latter factor relate to the direct
effects from the elevated carbon dioxide level itself and
to the indirect effects relating to an increase in blood
catecholamine levels with associated sympathomimetic
effects (8). The net effect of elevating $PaCO_2$ levels from
40 to 50 mm Hg includes an increase in stroke volume,
heart rate, cardiac output, and mean blood pressure
combined with a decrease in systemic vascular resistance
(9).

Hypotension may be caused by several factors.
Preload will be decreased by hemorrhage, venous gas
embolism, or a marked elevation of intra-abdominal
pressure that causes vena caval compression and a
decrease in venous return (e.g., excessive insufflation
pressure). Excessive anesthetic blood levels (e.g., volatile
anesthetics) can decrease cardiac contractility as well as
systemic vascular resistance. Vagal stimulation from peritoneal manipulation (e.g., with the insufflation needle,
trocar, or surgical instruments) can produce sudden cardiovascular collapse (10).

Hemorrhage can occur as a result of vascular damage
during the placement of the insufflation needle or trocar
(especially when placed away from the relatively avascular midline) (7) or during the surgical procedure itself.
The incidence of vascular injuries during laparoscopic
cholecystectomies is 0.25% (2). If bleeding is excessive or
uncontrolled, an open laparotomy may be indicated.

The increase in intra-abdominal pressure from the
pneumoperitoneum can affect venous return and systemic vascular resistance. Mild to moderate elevations in
intra-abdominal pressures (up to 20 mm Hg or 30 cm
H_2O) can increase the central venous pressure (CVP;
about one-third the rise in intra-abdominal pressure),
mean blood pressure, and usually heart rate; higher intra-
abdominal pressures (above 30 mm Hg or 40 cm H_2O)
can depress CVP and blood pressure (11, 12). Presum-
ably, at mild to moderate elevations in intra-abdominal
pressure, blood is forced out of the abdominal organs
and into the central circulation. As the intra-abdominal
pressure continues to rise and the abdominal capacitance
vessels empty, the venous return from the lower part of
the body declines. The increasing rise in intra-abdominal
pressure produces a corresponding rise in the femoral
venous pressure (11). Significant hypotension as the
result of excessive intra-abdominal pressures (e.g.,
40 mm Hg) can usually be treated by promptly lowering
the intra-abdominal pressure (13). Overdistention of the
peritoneal cavity has led to cardiac arrest and death (14).

Cardiac output changes reported to result from
increased intra-abdominal pressure vary from study to
study. Some investigators have shown an increase in
cardiac output as the intra-abdominal pressure increases
(11); others show no change in cardiac output (12) or a
fall in cardiac output (15, 16) with the recommended
intra-abdominal pressures. With excessive intra-
abdominal pressures (i.e., above 30 mm Hg or 40 cm
H_2O), however, most agree that cardiac output will
decrease (12, 15). Differences between studies may relate
to the following factors:

- The rate of intra-abdominal insufflation, with
  slower insufflation (distention produced in 15
  minutes) (11) showing less detrimental cardiovascular effects than faster insufflation (distention produced in 4 minutes) (12, 15).
- The type of insufflation gas (carbon dioxide versus
  nitrous oxide) (11, 16).
- The type of anesthesia used (general versus regional
  anesthesia).
- The type of respiratory control under general anesthesia (spontaneous versus controlled).
- The use or nonuse of muscle relaxants under
  general anesthesia.
- The level of anesthesia with regional anesthesia
  (T_{2-6} under epidural or spinal anesthesia) versus no
  significant level with local infiltration anesthesia.

Increased vagal tone from stretching of the peritoneum by manipulation of instruments or intra-abdominal pressure may result in marked slowing of the heart rate, nodal rhythms, and occasionally cardiac arrest (17, 18).

Cardiac arrhythmias, such as sinus tachycardia and premature ventricular contractions, are associated with elevated blood levels of both carbon dioxide and catecholamines (18, 19). Patients under general anesthesia have higher blood carbon dioxide levels when carbon dioxide is insufflated than patients who undergo nitrous oxide insufflation when similar minute ventilations are maintained. Patients under general anesthesia with spontaneous respirations exhibit higher blood carbon dioxide levels than patients with controlled respirations. In addition, halothane (but not enflurane, isoflurane, desflurane, or sevoflurane) sensitizes the myocardium to catecholamine-induced ventricular ectopy (20–22). Thus, the combination of halothane anesthesia with spontaneous respirations and carbon dioxide insufflation can lead to a high frequency of arrhythmias. In one study, cardiac arrhythmias were observed in 17% of spontaneously breathing patients under halothane anesthesia when carbon dioxide was used as the insufflating gas compared with 4% of patients for whom nitrous oxide was used as the insufflating gas (19).

Vascular gas embolisms can occur whenever the insufflation gas enters a blood vessel, although clinically significant gas embolisms are extremely rare (3, 23, 24). On the other hand, subclinical embolisms (with no signs of cardiorespiratory instability) are quite common. In one study with transesophageal echocardiography (TEE), 11 of 16 patients undergoing laparoscopic cholecystectomy experienced subclinical gas embolisms (25). The reported frequency of gas embolisms clearly depends upon the surveillance method used and the clinical significance of the embolism. The most sensitive monitors for detecting gas embolism are TEE (visualization of densities consistent with air) and precordial Doppler ultrasound (auditory change in frequency). The next most sensitive indicators are increased pulmonary artery pressures, decreased end-tidal CO_2 levels, and decreased arterial oxygen tensions. The least sensitive indicators consist of increased arterial CO_2 tensions and decreased systemic blood pressures (26).

The signs that develop as a result of a gas embolism depend upon whether the gas enters the arterial or venous systems, the type of gas injected (air or oxygen versus the more soluble carbon dioxide or nitrous oxide), the total volume and rate of injection of the gas, the position of the patient, and the efficacy of the respiratory excretion mechanism (27). Clinical signs of a large venous gas embolism developing from direct venous insufflation (if the insufflation needle is inserted in a vein) include a decrease in end-tidal carbon dioxide, a decrease in oxygen saturation, a loud churning sound known as a "millwheel" murmur, ST-segment depression, tachycardia, systemic hypotension, elevated CVP, cyanosis, and occasionally cardiac arrest. If an air lock occurs in the right side of the heart, death can occur. Treatment of a large venous embolus includes stopping the insufflation of gas, administering 100% oxygen, placing a central venous line to help aspirate the gas from the heart, and cardiovascular support (such as closed chest compressions and epinephrine) as indicated. Closed chest compressions may help break up the obstructing gas embolus (28). In one severe case, a median sternotomy followed by cardiopulmonary bypass and venting of gas from all four cardiac chambers was carried out successfully (29).

If the gas embolized is carbon dioxide, a noticeable rise in the blood carbon dioxide level may be accompanied by marked acidosis. In one case report of a venous gas embolism (3), an arterial blood gas sample was drawn shortly after a suspected carbon dioxide gas embolism demonstrating a $PaCO_2$ of 103 mm Hg, a PaO_2 of 44 mm Hg, and a pH of 6.93. Twenty milliliters of foamy blood was aspirated from a CVP line, confirming the venous gas embolism.

Wadhwa et al. (30) monitored 100 patients with a Doppler transducer placed over the right heart (which can detect a gas embolism as small as 0.1 mL) and found no evidence of venous gas embolism when nitrous oxide was used as the insufflating gas.

Recently, a case of a cerebral arterial gas embolism associated with laparoscopy was reported. In this patient, who had an atrial septal defect, a CO_2 venous gas embolism was followed by cerebral arterial embolism documented by transcranial Doppler probe and somatosensory evoked potentials. Fortunately, the patient recovered with no neurological dysfunction (31).

Because clinically significant gas embolisms are rare, elaborate routine monitoring for embolism (i.e., Doppler ultrasound) and the placement of a CVP line to aspirate for possible gas embolism does not seem to be indicated.

Respiratory complications

Both patient position and the gaseous distention of the abdomen alter lung compliance. In rare circumstances, insufflation of gas may lead to pneumothoraces (unilateral or bilateral) (32–36), mediastinal emphysema (35, 36), subcutaneous emphysema (35–38), or diaphragmatic rupture if excessive abdominal insufflation occurs (36). All of these events can result in respiratory compromise. In addition, when carbon dioxide is used for insufflation, absorption of the carbon dioxide affects blood gases.

For gynecological surgery, the Trendelenburg position (approximately 20° to 30° head down) is commonly used; this position decreases lung compliance. Once the pneumoperitoneum is established, a further decrease in lung compliance is incurred due to the increased intra-abdominal pressure. The decreased lung compliance can be easily demonstrated under general anesthesia (where airway pressures are monitored) by observing the increase in airway pressures. Under general anesthesia with muscle paralysis and a constant minute volume, airway pressures increase by approximately 5 to 7 cm of H_2O when intra-abdominal pressures rise to 20 mm Hg (11, 37).

More dramatic alterations of arterial blood gases are observed with carbon dioxide insufflation than with nitrous oxide insufflation. With controlled ventilation under general anesthesia, Alexander et al. (37) reported an increase in $PaCO_2$ from 27 to 36 mm Hg and a decrease in pH from 7.47 to 7.39 with carbon dioxide insufflation, but no change in $PaCO_2$ or pH when nitrous oxide was used (39).

In 1990, Ciofolo et al. (40) noted an increase in minute ventilation in patients under epidural anesthesia from 9.15 liters per minute to 10.4 liters per minute when the 20° Trendelenburg position was employed; this measurement reached 11.8 liters per minute when carbon dioxide pneumoperitoneum was established. This increase in minute ventilation was primarily due to a higher respiratory rate (increasing from 17 breaths per minute to 18 breaths per minute when the Trendelenburg position was obtained, and to 23 breaths per minute after carbon dioxide insufflation). Arterial blood gas levels of carbon dioxide remained the same throughout the procedures.

Under local anesthesia with mild sedation (fentanyl 2 µg/kg or a combination of diazepam 0.1 to 0.2 mg/kg and meperidine 0.8 to 1.3 mg/kg), patients in the Trendelenburg position with either nitrous oxide or carbon dioxide pneumoperitoneum and intra-abdominal pressures of less than 15 mm Hg do not usually develop hypercarbia. A few patients became apneic, however. Thus monitored anesthetic care must be provided (41, 42).

Gastrointestinal (GI) complications

Perforation of the GI tract rarely occurs during endoscopic procedures, with an incidence of 0.14% in laparoscopic cholecystectomies (2), but can occur during the introduction of the insufflation needle (43, 44) or the laparoscopic trocar (44, 45). In the reported cases, this injury was associated with mask ventilation in patients with a difficult airway, and unintentional esophageal intubation before proper endotracheal intubation followed by inadequate or no gastric suctioning.

If GI perforation occurs with the insufflation needle, the stomach should be emptied with a nasogastric tube, the insufflation needle reinserted, and the laparoscope introduced to observe the puncture site for injuries. If bleeding or visceral damage appears minimal, the scheduled procedure can often be completed. The nasogastric tube should be left in place with no oral intake for 24 to 48 hours, and the patient should be observed for signs of peritonitis. If bleeding or visceral damage appears excessive, an open laparotomy and repair may be necessary (43).

If GI perforation by the laparoscopic trocar occurs, the trocar should be left in place to facilitate localization of the perforation. Immediate laparotomy should be undertaken to repair the defect (36).

To minimize such complications, gastric suctioning should be performed prior to the introduction of the insufflation needle in patients where positive pressure mask ventilation or esophageal intubation has occurred. Some anesthesiologists perform gastric suctioning on all patients undergoing intra-abdominal laparoscopy.

Anesthetic management

The goals of anesthetic management during laparoscopic surgery are to provide adequate depth of analgesia or anesthesia for the patient, to provide optimal surgical conditions for the surgeon, and to safeguard and facilitate rapid recovery and ambulation of the patient.

Selection of anesthesia

The selection of the type of anesthesia (general, regional, or attended local) is based on the type and extent of the surgical procedure, the patient's medical condition, the desires of the patient and surgeon, and the skills of the anesthesiologist. For short, simple procedures (e.g., tubal ligations) where little muscle relaxation is needed, local anesthesia can often be safely administered. Patients undergoing regional or attended local anesthesia should be motivated, cooperative individuals with good respiratory function. Many patients and surgeons prefer general anesthesia for patient comfort, especially for lengthy procedures.

Monitoring

Standard anesthesia monitoring for all surgical procedures includes an electrocardiogram, blood-pressure, stethoscope, and pulse oximeter. With general anesthesia, a nerve stimulator, temperature probe, and end-tidal carbon dioxide monitoring or mass spectrometer are added.

Airway pressures should be monitored closely during administration of general anesthesia. Unexpected excessive airway pressures may signify light general anesthesia, bronchospasm, mainstem or endobronchial intubation, tension pneumothorax, or excessive overdistention of the abdomen. Obese patients and patients placed in the Trendelenburg position may also show an elevation of airway pressures. Once the patient and the endotracheal tube are properly positioned, the airway pressures should remain constant and should not increase as would be seen with a tension pneumothorax.

General anesthesia

The major advantage of general anesthesia is that it allows optimal control of the respiratory and cardiovascular status of the patient, especially during long surgical procedures.

Induction

Thiopental and propofol are the most commonly used intravenous induction agents. For outpatients, the short-acting agent propofol may be preferable, as patients tend to recover more rapidly and have less nausea; this choice is more expensive, however (46).

Sole use of mask ventilation carries the risk of hypoventilation, gastric distention leading to possible perforation with the laparoscopic instruments (43–45), or aspiration of gastric contents (47). As a result, most anesthesiologists prefer endotracheal intubation and controlled ventilation for safety. To avoid complications of gastric distention, many anesthesiologists institute a rapid-sequence induction with endotracheal intubation for all patients undergoing laparoscopic surgery. Others induce the patient after a few manual ventilations to ensure the ability to ventilate the patient prior to the administration of muscle relaxants. Gastric suctioning is then performed prior to insertion of the insufflation needle. Recently, some anesthesiologists have demonstrated the safe use of the laryngeal mask airway (LMA) for gynecological laparoscopy (48). The role of the LMA for non-gynecological laparoscopic surgery has yet to be determined.

Atropine (0.4–0.8 mg) or glycopyrrolate (0.2–0.4 mg) may be administered to decrease the incidence or severity of reflex (vagal) bradycardia or asystole during peritoneal stimulation (18).

Muscle relaxants

Muscle relaxants are used both to optimize conditions for endotracheal intubation and to allow for better visualization of the abdominal cavity during the surgery.

Succinylcholine (a depolarizing muscle relaxant) is the muscle relaxant of choice for rapid-sequence inductions because of its fast onset of action. Given the higher incidence of postoperative myalgias associated with its use alone, especially in outpatients, pretreatment with a nondepolarizing muscle relaxant is typically undertaken. Many anesthesiologists prefer to avoid succinylcholine and use a nondepolarizing muscle relaxant, such as short-acting mivacurium or the intermediate muscle relaxants rocuronium, atracurium, cisatracurium, or vecuronium, for both intubation and maintenance of relaxation. These nondepolarizing relaxants are not associated with postoperative myalgias but take longer (i.e., 60–120 seconds) to achieve muscle relaxation adequate for intubation. In this setting, manual ventilation is required prior to intubation, and gastric suctioning is

recommended to avoid the possibility of unrecognized gastric inflation.

After induction and during the surgical procedure, a decrease in abdominal muscle tone can be achieved by deep levels of general anesthesia or the use of muscle relaxants. This technique allows better visualization of the abdominal contents at the recommended intra-abdominal pressures. High intra-abdominal pressures with low insufflation volumes may reflect inadequate muscle relaxation.

The maintenance relaxant chosen often depends upon the duration of the procedure. For short-duration procedures, a succinylcholine drip or mivacurium can be used. For intermediate-duration cases, rocuronium, atracurium, cisatracurium, or vecuronium is commonly employed. In a long-duration procedure, the intermediate agents can be used and supplemented as needed, or a longer-acting agent, such as pancuronium, metubine, or d-tubocurare, may be chosen.

Maintenance

Several anesthetic combinations may be used. Although some studies suggest that maintenance nitrous oxide may cause more postoperative nausea and vomiting and perhaps should be avoided (49, 50), other studies found no such link (51–54). In addition, some investigations have suggested avoiding nitrous oxide because it may lead to bowel distention. In a recent study on laparoscopic cholecystectomy patients, however, no clinically apparent adverse effects were noted during the surgery; in the same study, surgeons guessed correctly only 44% of the time as to whether nitrous oxide was administered (54).

Currently, most anesthesiologists use a base of nitrous oxide with oxygen and then add either a volatile agent (halothane, enflurane, isoflurane, desflurane, or sevoflurane), a narcotic/tranquilizer combination, or propofol infusions for maintenance anesthesia. Some prefer to avoid halothane because it (unlike the other volatile anesthetics) sensitizes the myocardium to arrhythmias when carbon dioxide blood levels are elevated. If rapid awakening is desired, total intravenous anesthesia with propofol (46) or the newer volatile anesthetics desflurane or sevoflurane can be used.

Under general anesthesia, an increase in minute ventilation is needed to maintain normal blood carbon dioxide levels and pH values with carbon dioxide insufflation. To increase minute ventilation, the respiratory rate or the tidal volume can be increased. A rise in the respiratory rate will not increase the airway pressures and may be preferred over higher tidal volumes, which do increase the airway pressures. End-tidal carbon dioxide monitors can help monitor adequate ventilation.

When the insufflation needle or the trocar is introduced, it may be desirable to halt ventilation temporarily. This technique prevents the intestinal contents from being pushed toward the needle or trocar as they are inserted.

When significant hypotension arises, the surgeon should be notified, the intra-abdominal pressure reduced, and a rapid inspection for intra-abdominal bleeding performed. If no significant bleeding is seen and hypotension remains uncorrected, the procedure should be terminated with removal of any remaining intra-abdominal gas, and the etiology of the hypotension identified and treated.

If ventricular bradycardia or asystole develops, the abdomen should be deflated, the needle or trocar promptly removed, and atropine administered. In the case of cardiac arrest, CPR will be needed to circulate the atropine. In rare cases, epinephrine or external cardiac pacing may be required to treat the bradycardia.

If ventricular ectopy (ventricular tachycardia, premature ventricular beats) develops, hypoventilation or a light level of anesthesia with sympathetic hyperactivity may be implicated. If correction of these conditions does not resolve the ventricular ectopy, consider the administration of an antiarrhythmic drug (such as intravenous lidocaine at 1 mg/kg) or a change in the anesthetic maintenance (e.g., halothane to enflurane, isoflurane, desflurane, sevoflurane, or a nitrous-narcotic technique).

Regional anesthesia (epidural and spinal anesthesia)

Epidural and spinal anesthesia are both safe and effective for intra-abdominal laparoscopic surgery despite initial concerns related to the Trendelenburg position and abdominal distention (40, 55–57). Advantages of regional anesthesia include decreased postoperative nausea and vomiting as well as a decrease in postoperative sore throats.

Anesthetic levels have a cephalad dermatomal spread commonly attained to T_{2-6}. Slow insufflation of the distending gas and lower intra-abdominal maintenance pressures may decrease the discomfort from abdominal distention.

Arterial blood gas values remain within normal limits (40, 55, 57) by increasing minute ventilation (40). Patients undergoing regional anesthesia should therefore have good lung function. If a compromise in respiratory status exists, the patient may not be able to maintain the increased minute ventilation required to maintain adequate ventilation. Heavy sedation should be avoided if the patient is to maintain the increased minute ventilation. In addition, supplemental oxygen should be used as in the administration of all major regional anesthetics.

Commonly used agents for spinal anesthesia include lidocaine (duration about 60 minutes) or, if a longer duration is needed, bupivacaine (duration about 90 minutes). For epidural anesthesia, chloroprocaine (duration about 45 minutes) or lidocaine (duration about 60 minutes) can be used for short procedures; for longer procedures, an epidural catheter can be inserted and additional chloroprocaine or lidocaine injected, or a longer-acting local anesthetic such as bupivacaine (duration about 90 minutes) may be used. A small amount of epinephrine can be added to reduce the absorption of local anesthetic and to prolong its action. Recently, a small amount of narcotic, such as fentanyl, has been added to the local anesthetic to provide better analgesia.

Attended local anesthesia

When the procedure is of relatively short duration and involves minimal abdominal distention (e.g., tubal ligations or diagnostic laparoscopies), patients can often tolerate local anesthesia with mild intravenous sedation quite well (41, 58, 59). Supplemental oxygen should be administered to all patients receiving sedation. Sedation with short-acting drugs such as fentanyl, alfentanil, midazolam, or propofol may permit more rapid recovery at the end of the procedure and may be preferred over longer-acting drugs such as morphine, meperidine, and diazepam. An intravenous line should be established before beginning the procedure to allow the administration of intravenous sedative drugs and to permit introduction of atropine should a reflex bradycardia develop. Anesthesia personnel must be available to deal with any adverse effects such as apnea or cardiac arrhythmias should they develop (41, 42, 60).

Special clinical considerations
Patient considerations
Postoperative pain

In patients undergoing tubal ligation (a procedure more painful than a diagnostic laparoscopy), the topical application of local anesthetic to the fallopian tube can minimize postoperative pain. It also helps to reduce the number of patients admitted overnight from outpatient units due to postoperative nausea and vomiting (61, 62). Although several local anesthetics are safe for intraperitoneal application, etidocaine (greater lipid solubility) appears to provide better analgesia than either lidocaine or bupivacaine (62, 63).

Hypovolemia

Patients with a decrease in circulating blood volume may experience profound hypotenuse when the abdomen is distended. Hypovolemia should be corrected before beginning the procedure, particularly if regional anesthesia is being considered. Laparoscopy may be contraindicated if normovolemia cannot be obtained.

Pelvic surgery

Patients undergoing pelvic surgery are placed in 20° to 30° Trendelenburg (head down) position. The head-down position facilitates venous blood return but complicates ventilation slightly due to the decreased lung compliance indicated by higher airway pressures. When the patient is placed in the Trendelenburg position, the endotracheal tube can occasionally advance into the right mainstem bronchus. The position of the endotracheal tube should be checked and repositioned if indicated (64).

Special procedures

Assisted reproductive techniques (ART)

Laparoscopy has been performed as part of ART programs for oocyte harvest (now much less commonly performed because of advances in transvaginal ultrasound guided oocyte retrievals) and gamete or zygote intrafallopian tube transfers (GIFT or ZIFT). (Today, the zygote is more commonly transferred transvaginally without anesthesia, however.)

Because the fertilization and pregnancy rates for ART procedures are less than 50% per cycle in many series, factors that may affect success are currently being assessed. The use of nitrous oxide as part of the maintenance general anesthetic (known to have some toxic effects), the duration of general anesthesia, and the carbon dioxide pneumoperitoneum have recently been reviewed. Rosen et al. (65) noted similar rates of fertilization and pregnancy for women undergoing oocyte retrieval when general anesthesia was maintained with 60% nitrous oxide and 0.7% isoflurane in oxygen anesthesia compared with the use of 1.4% isoflurane in oxygen anesthesia.

When laparoscopy is performed for oocyte harvest under general anesthesia with a carbon dioxide pneumoperitoneum, a negative correlation exists between the duration of anesthesia and the fertilization and cleavage of the oocytes in vitro. Whether this effect is related to the general anesthetic agents or the carbon dioxide pneumoperitoneum is currently unclear (66, 67). As a result, patients are usually prepared and draped while awake, and general anesthesia is induced when the surgeon is ready to start the operation. Future studies comparing the success rates of cases performed under regional anesthesia with those carried out under general anesthesia may delineate whether the adverse effects on fertilization are due to the anesthetic drugs or to the carbon dioxide pneumoperitoneum.

Cholecystectomy

Cholecystectomy patients are first placed in the Trendelenburg position to establish the carbon dioxide pneumoperitoneum and to insert the four or five trocars to be used for the laparoscope and various surgical instruments (1, 68). The patient is then placed in a 30° to 40° reverse Trendelenburg (head up) position, sometimes with a left lateral tilt for the surgery. The head-up tilt facilitates ventilation (smaller increase in airway pressures) but increases the likelihood of hypotension (less venous return due to pooling of blood in the lower extremities). Light general anesthesia with adequate hydration helps to prevent significant falls in systemic blood pressure. Because the surgical field involves the upper abdomen, an oral gastric tube with constant suction may optimize the operating conditions (68, 69).

Hysteroscopy

Hysteroscopy, or the transvaginal approach to looking directly into the uterine cavity, is performed either alone or in combination with a laparoscopic procedure. The hysteroscope has channels to enable the infusion of a liquid or gaseous distention medium (to obtain good visualization of the intrauterine cavity) and the passage of instruments. Many distending media are used, including saline, Ringer's lactate, D5W, dextran, glycine, and CO_2 (70, 71).

When performing hysteroscopy, both the amount of distention medium used and the intrauterine pressures generated should be carefully monitored. Although absorption of the distention medium occurs primarily through the uterine wall and into the bloodstream, some fluid may leak through the fallopian tubes and enter the peritoneal cavity. Maintenance of intrauterine distention pressures that are lower than the patient's diastolic blood pressure has been recommended to decrease excessive absorption of the medium.

For diagnostic hysteroscopy, saline or CO_2 is commonly used. If electrocautery is needed, a nonelectrolyte solution such as glycine is preferred.

Another commonly used uterine distention medium is 32% dextran-70 in dextrose 10% in water (Hyskon; Medisan Pharmaceuticals, Inc., New Jersey) (72). The initial volume of Hyskon needed to distend the uterine cavity is typically 50 to 100 mL; it is introduced at a low pressure of 100 mm Hg. Occasionally, a lower concentration of dextran is instilled into the peritoneal cavity to help prevent postsurgical adhesions (73). Complications related to dextran usage are rare but include anaphylactic reactions (incidence about 1 per 10,000) (73, 74), pulmonary edema (75–78), electrolyte imbalances (e.g., hyponatremia, hypokalemia) (75), and coagulation disorders (75, 76). Pulmonary edema occurs in approximately 0.1% of all patients, but its incidence increases to 1.4% when more than 500 mL is instilled (72). This complication appears to be related to the absorption of the dextran into the circulation. The absorption of 100 mL of Hyskon will expand the circulating blood volume by approximately 800 mL (72, 75). The incidence of complications is greater with large volumes of Hyskon (exceeding 500 mL), high distending pressures (greater than 150 mm Hg), and long surgical procedures (longer than 45 minutes) (72, 75, 78, 79).

In addition, 1.5% glycine solution is used in hysteroscopic procedures. In one recent case report, excessive amounts of glycine (a neuroinhibitory transmitter) absorbed intravascularly produced complete and total blindness in a patient; the blindness resolved over a few hours (71).

If carbon dioxide is used, a special insufflator is required (not the insufflator used in laparoscopy) that delivers a flow rate of 25 to 100 mL/min (70).

Summary

Administering anesthesia for laparoscopic procedures requires a general knowledge of the surgical procedure, especially the effects and complications of producing and maintaining a pneumoperitoneum. This chapter reviewed basic aspects of the surgical procedure; some complications as they relate to the cardiovascular, respiratory, and gastrointestinal systems; basic anesthetic management under general and regional anesthesia; and some special clinical conditions.

REFERENCES

1. Reddick EJ, Olsen DO. Laparoscopic laser cholecystectomy. A comparison with mini-lap cholecystectomy. Surg Endosc 1989;3:131–133.
2. Deziel DJ, Millikan KW, Economou SG, Doolas A, Ko S-T, Airan MC. Complications of laparoscopic cholecystectomy—a national survey of 4,292 hospitals and an analysis of 77,604 cases. Am J Surg 1993;165:9–14.
3. Yacoub OF, Cardona I Jr, Coveler LA, Dodson MG. Carbon dioxide embolism during laparoscopy. Anesthesiology 1982;57:533–535.
4. Graff TD, Arbegast NR, Phillips OC, Harris LC, Frazier TM. Gas embolism. A comparative study of air and carbon dioxide as embolic agents in the systemic venous system. Am J Obstet Gynecol 1959;78:259–265.
5. Robinson JS, Thompson JM, Wood AW. Laparoscopy explosion hazards with nitrous oxide. Brit Med J 1975;3:764–765.
6. Greilich PE, Greilich NB, Froelich EG. Intra-abdominal fire during laparoscopic cholecystectomy. Anesthesiology 1995;83:871–874.
7. Hurd WW, Pearl ML, DeLancey JOL, Quint EH, Garnett B, Bude RO. Laparoscopic injury of abdominal wall blood vessels: a report of three cases. Obstet Gynecol 1993;82:673–676.
8. Price HL. Effects of carbon dioxide on the cardiovascular system. Anesthesiology 1960;21:652–663.
9. Cullen DJ, Eger EI II. Cardiovascular effects of carbon dioxide in man. Anesthesiology 1974;41:345–349.
10. Brantley JC III, Riley PM. Cardiovascular collapse during laparoscopy. A report of two cases. Obstet Gynecol 1988;159:735–737.
11. Smith I, Benzie RJ, Gordon NLM, Kelman GR, Swapp GH. Cardiovascular effects of peritoneal insufflation of carbon dioxide for laparoscopy. Brit Med J 1971;3:410–411.
12. Marshall RL, Jebson PJR, Davie IT, Scott DB. Circulatory effects of carbon dioxide insufflation of the peritoneal cavity for laparoscopy. Brit J Anaesth 1972;44:680–684.
13. Lee CM. Acute hypotension during laparoscopy: A case report. Anesth Analg 1975;54:142–143.
14. Arthure H. Laparoscopy hazard. Brit Med J 1970;4:492–493.
15. Lenz RJ, Thomas TA, Wilkins DG. Cardiovascular changes during laparoscopy. Studies of stroke volume and cardiac output using impedance cardiography. Anaesthesia 1976;31:4–12.
16. Marshall RL, Jebson PJR, Davie IT, Scott DB. Circulatory effects of peritoneal insufflation with nitrous oxide. Brit J Anaesth 1972;44:1183–1187.
17. Shifren JL, Adlestein L, Finkler NJ. Asystolic cardiac arrest: a rare complication of laparoscopy. Obstet Gynecol 1992;79:840–841.
18. Carmichael DE. Laparoscopy-cardiac considerations. Fertil Steril 1971;22:69–70.
19. Scott DB, Julian DG. Observations on cardiac arrhythmias during laparoscopy. Brit Med J 1972;1:411–413.
20. Johnston RR, Eger EI II, Wilson C. A comparative interaction of epinephrine with enflurane, isoflurane, and halothane in man. Anesth Analg 1976;55:709–712.
21. Joas TA, Stevens WC. Comparison of the arrhythmic doses of epinephrine during forane, halothane, and fluroxene anesthesia in dogs. Anesthesiology 1971;35:48–53.
22. Physician's Desk Reference, 51st ed. Montvale, NJ: Medical Economics Company, Inc., 1997, 2830.
23. Clark CC, Weeks DB, Gusdon JP. Venous carbon dioxide embolism during laparoscopy. Anesth Analg 1977;56:650–652.
24. Ostman PL, Pantle-Fisher FH, Faure EA, Glosten B. Circulatory collapse during laparoscopy. J Clin Anesth 1990;2:129–132.
25. Derouin M, Couture P, Boudreault D, Girard D, Gravel D. Detection of gas embolism by transesophageal echocardiography during laparoscopic cholecystectomy. Anesth Analg 1996;82:119–124.
26. Glenski JA, Cucchiara RF, Michenfelder JD. Transesophageal echocardiography and transcutaneous O$_2$ and CO$_2$ monitoring for detection of venous air embolism. Anesthesiology 1986;64:541–545.
27. Durant TM, Long J, Oppenheimer MJ. Pulmonary (venous) air embolism. Am Heart J 1947;33:269–281.
28. Gottlieb JD, Ericsson JA, Sweet RB. Venous air embolism—a review. Anesth Analg 1965;44:773–779.
29. Diakun TA. Carbon dioxide embolism: successful resuscitation with cardiopulmonary bypass. Anesthesiology 1991;74:1151–1153.
30. Wadhwa RK, McKenzie R, Wadhwa SR, Katz DL, Byers JF. Gas embolism during laparoscopy. Anesthesiology 1978;48:74–76.
31. Schindler E, Muller M, Kelm C. Cerebral carbon dioxide embolism during laparoscopic cholecystectomy. Anesth Analg 1995;81:643–645.
32. Doctor NH, Hussain Z. Bilateral pneumothorax associated with laparoscopy. A case report of a rare hazard and review of literature. Anaesthesia 1973;28:75–81.
33. FitzGerald TB, Johnstone MW. Diaphragmatic defects and laparoscopy. Brit Med J 1970;2:604.
34. Whiston RJ, Eggers KA, Morris RW, Stamatakis JD. Tension pneumothorax during laparoscopic cholecystectomy. Brit J Surg 1991;78:1325.
35. Batra MS, Driscoll JJ, Coburn WA, Marks WM. Evanescent nitrous oxide pneumothorax after laparoscopy. Anesth Analg 1983;62:1121–1123.
36. Steptoe PC. Laparoscopy in gynecology. Edinburgh and London: E.S. Livingstone, 1967:30–34.
37. Alexander GD, Noe FE, Brown WM. Anesthesia for pelvic laparoscopy. Anesth Analg 1969;48:14–18.
38. Bard PA, Chen L. Subcutaneous emphysema associated with laparoscopy. Anesth Analg 1990;71:100–106.
39. Alexander GD, Brown EM. Physiologic alterations during pelvic laparoscopy. Am J Obstet Gynecol 1969;105:1078–1081.
40. Ciofolo MJ, Clergue F, Seebacher J, Lefebvre G, Viars P. Ventilatory effects of laparoscopy under epidural anesthesia. Anesth Analg 1990;70:357–361.
41. Brown DR, Fishburne JI, Roberson VO, Hulka JF. Ventilatory and blood gas changes during laparoscopy with local anesthesia. Am J Obstet Gynecol 1976;124:741–745.
42. Diamant M, Benumof JL, Saidman LJ, Kennedy J, Young P. Laparoscopic sterilization with local anesthesia: complications and blood-gas changes. Anesth Analg 1977;56:335–337.
43. Endler GC, Moghissi KS. Gastric perforation during pelvic laparoscopy. Obstet Gynecol 1976;47:40S–42S.
44. Chiu HH, Ng KH. Complication of laparoscopy under general anaesthesia. Anaesth Intens Care 1977;5:169–171.

45. Whitford JHW, Gunstone AJ. Gastric perforation: a hazard of laparoscopy under general anesthesia. Brit J Anaesth 1972;44:97–99.

46. DeGrood PMRM, Harbers JBM, van Egmond J, Crul JF. Anaesthesia for laparoscopy. A comparison of five techniques including propofol, etomidate, thiopentone and isoflurane. Anaesthesia 1987;42:815–823.

47. Duffy BL. Regurgitation during pelvic laparoscopy. Brit J Anaesth 1979;51:1089–1090.

48. Verghese C, Brimacombe JR. Survey of laryngeal mask airway usage in 11,910 patients; safety and efficacy for conventional and nonconventional usage. Anesth Analg 1996;82:129–133.

49. Lonie DS, Harper NJN. Nitrous oxide anaesthesia and vomiting. The effect of nitrous oxide anaesthesia on the incidence of vomiting following gynaecological laparoscopy. Anaesthesia 1986;41:703–707.

50. Felts JA, Poler SM, Spitznagel EL. Nitrous oxide, nausea, and vomiting after outpatient gynecologic surgery. J Clin Anesth 1990;2:168–171.

51. Sengupta P, Plantevin OM. Nitrous oxide and day-care laparoscopy. Effects of nausea, vomiting and return to normal activity. Brit J Anaesth 1988;60:570–573.

52. Hovorka J, Korttila K, Erkola O. Nitrous oxide does not increase nausea and vomiting following gynaecological laparoscopy. Can J Anaesth 1989;36:145–148.

53. Sukhani R, Lurie J, Jabamoni R. Propofol for ambulatory gynecologic laparoscopy: does omission of nitrous oxide alter postoperative emetic sequelae and recovery? Anesth Analg 1994;78:831–835.

54. Taylor E, Feinstein R, White PF, Soper N. Anesthesia for laparoscopic cholecystectomy. Is nitrous oxide contraindicated? Anesthesiology 1992;76:541–543.

55. Bridenbaugh LD, Soderstrom RM. Lumbar epidural block anesthesia for outpatient laparoscopy. J Reprod Med 1979;23:85–86.

56. Burke RK. Spinal anesthesia for laparoscopy. A review of 1,063 cases. J Reprod Med 1978;21:59–62.

57. Caceres D, Kim K. Spinal anesthesia for laparoscopic tubal sterilization. Am J Obstet Gynecol 1978;131:219–220.

58. Peterson HB, Hulka JF, Spielman FJ, Lee S, Marchbanks PA. Local versus general anesthesia for laparoscopic sterilization: a randomized study. Obstet Gynecol 1987;70:903–908.

59. Wheeless CR Jr. Outpatient laparoscope sterilization under local anesthesia. Obstet Gynecol 1972;39:767–770.

60. Bordahl PE, Raeder JC, Nordentoft J, Kirste U, Refsdal A. Laparoscopic sterilization under local or general anesthesia? A randomized study. Obstet Gynecol 1993;81:137–141.

61. McKenzie R, Phitayakorn P, Uy NTL, Tantisira B, Wadhwa RK, Vicinie AF. Topical etidocaine during laparoscopic tubal occlusion for postoperative pain relief. Obstet Gynecol 1986;67:447–449.

62. McKenzie R. Postoperative pain after laparoscopic sterilisation. Anaesthesia 1989;44:450.

63. Spielman FJ, Hulka JF, Ostheimer GW, Mueller RA. Pharmacokinetics and pharmacodynamics of local analgesia for laparoscopic tubal ligations. Am J Obstet Gynecol 1983;146:821–824.

64. Heinonen J, Takki S, Tammisto T. Effect of the Trendelenburg tilt and other procedures on the position of endotracheal tubes. Lancet 1969;1:850–853.

65. Rosen MA, Roizen MF, Eger EI II, et al. The effect of nitrous oxide on in vitro fertilization success rate. Anesthesiology 1987;67:42–44.

66. Boyers SP, Lavy G, Russell JB, DeCherney AH. A paired analysis of in vitro fertilization and cleavage rates of first- versus last-recovered preovulatory human oocytes exposed to varying intervals of 100% carbon dioxide pneumoperitoneum and general anesthesia. Fertil Steril 1987;48:969–974.

67. Hayes MF, Magyar DM, Sacco AG, Endler GC, Savoy-Moore RT, Moghissi KS. Effect of general anesthesia on fertilization and cleavage of human oocytes in vitro. Fertil Steril 1987;48:975–981.

68. Zucker KA, Bailey RW, Scovill WA, Imbembo AL. Laparoscopic biliary tract surgery: Current status and outlook for the 1990s. Hosp Phys 1991;27:35–44.

69. Marco AP, Yeo CJ, Rock P. Anesthesia for a patient undergoing laparoscopic cholecystectomy. Anesthesiology 1990;73:1268–1270.

70. March CM. Hysteroscopy. J Reprod Med 1992;37:293–311.

71. Levin H, Ben-David B. Transient blindness during hysteroscopy: a rare complication. Anesth Analg 1995;81:880–881.

72. Physician's Desk Reference, 51st ed. Montvale, NJ: Medical Economics Company, Inc., 1997, 1633.

73. Borten M, Seibert CP, Taymor ML. Recurrent anaphylactic reaction to intraperitoneal dextran-75 used for prevention of postsurgical adhesions. Obstet Gynecol 1983;61:755–757.

74. Ahmed N, Falcone T, Tulandi T, Houle G. Anaphylactic reaction because of intrauterine 32% dextran-70 instillation. Fertil Steril 1991;55:1014–1016.

75. McLucas B. Hyskon complications in hysteroscopic surgery. Obstet Gynecol Surv 1991;46:196–200.

76. Jedeikin R, Olsfanger D, Kessler I. Disseminated intravascular coagulopathy and adult respiratory distress syndrome: life-threatening complications of hysteroscopy. Am J Obstet Gynecol 1990;162:44–45.

77. Peterson HB, Hulka JF, Phillips JM. American Association of Gynecologic Laparoscopists' 1988 membership survey on operative hysteroscopy. J Reprod Med 1990;35:590–591.

78. Golan A, Ron-El R, Siedner M, Herman A, Bahar M, Caspi E. High-output left ventricular failure after dextran use in an operative hysteroscopy. Fertil Steril 1990;54:939–941.

79. Diamond MP, Lavy G, DeCherney AH. Hysteroscopic use of dextran-70. Contemp Ob/Gyn 1989;34:29–38.

Insufflation Needle Insertion Techniques: Management of Perforation of Bowel and Bladder

3

Lisa D. Erickson

The creation of a pneumoperitoneum is the first step in laparoscopy. In this chapter, techniques and tips for insertion of the insufflation needle are discussed, and special emphasis is given to prevention and management of injuries to the bowel and bladder.

History

Various insufflation methods for establishing a pneumoperitoneum preceded the use of the Veress needle. In particular, techniques for viewing the abdominal cavity followed on the heels of cystoscopy developments. In 1902, Kelling was the first to produce an artificial pneumoperitoneum in dogs using filtered air through a separate needle (1). In 1910, Jacobaeus introduced air by means of a trocar used for the cystoscope (2). In 1924, Zollikofer used carbon dioxide for insufflation, promoting the rapid absorption properties (3).

A spring-loaded pneumoperitoneum needle with a blunt probe surrounded by a sharp outer sleeve was developed by Veress in Hungary in 1938 (4). It provides additional safety—that is, it prevents intra-abdominal perforations—because the spring behind the blunt, inner, metal piece is designed to push away nonfixed, intra-abdominal structures such as loops of bowel (5). As soon as the needle passes through the abdominal wall and into the peritoneal cavity, it automatically becomes blunt-ended (Fig. 3.1).

The Veress needle is most commonly used for insufflation of the abdominal cavity for laparoscopy. In the years since its introduction, many investigators have improved the instrumentation and technology of laparoscopic equipment, thereby increasing the safety of the procedure and decreasing operative complications.

Creating the pneumoperitoneum

Preparing the patient

Operative risks have been significantly reduced by improvements in surgical technique. Most accidents occur during the primary puncture with the Veress needle or the trocar for the laparoscope (6). To rule out hepatosplenomegaly and to ascertain the position of the bifurcation of the aorta, all preoperative examinations should include palpation of the abdomen. Previous abdominal incisions contain the hidden possibility of anterior peritoneal adhesions. One author suggested that the needle should be introduced in the side of the umbilicus opposite of any previous abdominal operation (7).

Before the needle is inserted, the insufflation equipment should be thoroughly examined. The patency of the needle and the spring-loaded snap mechanism are tested. The preinsertion manometer pressure is determined, and the flow ball is checked to ensure that it indicates patency of the system. It is extremely important to monitor the rate of flow, the amount of gas delivered, and intraperitoneal pressures.

Each insufflator offers various special features. For example, some insufflators include a maximal pressure setting mechanism that automatically shuts off the gas at a preset level; this feature prevents overdistention of the abdomen. Insufflator pressure gauges can indicate actual pressures and fluctuations, a feature that is helpful for diagnosing misplacement of the needle. If the pressures are high (more than 20 mm Hg), serious consideration should be given to withdrawing the needle (8).

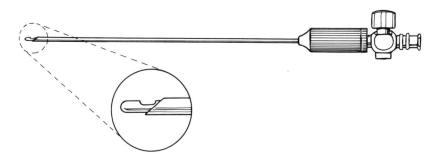

Fig. 3.1 The Veress needle. (By permission of Mayo Foundation.)

(a)   (b)

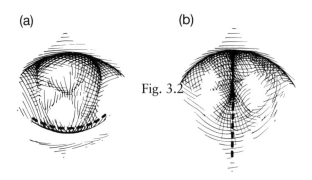

Fig. 3.2

Fig. 3.2 (a) Horizontal, semilunar, infraumbilical incision. (b) Vertical infraumbilical incision. (By permission of Mayo Foundation.)

Inserting the needle

The most common site for insertion of the Veress needle involves the infraumbilical region. Regardless of the patient's size, the umbilicus represents the thinnest portion of the abdominal wall. Extremely obese patients may require an extra-long Veress needle (9). The initial incision for placement of the needle, which has traditionally been infraumbilical and semilunar, provides variable cosmetic results. In selected patients, a vertical incision started in the center of the umbilicus is more anatomic, and after healing it remains concealed within the natural creases (Fig. 3.2). In Toth and Graf's study (10), the center of the umbilicus was the needle entry site in 217 patients; they noted good cosmetic results, less bleeding, and no hernia formation. Alternative abdominal sites for insertion are midline suprapubic, supraumbilical, left upper quadrant midclavicular, and left lower quadrant, McBurney's point (Fig. 3.3).

After the incision, the abdominal wall is elevated manually or with a towel clip or tenaculum. The needle, which is held in a dart-like fashion, is initially inserted perpendicular to the fascia, hooked and pulled inferiorly toward the pubis (away from the bifurcation of the aorta), and then redirected at a 45° angle toward the hollow of the sacrum (Fig. 3.4).

An issue that has inspired debate is whether the peritoneum is raised when the abdominal wall is elevated. Some surgeons support the use of an insertion technique

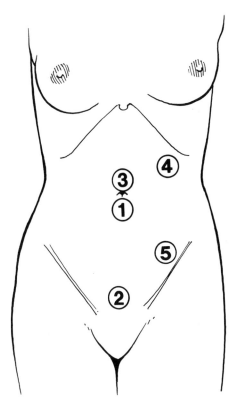

Fig. 3.3 Alternative abdominal insertion sites for insufflation. (1) Infraumbilical. (2) Midline suprapubic. (3) Supraumbilical. (4) Left upper quadrant midclavicular. (5) Left lower quadrant, McBurney's point. (By permission of Mayo Foundation.)

that does not involve lifting the abdominal wall. This approach would also eliminate any tearing of the tissue by the clamps or bruising of the abdominal wall.

Tests for placement

Several tests can be used to determine that the insufflation needle is properly positioned (Table 3.1). The usual signs of correct needle placement depend on the principle of negative intra-abdominal pressure.

Manometer test

After placement of the needle, the gas tubing from the insufflator is connected. The abdominal wall is elevated,

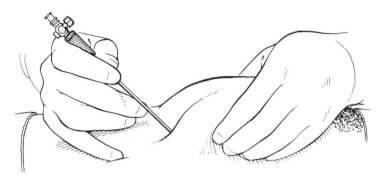

Fig. 3.4 Insertion of the Veress needle through the umbilical incision with manual elevation of abdominal wall. (By permission of Mayo Foundation.)

Table 3.1. Safety tests for correct placement of needle.
Manometer test
Hissing sound
Aspiration test
Hanging drop test
Disappearance of liver dullness

in a maneuver that causes the gauge to read a negative pressure.

Hissing sound

With the valve of the Veress needle in the off position, the abdomen is elevated and the needle is inserted. When proper positioning is suspected, the abdomen is released and the valve is opened. The abdominal wall is regrasped and elevated, which causes air to rush through the needle into the cavity and produce a hissing noise. When this sign was present, two different authors reported no complications in needle placement (11, 12).

Aspiration test

A syringe filled with saline is attached to the Veress needle. After placement of the needle, the syringe is pulled back. Aspiration of any material is considered a positive response, and the needle should be withdrawn. If no material is aspirated, 5 mL of saline is injected and reaspiration is attempted. If the needle tip is not correctly positioned, the fluid will be trapped and reaspiration cannot occur (6).

Hanging drop technique

This technique is similar to the aspiration test in that a small drop of water is placed on the end of the open Veress needle. As the abdominal wall is lifted, the water should disappear down the shaft if the needle is in the peritoneal cavity (13).

The presence of a foul odor, gas emitting from the rectum, eructations, and aspiration of intestinal contents or blood are indications to remove the needle immediately.

Some reassurance can be obtained by determining the opening abdominal pressures after directly connecting the gas insufflation tubing to the needle. Pressures less than 10 mm Hg are fairly consistent indicators of proper placement. Wide fluctuations in pressure may reflect misplacement in the omentum or bowel, and the needle should be removed. Steady, slow fluctuations consistent with respiratory variation are common.

Disappearance of liver dullness

The disappearance of liver dullness is a late and nonspecific finding. In such cases, general palpation of the abdomen can ensure uniform filling consistent with a successful pneumoperitoneum. The insufflation rate of flow should be set at 1 liter/minute or the low-flow setting until correct placement is completely assured.

It is sometimes difficult to judge whether the insufflation needle is in the peritoneal cavity. Various safety tests are available to assist in such cases. All of the tests described above have a low rate of specificity and sensitivity, so clinical judgment and experience are called into play.

Alternative sites of insertion

Most of the common operative complications occur during the early learning experience of the laparoscopist (14, 15). The willingness of the surgeon to remove the needle and reinsert it is critical. If all safety tips fail and proper positioning of the needle cannot be ensured, then alternative sites of insertion or stopping the procedure should be considered. Mintz (16) stated that, "in the case of unsatisfactory pneumoperitoneum . . . I still probably stop once a year and send a patient back to her bed. I must add that I learned from 13 colleagues that they did likewise 70 times out of a total of 30,000 laparoscopies." Neely *et al.* (17) examined the medical records for 1024 laparoscopies performed by 30 different operators during a six-year period; they noted that the principal cause of a failed laparoscopy was the inability to produce an adequate pneumoperitoneum, which occurred in 29 cases (2.8%).

Howard (18) had one failed laparoscopy in 125 cases. He attributed his success to the fact that in selected difficult cases—some due to obesity—the pneumoperitoneum was introduced via the cul-de-sac (Fig. 3.5). In 1975, Neely *et al.* tested the hypothesis that regular use of the posterior cul-de-sac as an insertion route should simplify the procedure in difficult cases. They noted fixed retroversion and previous vaginal vault operation as a contraindication to the use of this insertion site. In their study, a modified longer needle with a stop for depth control was used. The vaginal route produced a successful pneumoperitoneum in 103 of 107 cases; in four cases, a subumbilical insertion was used. In three of these four cases, the vaginal needle had caused extraperitoneal insufflation. In 1977, Mintz used a vaginal route for insufflation only when the pouch of Douglas was found to be free when the patient was examined under anesthesia; this situation occurred in 80% of patients.

In 1979, Morgan (19) described the use of transuterine insertion of the Veress needle in 1500 laparoscopies without known complications related to the site of the pneumoperitoneum puncture (Fig. 3.6). Wolfe and Pasic (20) used the transfundal approach in 100 patients who either were obese (*n* = 86) or had a previous unsuccessful attempt at transabdominal insufflation (*n* = 14). Preoperative evaluation consisted of cervical cultures, Pap smear, and pregnancy test. Two patients who had previously been the subject of unsuccessful attempts at transuterine insufflation underwent the transabdominal approach. No intraoperative complications were associated with this insufflation method.

Contraindications to transfundal insertion include situations that might be complicated by bowel adhesions to the uterus, such as previous abdominal operation, myomectomy, or history of extensive pelvic inflamma-

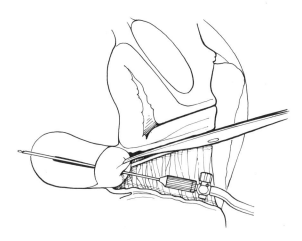

Fig. 3.6 Transuterine insertion of the insufflation needle. (By permission of Mayo Foundation.)

tory disease. Chromopertubation for infertility might cause dye to escape through the fundus and may not allow sufficient pressure to document patency of the fallopian tubes.

Preoperative consultation with the patient regarding the risks, benefits, and alternatives to laparoscopy should encompass concerns about anesthesia, allergic reactions, infection, damage to bowel and bladder, bleeding, and the possibility of laparotomy to repair any damage. In addition, in the high-risk patient, the discussion should include the possibility of canceling the procedure because of a failed pneumoperitoneum in order to prepare both the physician and the patient for this possible outcome.

No pneumoperitoneum

The first endoscopic procedures of the 1900s were performed without a pneumoperitoneum (3). In 1978, Dingfelder (21) reexamined the prerequisite of a pneumoperitoneum before insertion of the trocar by performing direct insertions in 301 laparoscopies. His procedure consisted of manually elevating the abdominal wall and direct placement of the trocar. The laparoscope was immediately inserted to verify position, and a pneumoperitoneum was then established. No technical failures occurred. The author concluded that direct insertion of the trocar with maximal elevation of the relaxed and undistended abdominal wall seems to allow better control of the thrusting maneuver of insertion.

In 1986, Saidi (22) published the results in 1108 cases of direct trocar insertion without prior pneumoperitoneum. Multiparity was noted as a positive factor in elevating the abdominal wall. In several nulliparous patients, towel clips were used. Obesity created no failures or major problems, and no technical failures or intraoperative complications were encountered. Postoperative complications showed an increased incidence of subcutaneous hemorrhage resulting in petechias and discoloration.

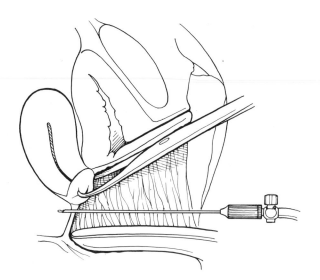

Fig. 3.5 Cul-de-sac insertion of the insufflation needle. (By permission of Mayo Foundation.)

In 1983, Copeland et al. (23) reported only three complications with direct trocar insertions in more than 2000 cases. In a retrospective review of 937 cases of direct trocar insertion performed in a teaching institution, Byron et al. (24) found that no major complications had occurred during the study. Minor complications consisting of more than three insertion attempts and failure to enter the abdomen were observed in 3.2% of the patients. Obesity was the only factor associated with complications because it was difficult to elevate the abdominal wall. In the opinion of Byron et al., all patients who are considered candidates for a laparoscopic procedure with a Veress needle insufflation technique are equally served with the technique of direct trocar insertion.

Gasless laparoscopy with mechanical peritoneal distention

As minimally invasive procedures continue to replace more traditional surgical methods, alternatives in laparoscopy continue to emerge. A new gasless technique called Laparolift involves a mechanical peritoneal lifting device that provides a view of the abdominal cavity without insufflation. This retracting system eliminates concerns about the effects of carbon dioxide on the patient who is having laparoscopic surgery (25).

The optical Veress needle

Complications related to the blind puncture with the Veress needle have inspired alternative techniques for laparoscopic access to the abdomen. A new endoscopic instrument designed to visualize all tissues in the cannular tract through the abdominal wall may achieve safer endoscopic access to the abdominal cavity. Although no surgical procedure can be absolutely injury-free, the main advantage of the optical Veress needle includes the immediate recognition of needle misplacement before insufflation (26).

Sonographic study of pneumoperitoneum

In an attempt to avoid bowel injuries related to the induction of pneumoperitoneum and insertion of the trocar, abdominal sonograms have been used after induction of pneumoperitoneum to indicate the presence of intestinal loops. The use of ultrasonography has been suggested to be extremely useful in cases of pseudomyxomas and other peritoneal diseases. In the case of ascites, it has been possible to insert the Veress needle into fluid collections under ultrasonographic guidance. Ultrasonography may be considered for patients who have previously experienced an abdominal operation or peritoneal abnormality (27).

Preperitoneum insufflation

Preperitoneum insufflation—a common complication of laparoscopy—can be difficult to correct and can result in abandonment of the procedure. A technique to avoid abandonment of the procedure was described by Kabukoba and Skillern (28):

. . . the laparoscope is left in situ. The gas should not be released because it is used to maintain the view. The laparoscope is advanced to a level about 4 cm from the symphysis pubis. A tiny incision is made at this level in the midline, and the Veress needle is introduced and directed toward the pouch of Douglas. The tip of the needle is visualized in the insufflated extraperitoneal space and must be kept in view until it is gently stabbed into the peritoneal cavity. Seeing the tip actually go through the peritoneum is a crucial step. The intra-abdominal pressure gauge may not be helpful. . . . The trocar valve is opened to release the extraperitoneal gas, and insufflation of the peritoneal cavity under direct vision begins. The increasing intra-abdominal pressure will force the extra-abdominal gas to escape. . . . When satisfactory pneumoperitoneum has been achieved, the laparoscope is withdrawn. The trocar is now introduced into the peritoneal cavity and the laparoscopic procedure is continued as normal.

Impact of body habitus on laparoscopic pneumoperitoneum

McDougall et al. (29) studied the relationship between pneumoperitoneum pressure and carbon dioxide insufflation volume in the clinical setting of laparoscopic urological procedures. Their goal was to determine whether a patient's height, weight, and body mass index had any direct effect on the pressure-volume relationship. In their study, they found that the delivered carbon dioxide volume can be predicted for a given insufflation pressure and that this delivered volume and pressure remain independent of the patient's height, weight, or body mass index. Of particular interest was the finding that increasing the intra-abdominal pressure from 15 mm Hg to 30 mm Hg increases the delivered volume of carbon dioxide insufflated by 50% even though the actual abdominal volume does not significantly change. Ninety-four percent of the abdominal volume is obtained at 15 mm Hg.

Injuries to bowel and bladder

Gastric injuries

Kelling and Jacobaeus suggested that the mobility of the intestines in the living subject prevents injury because of their ability to recede or slip aside from the trocar (1). Inadvertent perforation of the stomach usually occurs as a result of gastric distention resulting from either preoperative aerophagia or iatrogenic inflation of the stomach with artificial ventilation.

In 1972, Whitford and Gunstone (30) published the first case report of gastric perforation. In this case, which was complicated by intubation of the esophagus, the endotracheal tube was removed and correctly repositioned in the larynx. Manual decompression of the abdomen relieved the distention. The Veress needle was inserted twice because of unsatisfactory flow of carbon dioxide and left in place to reach a pressure of 22–24 cm H_2O. When the trocar was inserted, the abdomen immediately deflated, accompanied by the noisy regurgitation of its gaseous contents up the esophagus. Gastric rugae were seen through the laparoscope, which was left in situ, and a laparotomy was performed. Perforation into the lumen of the stomach was repaired with catgut. Postoperative treatment consisted of nasogastric tube placement and intravenously administered fluids. In this case, the absence of eructation of carbon dioxide was thought to reflect the competence of the cardia of the stomach. The authors concluded that should inadvertent esophageal intubation and inflation occur, a gastric tube should be passed to empty the stomach before attempting to establish a pneumoperitoneum.

In 1973, Reynolds and Pauca (31) reported a similar case of inadvertent intubation of the esophagus. After proper placement of the endotracheal tube, manual gastric decompression was attempted. The procedure began with the infraumbilical incision for the Veress needle. When the patient began to eruct gas, an oral suction catheter was placed down the esophagus and the needle was removed. The procedure was resumed when the stomach was decompressed, and laparoscopic examination of the stomach revealed some subserosal emphysema with no evidence of bleeding. The patient was placed on intravenously administered fluids with no oral intake and was observed; no further complications ensued.

Endler and Moghissi (32) reported two cases of conservative management of a gastric perforation with a Veress needle. One case occurred because of difficulties in ventilation, and the other was attributable to increased anxiety and aerophagia; both conditions caused overdistention of the stomach. According to these authors, when gastric perforation is suspected, a nasogastric tube should be inserted immediately and the stomach decompressed. The Veress needle can then be reinserted and laparoscopy can proceed in the usual fashion. It is important to visualize the site of perforation and assess the degree of damage and bleeding. In the absence of active bleeding, a conservative course is indicated. It should consist of gastric drainage by nasogastric tube for 24 to 48 hours, withholding of food and fluids, and close observation. In the event of undue bleeding or a greater degree of damage, surgical repair must be considered.

Loffer and Pent (33) reached a similar conclusion: If the Veress needle has been inserted into the stomach without tearing, no further therapy is indicated because its small diameter leaves no defect.

The routine use of a nasogastric suction tube to decompress the stomach before insertion of a Veress needle is a simple safeguard that can prevent perforation of the stomach.

Bowel injuries

Injuries associated with pneumoperitoneal needle insertion during laparoscopy occur despite increasing physician experience and safeguards. In their review of the large body of literature on this subject, Loffer and Pent (33) found that perforation injuries to the gastrointestinal system were mentioned 20 times. The overall prevalence was 0.6 per 1000 cases; 11 of these incidents were attributable to the insufflation needle. The authors suggested that no further therapy is indicated if the Veress needle has been inserted into the stomach, bowel, or bladder without tearing, as its small diameter leaves no defect. The needle's small size produces minimal contamination of the abdominal cavity with bowel contents and thus the chance of spreading peritonitis is small.

Kleppinger (34), in an 18-month series of 1098 laparoscopy cases, reported two cases of bowel injury. One unrecognized case presented within 24 hours with peritonitis; it required laparotomy, which revealed a small perforation in the ileum. A 10-cm section showed intense hyperemia, thick exudate, and hemorrhage of the serosa. A resection of the small bowel with end-to-end anastomosis was performed. Two additional cases (0.3%) were complicated with a needle in the stomach; they were managed conservatively.

Levy *et al.* (35) used microscopic characteristics of injuries obtained at laparoscopy to differentiate traumatic from electrical injuries. Inadvertent trauma to the bowel at the time of needle or trocar insertion can go unrecognized, especially if it is a through-and-through perforation of bowel adherent to the anterior abdominal wall. Trauma-related bowel injuries are characterized by the following developments: limited noncoagulation-type cell necrosis, more severe in the muscle coat than in the mucosa; rapid and abundant capillary ingrowth with rapid leukocyte infiltration; rapid fibrin deposition at the injury site followed by fibroblastic proliferation; and significant reconstitution of the injured muscle coat by 96 hours.

Vilardell *et al.* (36) reviewed air insufflation of intestinal loops, which in one series occurred eight times in 500 examinations. In these instances, the patients were described as feeling abdominal distention and a sudden desire for defecation. Foul-smelling gas through the pneumoperitoneum needle was noted. According to the authors, this kind of accident is not serious because it happens most often when intestinal loops are adherent to the abdominal wall and the perforation promptly seals itself off. In their own personal series, intestinal puncture occurred twice while the pneumoperitoneum was being completed. The peculiar smell of intestinal gas was noted and the procedure was halted. Both patients were placed under observation and recovered without treatment.

Birns (37) described inadvertent perforation of the bowel as a well-recognized potential complication of laparoscopy that had a low frequency—0.06% to 0.3%. If the injury is due to insertion of the Veress needle into a hollow viscus without tearing, no further therapy is indicated because the small diameter leaves no defect and the muscular wall closes over the puncture site.

Pneumoperitoneum associated with ruptured abdominal viscus is well known in the general surgery literature, and several authors have previously described the non-operative management of colonoscopic perforations (38, 39). Small perforations can be safely managed nonoperatively because the bowel preparation prior to colonoscopy reduces the amount of toxicity and contents spilled into the peritoneum.

Expectant management, copious irrigation and suction, and the consideration of prophylactic antibiotics represent reasonable treatment options for trauma to the gastrointestinal system with the insufflation needle. If active bleeding or peritonitis becomes apparent later, a laparotomy is indicated for primary closure.

Bladder injuries

Bladder injuries with the insufflation needle are rare unless the bladder is overdistended because of lack of catheterization before the procedure. In addition, misplaced transuterine insertion techniques can occasionally perforate the bladder anteriorly. The bladder is very forgiving, and many surgical procedures are actually performed through the bladder wall, including oocyte retrievals and multifetal selective reduction procedures. Urinary retention as a sequela of bladder trauma is a possibility, and affected patients can be taught self-catheterization. The need for an indwelling Foley catheter because of a Veress needle perforation is rare, unless hemorrhage accompanies the trauma.

The frequency of trauma to the urinary tract during laparoscopy is reported to be 0.5% (40). In a case report by Schanbacher et al. (41), urinary bladder perforation during laparoscopy was detected by distention of the collection bag with carbon dioxide. The authors speculated that gas distention of the urinary collection bag might serve as a reliable early sign of bladder perforation during laparoscopy; once recognized, this injury can be treated earlier.

Summary

Many different options and techniques exist for safe insertion of the Veress needle. Each case may offer its own unique challenges to initiating a pneumoperitoneum. If a hollow viscus such as bowel or bladder is perforated, the damage is usually minimal and self-contained. In most cases, conservative treatment measures can be initiated in conjunction with expectant management.

REFERENCES

1. Nadeau OE, Kampmeier OF. Endoscopy of the abdomen; abdominoscopy: a preliminary study, including a summary of the literature and a description of the technique. Surg Gynecol Obstet 1925;41:259–271.
2. Wittman I. Peritoneoscopy, vol 1. Budapest, Hungary: Publishing House of the Hungarian Academy of Sciences, 1966.
3. Gunning JE. The history of laparoscopy. J Reprod Med 1974;12:222–226.
4. Lukács D, Veress E Jr. Száz éve született Veress Elemér. Orv Hetil 1976;117:483–485.
5. Phillips JM, ed. Laparoscopy. Baltimore: Williams & Wilkins, 1977.
6. Semm K. Operative manual for endoscopic abdominal surgery. Friedrich ER, ed. and trans. Chicago: Year Book Medical Publishers, 1987.
7. Ahn YW, Owens B. Techniques for laparoscopy on patients with previous abdominal surgery. Int J Fertil 1979;24:264–266.
8. Ohlgisser M, Sorokin Y, Heifetz M. Gynecologic laparoscopy: a review article. Obstet Gynecol Surv 1985;40:385–396.
9. Loffer FD, Pent D. Laparoscopy in the obese patient. Am J Obstet Gynecol 1976;125:104–107.
10. Toth A, Graf M. The center of the umbilicus as the Veress needle's entry site for laparoscopy. J Reprod Med 1984;29:126–128.
11. Gupta SP. Positioning the Veress needle. Br J Surg 1989;76:381.
12. Lacey CG. Laparoscopy: a clinical sign for intraperitoneal needle placement. Obstet Gynecol 1976;47:625–627.
13. Fear RE. Laparoscopy: a valuable aid in gynecologic diagnosis. Obstet Gynecol 1968;31:297–309.
14. Cunanan RG Jr, Courey NG, Lippes J. Complications of laparoscopic tubal sterilization. Obstet Gynecol 1980;55:501–506.
15. Phillips JM. Complications in laparoscopy. Int J Gynaecol Obstet 1977;15:157–162.
16. Mintz M. Risks and prophylaxis in laparoscopy: a survey of 100,000 cases. J Reprod Med 1977;18:269–272.
17. Neely MR, McWilliams R, Makhlouf HA. Laparoscopy: routine pneumoperitoneum via the posterior fornix. Obstet Gynecol 1975;45:459–460.
18. Howard RE Jr. Laparoscopy: preliminary experience. Va Med Mon 1972;99:1063–1066.
19. Morgan HR. Laparoscopy: induction of pneumoperitoneum via transfundal puncture. Obstet Gynecol 1979;54:260–261.
20. Wolfe WM, Pasic R. Transuterine insertion of Veress needle in laparoscopy. Obstet Gynecol 1990;75:456–457.
21. Dingfelder JR. Direct laparoscope trocar insertion without prior pneumoperitoneum. J Reprod Med 1978;21:45-4-7.
22. Saidi MH. Direct laparoscopy without prior pneumoperitoneum. J Reprod Med 1986;31:684–686.
23. Copeland C, Wing R, Hulka JF. Direct trocar insertion at laparoscopy: an evaluation. Obstet Gynecol 1983;62:655–659.
24. Byron JW, Fujiyoshi CA, Miyazawa K. Evaluation of the direct trocar insertion technique at laparoscopy. Obstet Gynecol 1989;74:423–425.
25. Kenyon T, Lenker M, Underwood K. Gasless laparoscopy with mechanical peritoneal distention. Minimally Invasive Surgical Nursing 1994;8:62–67.
26. Schaller G, Kuenkel M, Manegold BC. The optical "Veress-needle"—initial puncture with a minioptic. End Surg 1995;3:55–57.
27. Salmi A, Lanzani G, Massimo G, Rangoni G, Vincenzi L. Sonographic study of pneumoperitoneum to avoid intestinal trocar injuries during laparoscopy. Gastrointest Endosc 1994;40:492–493.
28. Kabukoba JJ, Skillern LH. Coping with extraperitoneal insufflation during laparoscopy: a new technique. Obstet Gynecol 1992;80:144–145.

29. McDougall EM, Figenshau RS, Clayman RV, Monk TG, Smith DS. Laparoscopic pneumoperitoneum: impact of body habitus. J Laparoendosc Surg 1994;4:385–391.

30. Whitford JHW, Gunstone AJ. Gastric perforation: a hazard of laparoscopy under general anaesthesia. Br J Anaesth 1972;44:97–99.

31. Reynolds RC, Pauca AL. Gastric perforation, an anesthesia-induced hazard in laparoscopy. Anesthesiology 1973;38:84–85.

32. Endler GC, Moghissi KS. Gastric perforation during pelvic laparoscopy. Obstet Gynecol 1976;47(suppl):40S–42S.

33. Loffer FD, Pent D. Indications, contraindications and complications of laparoscopy. Obstet Gynecol Surv 1975;30:407–427.

34. Kleppinger RK. One thousand laparoscopies at a community hospital. J Reprod Med 1974;13:13–20.

35. Levy BS, Soderstrom RM, Dail DH. Bowel injuries during laparoscopy: gross anatomy and histology. J Reprod Med 1985;30:168–172.

36. Vilardell F, Seres I, Marti-Vicente A. Complications of peritoneoscopy: a survey of 1455 examinations. Gastrointest Endosc 1968;14:178–180.

37. Birns MT. Inadvertent instrumental perforation of the colon during laparoscopy: nonsurgical repair. Gastrointest Endosc 1989;35:54–56.

38. Taylor R, Weakley FL, Sullivan BH Jr. Non-operative management of colonoscopic perforation with pneumoperitoneum. Gastrointest Endosc 1978;24:124–125.

39. Winek TG, Mosely HS, Grout G, Luallin D. Pneumoperitoneum and its association with ruptured abdominal viscus. Arch Surg 1988;123:709–712.

40. Borten M. Laparoscopic complications: prevention and management. Toronto: Decker, 1986:331–350.

41. Schanbacher PD, Rossi LJ Jr, Salem MR, Joseph NJ. Detection of urinary bladder perforation during laparoscopy by distention of the collection bag with carbon dioxide. Anesthesiology 1994;80:680–681.

Insufflation of the Obese Patient

Gary Holtz

4

Significant obesity is the most commonly encountered relative contraindication to laparoscopy. Preperitoneal insufflation is the most frequent problem associated with these patients; it unquestionably arises because of the greater abdominal wall thickness involved.

Anatomy

Hurd and associates (1) reviewed the medical charts of women younger than age 65 who had undergone either abdominal magnetic imaging (MRI) with a sagittal view or computerized tomography (CT), and for whom height, weight, and age data were available. Patients with ascites, gross anatomical deformities, significant intra-abdominal masses, or the surgical absence of the umbilicus were excluded. Nineteen obese subjects met these criteria and weighed at least 73 kg. Fourteen subjects who weighed less were also evaluated and served as controls.

In each subject, four distances were measured (Fig. 4.1): (A) from the lower margin of the umbilicus to the anterior abdominal peritoneum at a 45° angle from horizontal (the most frequently employed site and angle of insertion of the Veress needle); (B) from the base of the umbilicus to the peritoneum at a 45° angle; (C) from the base of the umbilicus to the peritoneum at a 90° angle (a technique often advocated for use in the obese subject); and (D) from the base of the umbilicus to the great vessels at a 90° angle. The distance from the lower margin of the umbilicus to the peritoneum or the great vessels at a 90° angle (another site and angle of insertion frequently employed in obese patients) was not measured.

Body mass index (BMI = weight/height^2 = kg/m^2), also termed the Quetelet index, was employed to classify subjects as nonobese (BMI = <25), overweight (BMI = 25–30) or obese (BMI >30). Most of the nonobese subjects weighed less than 160 lb, those considered overweight weighed 160–200 lb, and the obese were heavier than 200 lb.

As would be expected, all four distances lengthened as BMI or weight increased, although distances A and B increased to a much larger degree. In the nonobese, minimal differences existed between distances A, B, and C. In the overweight group, distance A was more than twice distance B. In the obese, distance A was more than 16 cm in seven of ten women, and distance B exceeded 11 cm in half of these subjects. In contrast, distance C was 6 cm or less in all subjects.

All distances were derived in supine, unanesthetized women. Although the thickness of the abdominal wall did not change, the distance from the umbilicus to major retroperitoneal vessels and the angle of the peritoneum below the umbilicus might conceivably be altered with the subject in the dorsolithotomy position. Nezhat *et al.* (2) evaluated the position of the aortic bifurcation relative to the umbilicus in 64 consecutive women undergoing laparoscopy. Patients who were overweight or obese frequently exhibited a shift in the relative location of the aortic bifurcation when placed in steep Trendelenburg position, with the percentage having it at or below the umbilicus increasing substantially.

Manual elevation of the abdominal wall or elevation produced as a consequence of insufflation would also increase the distance from the umbilicus to the major vessels and alter the angle of the peritoneum below the umbilicus. The latter would increase the distance from the umbilicus to peritoneum if the needle was inserted at a 45° angle. It is unknown what differences might be noted in males.

Periumbilical insufflation

These observations have relevance for those surgeons inserting the Veress needle through the periumbilical region, particularly as the umbilicus often lies above or

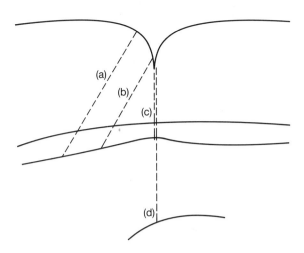

Fig. 4.1 Distances a–d from left to right. (Reproduced with permission from Hurd WW, Bude RO, DeLancey JOH, Gauvin JM, Aisen AM. Abdominal wall characteristics by MRI and CT imaging: the effect of obesity on laparoscopic approach. J Reprod Med 1992;36:473–476.)

at the level of the aortic bifurcation (1). If a standard-length (11.5–12 cm) Veress needle is employed in a nonobese individual, it may be inserted at a 45° angle, either in the lower margin of the umbilicus or at the base; this technique is associated with minimal likelihood of preperitoneal placement or major vessel injury.

Hurd and associates (1) recommended placement at a 45° angle through the base of the umbilicus in the overweight individual. In their study, the average distance from the lower margin of the umbilicus to the peritoneum was reported to be 6 ± 3 cm, suggesting this location should also permit a standard-length needle to traverse it, consistent with the author's experience. In three of nine subjects within this group, the average distance exceeded 10 cm—the basis for their recommendation. In the obese, they recommended placement of the needle at a 90° angle to the long axis of the patient through the base of the umbilicus so as to have a sufficiently long instrument to reach the peritoneal cavity. In contrast, the author was able to establish a pneumoperitoneum in 7 of 13 patients weighing more than 250 lb (maximum BMI = 50.6) with vertical placement of the Veress needle through the lower margin of the umbilicus (3). Unfortunately, Hurd *et al.* (1) did not measure this distance.

Clearly, usage of a longer (15–17 cm) needle alters these recommendations. Such instruments are long enough to reach the peritoneal cavity from the lower margin of the umbilicus in the overweight patient when inserted at a 45° angle, and usually can reach this location in the massively obese patient if directed somewhat more vertically. Their use also increases the risk of injury

to retroperitoneal blood vessels, however, placing even greater emphasis on appropriate techniques for elevating the abdominal wall.

Regardless of needle length, if vertical placement is planned, the umbilical area should be elevated by grasping on either side of this structure with the hands or towel clips. The abdomen should not be elevated in the usual manner by grasping below the umbilicus and lifting upward and caudal. The needle should be advanced only until the surgeon "senses" its entry into the abdominal cavity.

Alternative insertion sites

Several authors have described insertion of a Veress needle through alternative sites in an effort to avoid the difficulty associated with a thickened abdominal wall. The author has elected to employ these techniques only when dissection of peritoneum has hindered efforts to establish a pneumoperitoneum via preperitoneal insufflation.

Neely and colleagues (4) suggested placement of the needle through the posterior vaginal fornix. They recommended insertion 1.75 cm behind the cervical-vaginal junction (with a taut vagina). The needle was placed in the midline and advanced less than 3 cm. Clearly a longer needle would facilitate this technique given the length of the vagina. Neely *et al.* employed a specially designed needle that had a small hub limiting the potential depth of insertion.

Contraindications to such placement include a history or physical finding suggesting that the posterior cul-de-sac may be obliterated or involved with a significant disease process such as endometriosis. A mass located in this area—whether uterine, adnexal, or of other origin—or a posterior uterus that cannot be elevated with cervical traction are also contraindications.

The author has not had a favorable experience with this technique; a long Veress needle was not used and its absence may have partially accounted for the difficulties encountered. The inability to move the tip of the needle away from bowel or omentum filling the posterior cul-de-sac frequently resulted in high insufflation pressures and concern about inappropriate needle placement.

In 1979, Morgan (5) described insertion through yet another site, establishing the pneumoperitoneum via a transfundal puncture. Wolfe and Pask (6) subsequently reported the use of this technique in a group of obese patients, all having a BMI greater than 30. A tenaculum was used to straighten the uterus, and then sounded to determine the axis and assess length. A long Veress needle was then placed through the superior fundus.

The location of the large pelvic vessels, rectosigmoid, and sacral curve must be identified prior to puncture. To prevent injury to the structures enclosed within the broad ligament, lateral insertion should be avoided; an inappropriate anterior placement could perforate the bladder. In addition, a gas embolism could arise if the needle slips back into the endometrial cavity while being employed for insufflation.

Contraindications include uterine fibroids or suspected adhesions involving the uterine fundus. A relative contraindication is the inability to adequately straighten the long axis of the uterus. An intentional uterine perforation also complicates hydrotubation because of leakage through the defect created, although this problem can be minimized by applying pressure to the perforation site with a suprapubic probe. Clearly, however, subsequent hysteroscopy would be difficult at best.

Yet another technique for needle insertion is that described by Kleppinger (7). The uterus is elevated against the anterior abdominal wall and the needle passed through it into the fundus. Insertion can then be undertaken without risk of injury to the great vessels. It can be accomplished only if the fundus may be palpated abdominally when elevated, limiting its use in the obese. In many of these subjects, however, the lower abdominal wall is relatively thin. A slight risk of bowel or bladder injury remains if these organs are adherent to the fundus. To reduce the risk of the latter complication, the bladder should be emptied before surgery. (The author has no experience with this technique.)

Regardless of site or technique of insertion, it is crucial that the surgeon be confident of appropriate needle placement before insufflating significant volumes of gas. Although many techniques used to confirm correct placement are valid in the obese, a few are less reliable in these patients. Initial pressures should be less than 10 mm Hg in any patient with good abdominal wall relaxation and the usual increase in pressure should be seen with inspiration. Checking for liver dullness is much less reliable in these patients, as is the surgeon's ability to recognize asymmetric distention. Operating on the obese subject places particular emphasis on the surgeon's experience and ability to "sense" whether needle placement is correct. If any doubt exists, the needle should be removed and replaced prior to insufflation of a significant volume of gas. To avoid this problem, some surgeons employ direct trocar insertion in all patients, including obese subjects.

The availability of microendoscopes that may be inserted through an insufflation needle permits the direct visualization of the needle's location. Unfortunately, most operating rooms do not currently have such systems available.

Open laparoscopy

Open laparoscopy eliminates several problems encountered when performing laparoscopy in the massively obese. Preperitoneal insufflation is precluded and the risk of great vessel injury reduced. This surgical technique also facilitates entry to the abdominal cavity when preperitoneal emphysema has already occurred. Lastly, it "lengthens" the laparoscopic cannula.

Despite establishment of an adequate pneumoperitoneum, the laparoscopic trocar and sleeve may prove too short to reach and enter the abdominal cavity in the massively obese patient. It has been suggested that the use of higher than usual intra-abdominal pressure will push the peritoneum against the abdominal wall and facilitate placement of the trocar. The author has found this tactic to be ineffective. In three of seven subjects weighing more than 250 lb in whom the Veress needle was successfully inserted and an adequate pneumoperitoneum established, the trocar could not be placed into the abdominal cavity because it was too short (3).

When using the open technique, the length of the sheath ceases to be a limiting factor. The telescope may be placed through the cannula and this combined instrument used to align the defects in skin/fascia/peritoneum.

The open laparoscopy technique used by the author in obese patients represents a modification of the more general technique. After incision of the fascia, no sutures are placed to secure the Hasson cannula—this instrument is not used in the procedure. All dissection beneath this layer is performed bluntly with a Kelly clamp, and no effort is made to place retractors through the incision into the peritoneal cavity due to its depth. Instead, a finger is inserted into the abdomen to ensure that no bowel is adherent near the site of blunt entry and to confirm that all layers of the abdominal wall have been traversed. The standard laparoscopic cannula, with the telescope placed through it, is introduced. Appropriate placement is confirmed by observation through the endoscope, and the skin is then secured about the cannula with two Allis clamps. The technique for closure has been modified since publication; no effort is made to close the small defect in the fascia. The thickness of the preperitoneal fat and the lack of perfect vertical alignment in the sites of entry prevent herniation through this minimal defect. To date, the author has successfully performed open laparoscopy in all obese patients attempted, with the heaviest being 365 lb.

Conclusion

Obese patients are at significantly greater risk for complications when undergoing laparotomy. As a consequence, laparoscopic surgery may be of particular benefit to these individuals. It may be performed safely in virtually all obese subjects if appropriate modifications in technique are utilized.

REFERENCES

1. Hurd WW, Bude RO, DeLancey JOH, Gauvin JM, Aisen AM. Abdominal wall characteristics by MRI and CT imaging: the effect of obesity on laparoscopic approach. J Reprod Med 1992;36: 473–476.
2. Nezhat F, Nezhat C, Nezhat CH, Seidman D, Ashrafria M, Nezhat A. A laparoscopic appraisal of the anatomic relationship of the umbilicus to the aortic bifurcation. J Am Assoc Gynecol Lap 1995;2:536–537.
3. Holtz G. Laparoscopy in the massively obese female. Obstet Gynecol 1987;69:423–424.
4. Neely MR, McWilliams R, Makhlove HA. Laparoscopy: pneumoperitoneum via the posterior fornix. Obstet Gynecol 1975;45: 459–460.
5. Morgan HR. Laparoscopy: introduction of pneumoperitoneum via transfundal puncture. Obstet Gynecol 1979;54:260–261.
6. Wolfe WM, Pask R. Transfundal insertion of Veress needle in laparoscopy. Obstet Gynecol 1990;75:456–457.
7. Kleppinger RK. Closed techniques for equipment insertion. In: Martin DC, Holtz GL, Levinson CJ, Soderstrom RM, Phillips JM, eds. Manual of endoscopy. Santa Fe Springs, Calif.: The American Association of Gynecologic Laparoscopists, 1990.

Perforation of the Large Vascular Structures | 5

Barbara S. Levy

Introduction

One of the most devastating and life-threatening injuries to occur during diagnostic or operative laparoscopy is laceration of a major abdominal blood vessel. Reports have surfaced of perforations of the following vessels: aorta; vena cava; common, right, and left iliac arteries and veins; superior mesenteric vessels; inferior epigastric; and patent umbilical veins. The true incidence of great vessel injury is unknown, as the vast majority of cases go unreported. In 1989, Baadsgaard *et al.* (1) reviewed published cases of vascular injury and added one from their institution. Penfield (2), in a survey of 25 experienced laparoscopists from the United States, Canada, the United Kingdom, and the Netherlands, found 19 known episodes of needle and trocar injuries to the vascular system in more than 30,000 cases. In 1980, Hulka (serving as chairman of the American Association of Gynecologic Laparoscopists' Complications Committee) knew of more than 100 cases in the United States alone. Whatever the true incidence has been in the past, as more complex intra-abdominal surgical procedures are performed endoscopically, all with multiple trocar insertions, the risk of major vessel injuries will undoubtedly increase.

Historically, patients at highest risk for vascular injury have been young, thin, nulliparous women with well-developed abdominal musculature. The aorta may lie less than an inch (2.5 cm) below the skin in these women (3, 4). Obesity may play a role as well, as a surgeon trying to avoid properitoneal placement of the insufflating needle may overzealously thrust the instrument in a perpendicular fashion and impale the retroperitoneal vessels against the sacral promontory. Because laparoscopic procedures are being performed on a much more diverse patient population than ever before, other risk factors for vessel injury may surface as older and more medically complicated patients undergo this type of surgery.

Several technical factors have been identified as contributing to injuries of the great vessels. Operator inexperience clearly represents an important factor; most complications are known to occur in a surgeon's first 100 cases. Other commonly cited causative factors are a dull trocar, disposable trocars (5, 6), inadequate pneumoperitoneum, failure to stabilize the abdominal wall, perpendicular or lateral insertion of the needle or trocar, forceful thrusting motion for insertion, failure to note anatomical landmarks, and abnormal or inappropriate patient positioning. Each of these technical problems will be addressed in detail in this chapter with the hope that many vascular injuries can be avoided.

Anatomy

Knowledge of the anatomy of the retroperitoneal space and the corresponding abdominal wall landmarks is critical in carrying out this type of surgery. The aortic bifurcation occurs at the level of L4 in 75% of patients. L4 can be consistently located at the level of the summits of the iliac crests. In 9% of patients the bifurcation will lie above L4 and in 11% of patients it will be below 14–5. In 80% of patients, however, the bifurcation will appear within 1.25 cm above or below the iliac crests (7). Even in markedly obese patients the iliac crests are usually palpable.

The position of the umbilicus varies widely and should not be used to predict the location of the underlying great vessels. The Trendelenburg position rotates the sacral promontory and the lower aorta into a location closer to the umbilicus (8) and a much shallower angle (Figs. 5.1 and 5.2). In patients with such a diminished margin of safety, both vascular injury and preperitoneal insufflation will be more common. The operator (surgeon) should be present in the operating room when the sterile drapes are being applied and the patient is positioned. Many anesthesiologists, in an effort to expedite the case, will place the patient in a steep Trendelenburg position. After the drapes are applied, ascertaining the patient's true position may prove difficult.

Abdominal entry techniques

Once the patient is placed in the supine position, prepared, and draped, the superior aspect of the iliac crest should be palpated and an effort made to trace the aorta and its bifurcation by palpitation. This maneuver will also allow the surgeon to assess the adequacy of general anesthesia and abdominal wall relaxation before beginning the procedure. Next, a superficial skin incision is made. In multiparous, thin patients, an effort must be made to avoid peritoneal penetration. One case of superior mesenteric vein laceration has been reported (9) involving a perforation that occurred with the initial skin incision in a patient with a large rectus diastasis. The type of blade used for the incision was not discussed. Use of a No. 12 blade may help to avoid inadvertent incision of the peritoneum.

Before attempting to place the Veress needle, this instrument should be inspected and tested for proper function. Occasionally the operating personnel may reassemble the equipment improperly, forgetting the spring or combining a long needle with a short obturator.

During insertion the valve on the needle must remain open to allow room air to enter the abdominal cavity immediately upon peritoneal entry, thereby allowing the bowel to fall away from the needle tip. The technique also permits immediate recognition of the intravascular placement and prevents gas insufflation into the circulation.

Elevation of the entire abdominal wall may be attempted prior to needle insertion, but only by manual elevation or by placing sutures directly into the fascia. Attempts to elevate the abdominal wall with towel clips merely give the illusion of safety. They elevate the skin and subcutaneous space, but have no effect on the peritoneum (10). Elevating the skin will increase the distance over which the needle must travel and may distort the surgeon's perception of the angle of entry. Vigorous bites with towel clips intended to raise the full thickness of the abdominal wall may result in bowel perforation.

With the abdominal wall manually stabilized or elevated by the surgeon's nondominant hand, the Veress needle should be grasped between the thumb and forefinger of the dominant hand like a pencil. It is then firmly but gently guided at 45° toward the middle of the pelvic cavity, or toward the fundus of the elevated uterus if palpitation of the anatomy has proved difficult. Peritoneal placement should be verified by placing a syringe with 10–20 mL of saline on the hub of the needle. The fluid should drop freely into the peritoneal cavity. Reaspiration can be used to test for peritoneal or intravascular placement. In addition, a return of small bowel or stomach contents demonstrates inappropriate placement. A blood return from the needle should prompt the immediate suspicion of vascular injury unless hemoperitoneum was previously identified. If difficulty is encountered with Veress needle placement at the umbilicus, the instrument may be repositioned safely in the left upper quadrant under most circumstances.

Once proper intraperitoneal position has been established, insufflation may begin. Intraperitoneal pressure of greater than 15 mm Hg may indicate obstruction of the needle by the small bowel or the omentum. The needle tip may be freed by lifting and bouncing the anterior abdominal wall manually. This tactic causes a pocket of gas to accumulate around the needle tip and may force the small bowel and omentum away from it. The Veress needle itself should not be moved from its plane of insertion. Several reports indicate that further vascular injury occurred when the Veress needle was maneuvered after increased insufflation pressure had been noted. If the needle has been inserted into the retroperitoneal space, further manipulation of the needle could cause a great vessel perforation or laceration. If elevation of the abdominal wall does not decrease the insufflation pressure, the needle should be gently removed and replaced, taking care to repeat all the initial safety maneuvers.

More than half of all reported major vessel injuries were caused by either the primary or secondary trocar. Dull instruments have been implicated in contributing to this type of complication. For example, dull trocars require increased force to penetrate the fascia. Surgeons who are accustomed to reusable instruments may develop insertion techniques that prove hazardous when the less forgiving razor-sharp disposables are substituted. With all primary trocars, the depth of penetration of the trocar tip can be best controlled by stabilizing guidance of the surgeon's nondominant hand.

Preperitoneal insufflation with the consequent tenting of the peritoneum away from the abdominal wall, necessitating multiple attempts at trocar insertion, can be problematic. Corson (10) has demonstrated that the force necessary to pass a reusable trocar is twice as great as that needed to pass a disposable one. The safety shield most likely does not provide much additional protection. Instead, a drop of saline can be placed in the insufflation port of the trocar sleeve with the stopcock closed. Using a "Z" technique, the trocar and the most distal end of the sleeve are tunneled horizontally under the skin for a distance of 1 to 2 cm. Once the small insufflation ports in the trocar sleeve are subcutaneous, the stopcock is opened, allowing saline to travel to the end of the sleeve. When a gas-filled cavity is entered, saline will "spit" from the port, signaling to the surgeon that the trocar sleeve lies within the insufflation area.

The safety shield is designed to lock after release of the initial resistance. Not infrequently, it becomes hung up on the peritoneum, necessitating several passes with the trocar. As with any device, a smooth, steady gentle pressure should be applied to the instrument.

Once the pneumoperitoneum has been established, no further elevation of the anterior abdominal wall is possible. Rather than attempting to lift the skin, the surgeon's nondominant hand should be used to guide the depth of trocar insertion and steady the abdominal wall, ensuring the appropriate direction of insertion. This technique is particularly useful for surgeons with small hands who are attempting to control large trocars. If resistance to penetration of the fascia is encountered, either due to an inadequately sharpened trocar, inadequate muscle relaxation, or scarred fascia from previous surgery, the solution is not to twist and thrust the trocar repeatedly. Instead, a disposable or properly sharpened trocar should be substituted. If additional equipment is unavailable, the fascia may be nicked with a knife blade at the point of intended penetration. Safe, gentle, and controlled entry of the trocar is thereby facilitated, and multiple passes with the trocar avoided.

When the laparoscope is introduced through the trocar sheath and peritoneal fat is visualized, a small traumatic grasping forceps may be introduced through an operating channel and the peritoneum entered under direct vision. Once a small opening has been made in the peritoneum, it is an easy matter to guide the laparoscope and trocar sleeve through the opening and immediately insufflate the appropriate space to facilitate secondary trocar placement.

Some have argued that the "Z" technique may lead to iliac injury (11) by making the operator unaware of his or her actual angle of insertion. In reality, burrowing 1 to 2 cm below the umbilicus should allow the trocar to begin its entry into the pelvic cavity well below the dangerous area of the sacral promontory.

The surgeon should be familiar with multiple techniques for insufflation and abdominal access. When difficulty is encountered in penetrating the fascia or insufflating the abdomen, the open Hasson technique may be used. Minilaparotomy may always be considered.

All additional trocars must be placed under direct vision. Through transillumination, the inferior epigastric vessels can often be identified and avoided. The direction of secondary trocar insertion in the pelvis must be away from the sacral promontory and pelvic side walls and toward the fundus of the uterus—an acknowledgment that a small laceration of the uterine serosa is more readily controlled than a major vessel tear. Consequently, the surgeon should use the smallest ancillary trocar possible to decrease the risk of injury to the inferior epigastric.

Major vessel injury should be suspected whenever blood returns from the open insufflating needle. In addition, the sudden deterioration in vital signs (decreased end-tidal CO_2, decreased blood pressure, and increased heart rate) of a previously stable patient after needle or trocar insertion should be considered a vascular accident until proved otherwise. Peterson *et al.* (12) reported a case in which a 38-year-old healthy woman died due to an unrecognized aortic laceration. After initial insertion of the Veress needle, the insufflating pressure exceeded 20 mm Hg. The needle was manipulated until a normal pressure reading was obtained, and the abdomen insufflated with carbon dioxide. Four minutes after trocar insertion the patient's blood pressure could not be obtained. The surgeon searched the peritoneal cavity but found no sign of bleeding. Resuscitation efforts therefore focused on an anaphylactic reaction to anesthetic medication rather than exsanguination, and the patient died.

Whenever any additional manipulation of the needle or trocar is required and the patient becomes unstable, a vascular injury must be suspected. A large hematoma may accumulate in the retroperitoneal space before any intraperitoneal sign of hemorrhage becomes evident. Management includes notifying the anesthesiologist of the possibility of massive hemorrhage so that central lines can be placed and blood acquired. In such cases, laparotomy should be performed immediately through a midline incision; adequate exposure of the retroperitoneal vessels cannot be accomplished readily via a Pfannenstiel incision. Control of large bleeding vessels can be obtained by digital pressure or with sponge packs until the patient is stabilized and the appropriate surgical help has arrived. An additional anesthesiologist and a surgeon trained to manage vascular complications should be summoned immediately to the operating room. Once the patient has been stabilized, retractors can be placed for visualization, the peritoneum overlying the vessel incised, the vessels isolated and the injuries repaired with vascular sutures, clips, or patches. After the vascular repair is complete, a thorough abdominal exploration should be performed to search for concomitant injuries—especially to the bowel. Few sequelae have been reported when rapid and appropriate measures were initiated after vascular injury.

Summary

Major vessel injuries during laparoscopy are, for the most part, preventable (13). In the past most injuries reported in the literature were related to Veress needle trauma. More recent reports (14) demonstrate an increasing incidence of vascular injury caused by trocars. To minimize the likelihood of this type of injury, the surgeon must palpate the abdomen and review the anatomy in each patient. The position of the patient should be verified and the equipment inspected. The Veress needle should be open to the air during insertion and directed at 45° toward the hollow of the pelvic cavity. Each trocar must be sharp and inserted at the proper angle with careful, controlled descent. Finally, positive identification of abdominal wall vessels and insertion of all additional trocars under direct vision will prevent most major vessel perforation.

REFERENCES

1. Baadsgaard SE, Billie S, Egeblad K. Major vascular injury during gynecologic laparoscopy. Acta Obstet Gynecol Scand 1989;68: 283–285.
2. Penfield AJ. Trocar and needle injury. In: Phillips JM, ed. Laparoscopy. Baltimore: Williams & Williams, 1977:236–241.
3. Hulka JF. Major vessel injury during laparoscopy. Am J Obstet Gynecol 1980;138:590.
4. Kurzel RB, Edinger DD. Injury to the great vessels. A hazard of transabdominal endoscopy. South Med J 1983;76:656–657.
5. McDonald PT, Rich NM, Collins CJ, Anderson CA, Kozloff L. Vascular trauma secondary to diagnostic and therapeutic procedures: laparoscopy. Am J Surg 1979;136:651–655.
6. Shin CS. Vascular injury secondary to laparoscopy. NY State J Med 1982;82:935–936.
7. Gray H. In: Goss GM, eds. Anatomy of the human body, 28 ed. Philadelphia: Lea and Febiger, 1966:646–647.
8. Lynn SC, Katz AR, Ross PJ. Aortic perforation sustained at laparoscopy. J Reprod Med 1982;27:2;17–19.
9. Bartsich EG, Dillon TF. Injury of superior mesenteric vein laparoscopic procedure with unusual complication. NY State J Med 1981;81:933.
10. Corson SL. Major vessel injury during laparoscopy. Am J Obstet Gynecol 1980;138:589.
11. Katz M, Beck P, Tancer ML. Major vessel injury during laparoscopy: anatomy of two cases. Am J Obstet Gynecol 1979;135:544–545.
12. Peterson HB, Greenspan JR, Ory HW. Death following puncture of the aorta during laparoscopic sterilization. Obstet Gynecol 1982;59:133–134.
13. Yuzpe AA. Pneumoperitoneum needle and trocar injuries in laparoscopy. A survey on possible contributing factors and prevention. J Reprod Med 1990;35:485–490.
14. Nordestgaard AG, Bodily KC, Osborne RW, Buttorff JD. Major vascular injuries during laparoscopic procedures. Am J Surg 1995;169:543–545.

Perforation of the Inferior Epigastric Vessels | 6

D. Alan Johns

Major vascular injuries in gynecologic laparoscopy are rare, but bleeding in the abdominal wall caused by trocar placement has been encountered by every surgeon using a laparoscope. Of all laparoscopic complications, perforation of the inferior and superficial epigastric vessels is the most frequently encountered (and least likely to be reported). Both vessels are large and bleed profusely when injured. Perforation of the inferior epigastric artery will produce retroperitoneal or intraperitoneal bleeding; damage to the superficial epigastric will result in intramuscular or subcutaneous bleeding. Unfortunately, every laparoscopic surgeon will eventually encounter one of these bleeding vessels, an experience that is both terrifying and challenging.

Anatomy of the inferior epigastric vessels

Obviously, the best method of preventing complications related to these vessels is to avoid them altogether. Knowledge of the anatomy and normal course of the inferior and superficial epigastric arteries can substantially reduce the risk of vessel injury. Knowing where to look for these vessels aids in their identification, permitting the surgeon to direct the trocar spike away from trouble.

The inferior epigastric artery arises from the external iliac artery and anastomoses with the superior epigastric artery. It can usually be identified at the junction of the round ligament and the umbilical ligament (obliterated umbilical artery) at the inguinal canal. It lies *beneath* the rectus muscle and immediately above the peritoneum, coursing cephalad just medial to the lateral edge of the rectus muscle. Generally, the artery does not traverse the rectus muscle toward the midline. Because the course of the inferior epigastric artery follows the lateral aspect of the rectus muscle, any secondary punctures should be made medial or well lateral to the lateral edge of the rectus muscle (if it is identifiable).

The superficial epigastric artery arises from the femoral artery near the inguinal ring and courses medially *over* the rectus muscle toward the midline. Because it is not always visible (either directly or by transillumination of the abdominal wall), this vessel is more difficult to avoid.

Causes of vessel injury

Although laceration of the superficial or inferior epigastric vessel may occur during any laparoscopic procedure, certain factors increase the risk of this complication. In patients who have undergone previous abdominal surgery—particularly those with Pfannenstiel incisions—the course of either vessel may be altered or obscured by the incisional scar. Additionally, the density of these scars hinders directional control during trocar insertion.

The abdomen of the obese patient is impossible to transilluminate, making direct transabdominal visual identification of these vessels unlikely. In addition, working around a panniculus makes precise placement of the secondary trocar very difficult. In such situations, misdirection of the trocar (either medial or lateral to its intended path) may occur, placing the epigastric vessels at greater risk.

Obviously, the more attempts required to attain intraperitoneal placement of the trocars, the greater the risk of vessel injury. Once the trocar spike has traversed the fascia and the trocar sleeve has been placed, the trocar spike need not be used to replace a sleeve that has slipped out of position or been intentionally removed. Simply pass a blunt irrigating probe through the laparoscopic sleeve and direct the probe through the skin, fascial, and peritoneal incisions into the peritoneal cavity. Using the irrigation probe as a guide, push the sleeve through the abdominal wall and into place. The use of a trocar spike to *replace* a secondary trocar sleeve increases the risk of vessel injury and is unnecessary.

Patients requiring more than two secondary puncture sites are at greater risk for vessel injury. The more times that the surgeon must attempt to avoid the vessels, the more likely that a mishap will occur. In addition to the intraumbilical site, most laparoscopic procedures require two 5-mm secondary ports (and sometimes a third port). As the endoscopic surgeon becomes more familiar with suturing and electrosurgical techniques, the necessity for three or four secondary ports larger than 5.5 mm in size will decrease.

Obviously, the larger the trocar and sleeve, the greater the risk of abdominal wall vessel injury. Large trocars (10 and 11 mm) used for secondary ports are associated with a greater risk of perforation of the epigastric vessels than 5- and 3-mm sleeves. In addition, these larger trocars carry an increased risk of incisional hernia. One should always use the smallest possible trocar necessary to complete the procedure.

Minimizing the risk of injury during laparoscopic procedures

Identification of inferior epigastric vessels

Efforts to avoid injury to the epigastric vessels should begin as soon as the laparoscope is in place. In the slender patient, the edge of the rectus muscle and the epigastric vessels are occasionally visible by transillumination of the abdominal wall. This technique should never be exclusively used to identify and avoid the inferior epigastric artery, however. Instead, transillumination simply allows the surgeon to locate and stay away from more superficial branches of these vessels.

When the surgical procedure does not require placement of secondary trocars lateral to the border of the rectus muscle, the epigastric vessels can be avoided by remaining within a triangular area bounded by the oblit-erated umbilical arteries laterally and the dome of the bladder (Fig. 6.1). The obliterated umbilical artery (umbilical ligament) courses from the umbilicus along the anterior abdominal wall to the inguinal ring. Secondary puncture trocars positioned within the margins of this triangle should not place the inferior epigastric artery at risk.

More commonly, trocar sleeves must be located in a more lateral position, placing the inferior epigastric artery (and the iliac vessels) at greater risk. Careful inspection of the peritoneal surface of the anterior abdominal wall permits direct identification of the inferior epigastric artery, but the surgeon must be familiar with several anatomic landmarks (the obliterated umbilical artery, the inguinal canal, and the round ligament). The epigastric vessels are most easily identified at the inguinal ring where the obliterated umbilical artery and the round ligament meet. The pulsations of the inferior epigastric artery allow the surgeon to visually mark its course and place trocars accordingly.

Insertion of trocars

Knowing the exact location of the epigastric vessels is useless if the surgeon is unable to direct the trocar spike accurately. Once the relevant vessels have been identified, the proposed path of the trocar is established by pushing on the abdominal wall and marking the location for the skin incision. In the more obese patient, the path can be traced with a spinal needle to ensure that it remains at a distance from the vessels.

The tip of the trocar spike is pushed into (but not through) the fascia. The trocar is then passed through the fascia at a 90° angle to the abdominal wall and fascia. This angle of insertion is critical in minimizing the amount of tissue through which the trocar must pass and predicting its ultimate path.

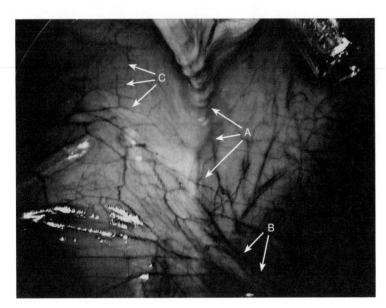

Fig. 6.1 Anatomical location of the inferior epigastric artery. A = umbilical ligament; B = round ligament; C = inferior epigastric artery.

Insertion of the secondary trocar is best accomplished while holding up the abdominal wall with the tip of the laparoscope, which is positioned lateral to the peritoneal entry site (thereby protecting the iliac vessels). Effectively, the surgeon pushes against the abdominal wall, the CO_2, and the laparoscope. Using this technique, it is not necessary to visualize the trocar spike coming through the fascia. Once the fascia has been traversed, the spike can be directed through the peritoneum under direct vision.

Control of bleeding upon vessel injury

When meticulous attention to preventive measures fails to avoid vascular injury (as occasionally happens), the surgeon must be prepared to control the resultant bleeding immediately. Rapid, definitive management is mandatory to prevent significant blood loss.

The first and most important rule is: **Do not remove the sleeve.** Immediately following the injury, a hematoma forms and quickly obscures the bleeding vessel. The trocar sleeve provides the only accurate marker for the location of the injured vessel. If the sleeve is removed, it becomes extremely difficult to identify the bleeding vessel within the large hematoma.

The magnitude of the bleeding dictates the first corrective action. If the hemorrhage is brisk and not *immediately* controllable, the skin and fascial incision should be enlarged and the vessel controlled by conventional means. In such a case, none of the methods mentioned later in this chapter should be attempted because of the risk of hypovolemic hypotension. The epigastric vessels run cephalad to caudad, and have significant anastamotic connections. For adequate hemostasis, both ends of the transected vessel usually require control.

Immediately after the injury, an attempt should be made to visually identify the vessel and control bleeding with electrosurgery. Using any 5-mm instrument, tilt the sleeve (i.e., the one that injured the vessel) toward the abdominal wall and away from the bleeding. This action should expose the lacerated vessel, which can then be controlled with electrosurgical coaptation. Because the developing hematoma will quickly obscure the bleeding vessel, this technique requires that all electrosurgical instruments be assembled, tested, and immediately available on the operative field. For this reason, no secondary trocar should be inserted unless every bipolar and unipolar forceps is ready for immediate use.

If electrosurgical instrumentation is not available or the damaged vessel is not obvious, suturing techniques may be attempted. A large curved or straight needle with 0-gauge (or larger) suture is passed into the abdomen and brought out lateral to the bleeding vessel. If the surgeon can secure the injured epigastric vessel within this ligature, bleeding is easily and quickly controlled. This "retention" suture is tied over a temporary "bridge"

consisting of a cloth sponge. The suture is removed 4 to 24 hours later, depending on the magnitude of the bleeding.

Although effective, suture methods are cumbersome and somewhat slow; they also require a significant amount of luck to achieve success with vessel injuries. Newer devices have greatly simplified this technique. The "J-Needle" (Unimar, Inc., Wilton, Connecticut), for example, uses a J-shaped needle to pass a suture through the trocar wound and back through the abdominal wall, encircling the bleeding vessel. The "Carter-Thomason Needle-Point Suture Passer" (Inlet Medical, Inc., Eden Prairie, Minnesota) utilizes a pointed instrument (Fig. 6.2) that functions as both a needle and grasper, permitting the surgeon to accurately direct it through the abdominal wall.

If immediate control of bleeding is required and none of these instruments is readily available, temporary hemostasis can be quickly achieved with a No. 12 Foley catheter, which will easily pass through a 5.5-mm trocar sleeve. Once the catheter has been passed through the sleeve and into the abdominal cavity (Fig. 6.3), it is inflated with 5 to 8 cc's of fluid; because it is less compressible than air, this fluid will better tamponade the bleeding vessel.

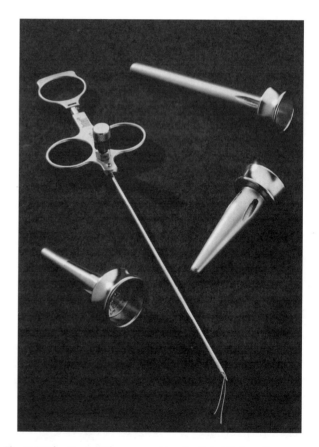

Fig. 6.2 The Carter-Thomason Needle-Point Suture Passer.

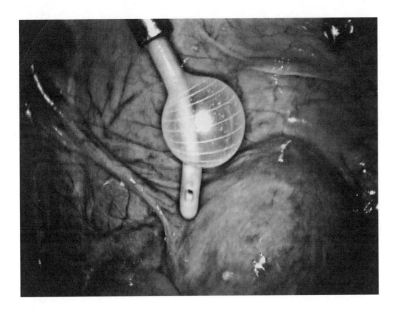

Fig. 6.3 The Foley catheter passed through the 5.5-mm suprapubic sleeve.

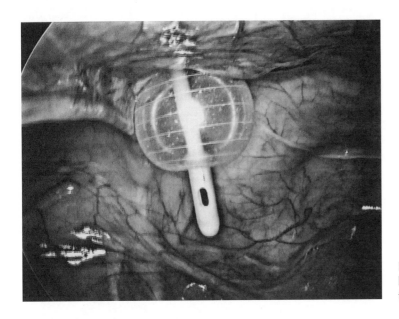

Fig. 6.4 Trocar sleeve removed and inflated Foley bulb pulled against the abdominal wall, compressing the injured inferior epigastric artery.

After the Foley bulb is inflated, the secondary trocar sleeve is removed from the abdominal wall. The Foley balloon is then pulled against the abdominal wall and secured by applying a hemostat to the catheter as it exits the skin incision (Fig. 6.4). Occlusion of the vessel should occur immediately. As soon as hemostasis is attained, another secondary trocar can be inserted and the operation continued.

The Foley catheter is a quick, temporary method of control, and should be removed before the patient leaves the operating room. If bleeding recurs after the catheter is removed, permanent control can be attained under more controlled circumstances.

Regardless of the technique used for control of epigastric vessel hemorrhage, a subcutaneous, subfascial, or retroperitoneal, hematoma usually develops. It will produce a large area of discoloration of the abdominal wall, often extending down into the labia.

On rare occasions, the clot may lyse and drain through one of the suprapubic incisions, typically 18 to 36 hours after development of the hematoma. The leakage of such a large amount of blood through the secondary puncture site will certainly alarm the patient unless he or she has been forewarned. Drainage of this hematoma, however, is usually associated with an immediate decrease in abdominal pain. The patient should be informed of these possibilities to avoid a panicked trip to the emergency room.

Conclusion

Given the increasing frequency of laparoscopic surgery, hemorrhagic complications from injury to the epigastric vessels will be a recurrent problem. It is imperative that the surgeon performing such procedures become familiar with all methods by which these injuries can be controlled, and that both the surgeon and the operating room staff be prepared to avoid a potentially serious hemorrhage. Rapid, efficient control of a hemorrhagic complication early in the laparoscopic procedure allows the surgeon to complete the operation with little associated morbidity.

7 Trocar Injuries to the Large Intestine

Steven R. Bayer

Injury to the intestinal tract during laparoscopy is an uncommon event. However, if this complication is not immediately recognized and managed appropriately, significant morbidity will most likely occur. At laparoscopy the intestines are most vulnerable to injury during trocar insertion. As insertion of the primary trocar is a blind procedure, it is amazing that trauma to the intestinal tract is not the rule rather than the exception. However, the establishment of a pneumoperitoneum and placement of the patient in the Trendelenburg position help to reduce the chance of bowel injury. Furthermore, the intestinal tract is not fixed, allowing it to move out of the way if it comes in contact with the advancing trocar.

While injury can occur to any segment of the intestinal tract, this chapter will be confined to a discussion on trocar injuries to the large intestine. The diagnosis, treatment, and prevention of this complication will be discussed.

Incidence

Injury to the colon during trocar insertion is a relatively rare complication, with an incidence of approximately 0.1% (1–3). The transverse colon is the segment of the large intestine that is most commonly traumatized.

Anatomic considerations

The large intestine begins in the right lower quadrant and encircles the abdominal cavity in a clockwise fashion as it ends in the rectum. The first part of the large intestine is the ascending colon, which begins at the ileocecal valve, the terminal segment of the small intestine. The ascending colon assumes a retroperitoneal location and extends superiorly up to the hepatic flexure. The transverse colon is the most mobile portion of the colon and extends between the hepatic and splenic flexures of the large intestine. Throughout its entire length the transverse colon is attached to the greater curvature of the stomach by the gastrocolic ligament. The omental apron drapes over and is attached to the anterior aspect of the transverse colon. The descending colon begins at the splenic flexure and extends inferiorly, assuming a retroperitoneal location. The next segment, which is also retroperitoneal, is the sigmoid colon, which distally turns into the rectum.

The ascending and descending segments of the colon are unlikely to be injured during trocar placement, not only because they are displaced laterally, but also because their retroperitoneal location prevents any intraperitoneal adhesions from displacing their position. From an anatomic standpoint the transverse colon is most at risk for injury for several reasons. First, it is intimately attached to the greater curvature of the stomach; gastric distention that can occur during mask ventilation can move the transverse colon inferiorly to a vulnerable position. Second, omental adhesions, either to the abdominal wall or to the pelvis, can result in displacement of the transverse colon to a location that can put it at risk for injury. The rectum and sigmoid colon are at a theoretical risk since they are fixed in the midline and in the path of the advancing trocar. Although their distant location from the trocar insertion site reduces their chance of injury, uncontrolled insertion of the primary or secondary trocar could result in injury to the distal colon. In addition, endometriosis involving the posterior cul-de-sac can result in attachment of the sigmoid colon to the posterior uterus, making it more vulnerable to injury during trocar placement.

Predisposing factors

Injury to the large colon by an experienced laparoscopist is usually avoided. However, if the surgeon deviates from proper surgical technique, intraabdominal injury can result. There are several situations that are associated with an increased incidence of injury to intraabdominal organs including the colon.

Failure to establish a pneumoperitoneum

The first step of laparoscopy is the establishment of a pneumoperitoneum. After insertion of the Veress needle into the peritoneal cavity, carbon dioxide insufflation is begun. On occasion the needle is not in the proper location and instead the preperitoneal space is insufflated. This situation is confirmed when on initial laparoscopic examination only loose areolar tissue is seen in a confined space. Insufflation of the preperitoneal space can complicate any laparoscopy, but is more common when this procedure is performed on the obese patient. After the problem is identified it is tempting to reinsert the trocar, but the risk of intraabdominal trauma is higher because the ballooned-out peritoneum is now in close proximity to the abdominal organs. The author's approach to this problem is to first empty the gas from the preperitoneal space through the laparoscopic sleeve and start over. Another attempt can then be made to reinsert the Veress needle through the original infraumbilical incision while making an adjustment in the angle of insertion. Because the previous insufflation of the preperitoneal space has separated the peritoneum from the abdominal wall, it may be more difficult to pierce the peritoneum with the Veress needle. If insufflation of the preperitoneal space occurs again or one cannot be assured that the needle is in the peritoneal cavity, then the surgeon has two options. First, the Veress needle can be inserted through an alternative port of entry (i.e., transcervical through the uterine fundus, transvaginally through the pouch of Douglas, or suprapubically). The other alternative is to perform an open laparoscopy.

During training it is taught that a prerequisite to trocar insertion is the establishment of a pneumoperitoneum. In the majority of patients this process is carried out without difficulty, but if the preperitoneal space is inadvertently insufflated the safety of the procedure is jeopardized. Several investigators have advocated direct trocar insertion without establishment of a pneumoperitoneum (4, 5). It is of interest that this approach is not associated with an increased incidence of intraabdominal trauma, suggesting that a pneumoperitoneum may not be necessary and may merely give the surgeon a false sense of security.

Dull instruments

Insertion of a dull trocar can also increase the chance of intraabdominal trauma. The excessive force that is necessary to insert a dull trocar not only makes it difficult to keep the abdominal wall elevated during the insertion, but also makes it hard to restrain the inertia of the advancing trocar when the peritoneum is finally penetrated. For this reason, these instruments must be sent out for sharpening on a regular basis.

Several surgical supply companies market disposable trocars. Even though they are expensive the surgeon is always guaranteed a sharp instrument.

Gastric distention

The transverse colon is attached to the greater curvature of the stomach, and gastric distention will cause displacement of the stomach and colon inferiorly to a location where both organs are at greater risk of being injured by the advancing trocar. Gastric distention occurs during mask ventilation, which in the past was a method of administration of anesthesia during the laparoscopic procedure. However, the currently accepted method is general endotracheal anesthesia, which decreases the possibility of gastric distention and prevents aspiration if regurgitation occurs. Nevertheless, prior to intubation mask ventilation is required. In our institution, a nasogastric tube is inserted to empty the stomach before the procedure is begun.

Pathologic conditions

Several pathologic conditions can put the intestinal tract at increased risk of trauma during trocar insertion. The risk of injury is increased in patients with intestinal obstruction, previous intestinal surgery (i.e., bowel resection, colostomy), or history of inflammatory bowel disease. A previous uncomplicated appendectomy is not a contraindication to trocar insertion, but if the appendix was ruptured bowel adhesions may have resulted, placing the intestinal tract at increased risk for injury. Other relative contraindications to trocar insertion are a previous midline incisional scar and obesity. In situations associated with an increased risk of traumatic trocar insertion, an open laparoscopy is a much safer alternative. Nevertheless, performance of an open laparoscopy reduces but does not eliminate the possibility of bowel injury because some sharp dissection is necessary (6). If the patient is at higher risk for gastrointestinal injury, a bowel preparation prior to the procedure may be prudent to reduce the chance of complications if indeed the bowel is injured.

Diagnosis

Immediate

The diagnosis of colon injury is obvious if stool is noted on the tip of the trocar or feculent material is seen in the abdominal cavity during the procedure. If the injury occurs to an empty colon, the only sign may be bleeding from the site of injury or a rent in the bowel. It is good practice during the initial viewing through the laparoscope to perform a systematic and thorough examination of the abdominal cavity to rule out any injury that might have been sustained during trocar insertion.

Delayed

A small rent in the colon may go unnoticed at the time of surgery. These patients will present in the early postoperative period with complaints of fever, chills, and abdominal pain. Physical findings may vary from a rigid abdomen to only localized tenderness, depending on the extent of abdominal contamination with feces. While different etiologic causes may explain this presentation, intestinal injury must always be considered in the differential diagnosis.

The diagnosis of colon injury can be somewhat difficult. A flat plate of the abdomen that demonstrates free air suggests a ruptured viscus; however, if the X ray is obtained in the immediate postoperative period, the free air may be residual carbon dioxide left over from the procedure. Contrast studies in a patient who is suspicious of an injury to the large bowel is contraindicated because infusion of barium and stool into the abdominal cavity is associated with significant morbidity. Any patient with an acute abdomen of uncertain etiology requires surgical exploration with examination of the entire abdominal cavity, including the intestinal tract, to identify the source.

Management

The management of colon injuries is by a surgical approach, and treatment is dependent on the site and extent of injury, the length of time since the injury occurred, and the extent of fecal contamination within the abdominal cavity. After the diagnosis is made, broad-spectrum antibiotics should be administered and a general surgeon consulted. Small wounds to any segment of the colon (except the rectum) with minimal peritoneal contamination can be adequately managed with a two-layer closure. Some have advocated primary closure with exteriorization of the repaired segment through an abdominal incision (7). If healing occurs normally, then the colon is returned to the abdominal cavity an average of 10–14 days later. If the exteriorized segment of colon fails to heal appropriately, then a colostomy can easily be performed. For more significant injuries to the colon when the trocar has completely penetrated two walls of the large intestine or the mesentery is involved, the fecal stream must be diverted. If the ascending colon is the injured segment, then it is repaired (either with a primary closure or resection) and a diverting ileostomy should be performed. For injuries to the other segments of the colon, the same approach is taken except that a double-barrel colostomy is performed. Intraperitoneal drains are put in place and antibiotics are continued during the postoperative period. When the patient has recovered the colostomy or ileostomy can be closed several weeks later.

Conclusion

The overall complication rate following laparoscopy is low, which unfortunately can provoke a relaxed attitude toward the procedure. There is no question that adherence to proper surgical technique will help to prevent intestinal injury during trocar insertion. In addition, a thorough history will identify those patients at greater risk for intestinal injury; in these cases an open laparoscopy is a better alternative. Nevertheless, if injury does occur, prompt recognition and proper managment will result in a good outcome.

It is also important to properly consult the patient. At the preoperative visit the author discusses with his patients the possibility of bowel injury and the potential consequences, including a colostomy. This discussion can be alarming to a patient who is undergoing the procedure for enhancement of fertility; however, the emotional impact as well as the medicolegal implications of an uninformed patient waking up with a colostomy are obvious.

REFERENCES

1. Baggish MS, Lee WK, Miro SJ, Dacko L, Cohen G. Complications of laparoscopic sterilization. Obstet Gynecol 1979;54:54–59.
2. Jordan JA, Edwards RL, Pearson J, Maskery PJK. Laparoscopic sterilization and follow-up hysterosalpingogram. J Obstet Gynaecol Br Commonw 1971;78:460–466.
3. Krebs HB. Intestinal injury in gynecologic surgery: a ten-year experience. Am J Obstet Gynecol 1986;155:509–514.
4. Jarrett JC Jr. Laparoscopy: direct trocar insertion without pneumoperitoneum. Obstet Gynecol 1990;75:725–727.
5. Byron JW, Fujiyoshi CA, Miyazawa K. Evaluation of the direct trocar insertions technique at laparoscopy. Obstet Gynecol 1989;74:423–425.
6. Penfield AJ. How to prevent complications of open laparoscopy. J Reprod Med 1985;30:660–663.
7. Kirkpatrick JR, Rajpal SG. The injured colon: therapeutic considerations. Am J Surg 1975;129:187–191.

Trocar Injuries to the Small Intestine | 8

Deborah A. Metzger

Injuries associated with trocar insertion still occur despite increasing physician experience and the use of standardized techniques. It has been estimated that 1.6–1.8 small bowel injuries occur per 1000 laparoscopic procedures as a result of trocar injury (1, 2). In a recent survey of Canadian gynecologists, one-quarter of the respondents reported at least one case of sharp trocar injury (3). The actual frequency of small bowel injury is difficult to determine because only large lacerations or those that become symptomatic postoperatively are included in the statistics. Injury to the gastrointestinal tract is a serious complication of trocar insertion. Whether discovered intraoperatively or several days following surgery, small bowel injuries result in unplanned laparotomy in half the cases and may be associated with other sequelae as well (3).

Predisposing conditions

In general, trocar injuries to the small bowel occur through careless technique or when the bowel is immobilized by adhesions. Patients with a history of multiple laparotomies, prior ruptured appendix, overdistended bowel, or disseminated carcinoma are particularly at risk for the presence of bowel adhesions to the anterior abdominal wall (Fig. 8.1). In the absence of adhesions or other predisposing conditions, the use of excessive force when inserting the trocar leads to displacement of the anterior abdominal wall in close proximity to the small bowel even with an adequate pneumoperitoneum (Fig. 8.2). Factors such as an inadequate umbilical incision, scar tissue from a prior laparoscopic or surgical procedure, uncontrolled sudden entry of the trocar, and a dull trocar contribute to small bowel injury in the absence of adhesions or other predisposing pelvic pathology. Extreme thinness and obesity may also make trocar insertion difficult.

Identification of the injury

If the trocar has made a large laceration in the small bowel, the surgeon may initially view a mucosal surface or notice a foul smell when the laparoscope is inserted. Alternatively, small bowel contents may be observed leaking from the laceration or a hematoma may be present on the small bowel serosa. If a small bowel injury is suspected, it is imperative that the bowel be examined as thoroughly as possible, even if it means performing a laparotomy to run the bowel. If the laparoscope is inserted into the bowel lumen, then the surgeon should leave the laparoscope in place to seal the puncture and to allow identification of the site of trauma. A laparotomy is then performed, the defect is identified, and a purse-string suture is placed and tied as the laparoscope is withdrawn to minimize peritoneal contamination (4, 5).

Injuries to the small bowel can be treacherous because they may not be recognized at the time of surgery. Under these circumstances, the patient generally presents on the third or fourth postoperative day with lower abdominal pain, mild fever, slight nausea, and anorexia. By the fifth or sixth postoperative day, these symptoms progress to include fever, severe abdominal pain, nausea, vomiting, obstipation, increased white blood cell (WBC) count, and abdominal tenderness with rebound and guarding (6).

Pertinent anatomy of the small intestine

The small intestine is covered by a continuation of the peritoneum that forms the covering of the intestinal mesentery. The intestine is a long, muscular tube composed of two layers of muscle oriented at right angles to one another: a thin, continuous, longitudinal outer layer and a thicker, circular, inner layer. The mucosa forms the innermost layer. This two-layer muscular arrange-

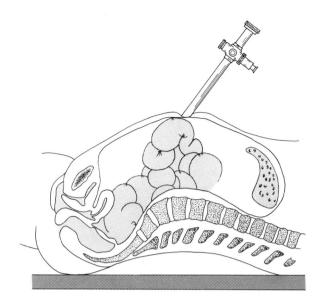

Fig. 8.1 Mechanism of trocar injury to the small bowel in the presence of adhesions to the anterior abdominal wall.

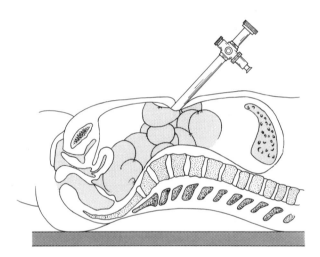

Fig. 8.2 Excessive force on the trocar decreases the distance from umbilicus to bowel, increasing the probability of bowel injury.

ment provides a safeguard against small, perforating injuries, as the contraction of the bowel musculature readily seals off small punctures.

The arterial supply to the small intestine comes from branches of the superior mesenteric artery, which enters through the root of the intestinal mesentery. The intestinal branches arise from the artery and anastomose with one another to form a series of arcades (Fig. 8.3). However, each branch of the arcade supplies a small segment of intestine with little overlap of blood supply. Thus, interruption of a small, perforating artery may significantly compromise a portion of intestine, resulting in necrosis and perforation.

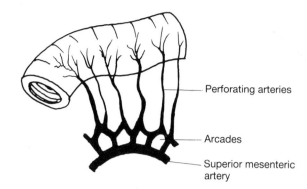

Fig. 8.3 Vascular anatomy of the small intestine. Note that the perforating arteries supply a small segment of bowel without overlap of blood supply.

Management

Complications of small bowel injury are related to the extent of damage and the point at which the injury is discovered. Sharp trocar injuries to the bowel can be superficial, limited to the serosa, or deep, involving the entire wall thickness. Small punctures or superficial lacerations of the small bowel seal readily and require no further treatment, assuming that careful inspection of the affected bowel reveals no leakage of bowel contents or bleeding. Small (<5 mm) superficial lacerations need to be inspected carefully to ensure that they involve only the serosa. In either case, the patient may be treated conservatively and discharged the day of surgery with instructions to report any untoward reaction over the subsequent seven days.

In contrast, patients with significant small bowel injury or obvious peritoneal soiling require immediate laparotomy. On initial inspection of the damaged bowel, particular attention should be paid to the existence of through-and-through injuries. Both sides of the bowel should be inspected, as the trocar may have punctured the side opposite the laceration, and if missed, peritonitis may develop postoperatively despite repair of the apparent injury.

The small bowel should be repaired in two layers, placing an initial row of interrupted sutures of 3/0 chromic catgut to approximate the mucosa and muscularis. A reinforcing layer of 3/0 silk Lembert sutures is used to approximate the muscularis and serosal edges (7). All lacerations should be closed transversely to minimize the occurrence of stenosis of the bowel lumen. This type of closure is appropriate only if the laceration is less than one-half the diamerer of the bowel. If the laceration exceeds one-half the diameter of the lumen, a segmental resection and anastomosis should be performed. If the mesenteric blood supply is interrupted by the puncture, a resection must be performed regardless of the size or

laceration to maintain blood supply to
segment of bowel (4). A timely intraoperation
ation with a general surgeon would be
ate in the presence of significant bowel

repair of a bowel laceration, it is most
thoroughly lavage the entire abdomen. A
ube should be placed and removed postoperatively
when drainage has decreased indicating resumption
of bowel function. The patient is not given anything
by mouth until he or she passes flatus.

When symptoms of a possible bowel laceration are
not apparent until after the patient has been discharged,
conservative management is successful in patients who
have not yet developed signs and symptoms of peritonitis
(6). In-hospital management consists of hydration,
nothing by mouth, and close observation with WBC
counts and physical examination every six hours. Clearly,
this type of conservative management is appropriate only
in those institutions where diligent observation of the
patient is available. Wheeless reported that over half of
all patients treated conservatively required no surgical
intervention (6). Those whose condition deteriorated
during the period of observation promptly underwent
laparotomy and had no complications attributable to
the delay in surgery.

Immediate laparotomy is indicated in those patients
initially presenting with fever, severe abdominal pain,
nausea, vomiting, obstipation, or peritoneal signs, or in
those conservatively managed patients who undergo a
deterioration in any of the laboratory or clinical parameters.
Surgical considerations for the management of
bowel injuries manifesting themselves during the postoperative
period differ somewhat from those managed
immediately after the injury. Clearly, the damaged bowel
must be repaired or resected as described earlier. In
addition, resection of all necrotic tissue in the pelvis is
mandatory, even if it requires a total abdominal hysterectomy
and bilateral salpingo-oophorectomy (6). If
burned or necrotic tissue that has been bathed in intestinal
contents, blood, and serum for hours or days is not
excised, a pelvic abscess with all its sequelae will develop
(6).

Wheeless presented a seven-point plan for the management
of patients with peritonitis secondary to bowel
perforation (6):

1. Preoperative stabilization with fluids, electrolytes,
   and nasogastric suction.
2. Exploratory laparotomy with repair or resection of
   the injured bowel.
3. Resection of all necrotic tissue.
4. Copious and repeated saline lavage of the
   abdomen.
5. Pelvic drainage through the vagina using a closed
   drainage system.
6. Aggressive antibiotic therapy.
7. Embolus prophylaxis with minidose heparin (5000
   units t.i.d.).

A recent American Association of Gynecologic
Laparoscopists' (AAGL) membership poll attests to the
seriousness of bowel injury in general and delay in diagnosis
in particular. The two deaths reported from 36,928
procedures were attributed to bowel injuries. In one
instance the patient had extensive adhesions from the
abdominal wall to the bowel. Although the bowel injury
was recognized and repaired, the patient developed a
persistent postoperative ileus and died of peritonitis. The
second death was attributable to sepsis after an unrecognized
small bowel perforation (1).

Avoiding injuries

The methods of avoiding trocar injuries to the small
bowel logically follow from the predisposing conditions
associated with an increased risk of bowel injury. Since
injury is generally attributable to poor technique or
bowel adhesions and distention, efforts to avoid injury
should concentrate on these two areas.

Trocar insertion technique should not deviate from the
surgeon's standard procedure without good cause. The
trocar should be pyramidal tipped and well sharpened to
facilitate penetration of muscle and fascia. Soderstrom
and Butler (8) demonstrated in a program for laparoscopic
sterilization that the complication rate could be
reduced 10-fold when a consistent operating format was
adopted. Establishment of a large pneumoperitoneum
before trocar insertion and elevation of the abdominal
wall to increase the distance between the abdominal wall
and viscera have been suggested as ways of decreasing
the chance of bowel injury. However, the literature fails
to support any of these techniques as being safer than
others.

Much attention has been given recently to the disposable
trocar because of its sharp tip and spring-loaded
safety-shield. Theoretically, a permanently sharp trocar
that provides controlled entry should decrease the risk of
injury to intraabdominal structures (9). However, there
have been no large-scale clinical trials to prove this
advantage of single-use trocars and, in fact, a surgeon
using these new devices may risk injury because of the
unexpected ease of insertion. At the University of Connecticut
Health Center, the first use of a disposable trocar
was associated with laceration of a mesenteric artery,
which was not discovered until several hours postsurgery.
This experience underscores the importnce of consistency
of technique and instruments as well as the potential
hazards of alterations in procedure.

The trocar should be inserted with the patient in a
completely horizontal position. Premature Trendelenburg
positioning does nothing to avoid bowel injuries,

particularly if bowel adhesions are present, and may significantly alter important landmarks such as the sacral promontory and sacral hollow. It is important to insert and advance the trocar toward the hollow of the sacrum to provide the greatest distance between the point of the trocar and unyielding, solid tissue. Using this technique, the bowel easily slides out of the way of the advancing trocar.

Special considerations are required for patients at the extremes of body weight. In the obese patient, the trocar may need to be angled close to the vertical, which means that the distance between sacral promontory and trocar is relatively small, leaving little room for error (i.e., uncontrolled entry). The very thin patient may be at even greater risk. The distance between the anterior abdominal wall and sacral promontory is often very small. Furthermore, the force required to introduce the trocar is often less than anticipated because the fascia is thin and offers little resistance (10).

Bowel distention secondary to obstruction is a relative contraindication to laparoscopy unless there are compelling reasons for the procedure such that the benefits outweigh the risks. However, bowel distention may be iatrogenic, resulting from intraluminal placement of the Veress needle. The surgeon may be unaware of this problem because of the lack of difference in filling pressures between the abdominal cavity and the bowel and the large capacity of the small bowel. Once an apparent pneumoperitoneum is created and the Veress needle is removed, the distended bowel serves as an easy target for a significant laceration by the trocar.

The presence of small bowel adhesions to the anterior abdominal wall is associated with a high risk of trocar injury. Patients with previous uncomplicated abdominal surgery are generally not at increased risk and do not require special considerations. In contrast, those who have had a bowel resection or exploratory laparotomy for trauma probably have an increased risk. Similarly, women who undergo a second-look laparoscopy for carcinoma of the ovary not only have risks of adhesions from previous abdominal surgery, but also generally have had an omentectomy and a disease process associated with adhesion formation (11).

Patients at high risk for bowel adhesions (i.e., those with previous bowel surgery) may be more appropriately managed utilizing open laparoscopy, rather than closed laparoscopy. In spite of this precaution, bowel lacerations can still occur upon entering the peritoneum (12). Moreover, it is difficult to determine which patients who have undergone pelvic surgery should have an open laparoscopy.

Several procedures have been described to assess the anterior abdominal wall for the presence of bowel adhesions. DeCherney (4) advocates the use of a small-gauge laparoscope called a needlescope, which is a 2–3-mm diameter endoscope. It can be advanced, instead of the Veress needle, under direct visualization of the umbilical, preperitoneal, and immediately subperitoneal structures. Thus, the needle can be placed intraabdominally and insufflation can proceed under direct visualization. Exploration of the periumbilical area with an 18-gauge needle attached to a syringe after the pneumoperitoneum has been established has also been advocated as a method of detecting bowel adhesions. By either aspirating (to look for bowel contents) or moving the needle at different angles (feeling for tissue that is resistant and adherent to the anterior abdominal wall), the presence of periumbilical adhesions can be ascertained (Fig. 8.4). The third method is to insert the Veress needle and inject 5 cm³ of Ringer's lactate solution. If aspiration reveals fluid, then adhesions are probable. It should be emphasized that none of these methods is fool-proof.

Should the presence of adhesions be detected by these relatively atraumatic techniques, the options for surgical approach include switching to laparotomy or insufflating at an alternative site (midline, right or left McBurney's point, below the left costal margin, or transvaginally (10). The trocar can then be inserted at any point in the midline between the xyphoid and the pubic symphysis, provided care is taken to remain at least 5 cm below the xyphoid and 5 cm above the pubic symphysis (10).

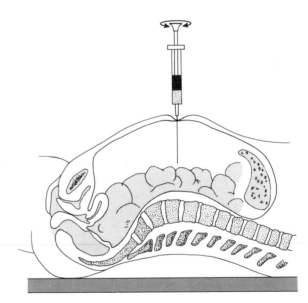

Fig. 8.4 Exploration of the anterior abdominal wall with syringe and needle to assess for the presence of bowel adhesions. After a penumoperitoneum is established, a 10-cm³ glass syringe containing 3 cm³ of normal saline is connected to a short, 18-gauge spinal needle that is inserted through the umbilicus. If there is adequate peritoneal space to accept the trocar, gas bubbles will appear in the saline and will elevate the plunger of the glass syringe. The limits of the potential space can be further defined by gradually advancing the needle and moving it from side to side until the surgeon is satisfied that sufficient room exists for introduction of the trocar.

When managing a patient at risk for bowel adhesions, it is prudent to perform a mechanical and antibiotic bowel preparation, preoperatively. This process will effectively eliminate bowel contents, decompress the bowel, and serve as prophylaxis against infection should perforation occur.

Summary

Although relatively uncommon, trocar injury to the small intestine requires prompt surgical intervention. Delay in identification of this injury can result in significant morbidity and mortality. Factors that are associated with an increased risk of bowel perforation include poor technique and bowel adhesions. Attention to consistency of technique and proper selection of patients can minimize the probability of trocar injury.

REFERENCES

1. Peterson HB, Halka JF, Phillips JM. American Association of Gynecologic Laparoscopists' 1988 Membership Survey on operative laparoscopy. J Reprod Med 1990;35:587–589.
2. Chamberlain G, Brown JD, eds. Gynaecologic laparoscopy report on the confidential enquiry into gynaecologic laparoscopy. London: Royal College of Obstetricians and Gynaecologists, 1978.
3. Yuzpe AA. Pneumoperitoneum needle and trocar injuries in laparoscopy. J Reprod Med 1990;35:485–490.
4. DeCherney AH. Laparoscopy with unexpected viscus penetration. In: Nichols DH, ed. Clinical problems, injuries and complications of gynecologic surgery. Baltimore: Williams & Wilkins, 1988: 62–63.
5. Corson SL, Soderstrom RM, Levy BS. Emergencies and laparoscopy. AAGL manual. Sante Fe Springs, California: American Association of Gynecologic Laparoscopists, 1990.
6. Wheeless CR. Gastrointestinal injuries associated with laparoscopy. In: Phillips JM, ed. Endoscopy in gynecology. Sante Fe Springs, Cal.: American Association of Gynecologic Laparoscopists, 1978:317–324.
7. Borton M. Gastrointestinal injuries. In: Borton M, ed. Laparoscopic complications: prevention and management. Philadelphia: BC Decker, 1986:317–329.
8. Soderstrom RM, Butler JC. A critical evaluation of complications in laparoscopy. J Reprod Med 1973;10:245–248.
9. Corson SL, Batzer FR, Gocial B, Maislin G. Measurement of the force necessary for laparoscopic trocar entry. J Reprod Med 1989;34:282–284.
10. Gomel V, Taylor PJ, Yuzpe AA, Rioux JE. The technique of endoscopy. In: Gomel V, Taylor PJ, Yuzpe AA, Rioux JE, eds. Laparoscopy and hysteroscopy in gynecologic practice. Chicago: Year Book Medical Publishers, 1986:56–74.
11. Loffer FD. Endoscopy in high risk patients. In: Martin DC, ed. Manual of endoscopy. Sante Fe Springs. Cal.: American Association of Gynecologic Laparoscopists, 1990:43–46.
12. Penfield AJ. How to prevent complications of open laparoscopy. J Reprod Med 1985;30:660–663.

9 Trocar Injuries to the Bladder

Dan C. Martin

Introduction

Trocar and Veress needle damage during laparoscopy is an uncommon occurrence, but still a significant concern (1). Damage to the bladder can arise in both high- and low-risk situations. High-risk factors include a full bladder, previous pelvic surgery that may have affected the anatomic relationships of the bladder, and distortion of the anatomy by an identified disease.

Although postoperative anuria can aid in the diagnosis of trocar injury, intraoperative recognition is important as no readily identifiable postoperative presentation characterizes all patients. This variability is particularly true when the patient is contaminated with sterile urine, which causes few—if any—peritoneal signs. Delay in recognition can result in abdominal distention and azotemia.

Both the intraperitoneal and extraperitoneal components must be diagnosed and treated. Treatment consists of 7 to 30 days of drainage, which is routinely followed by a cystogram performed prior to removal of the catheter for nonsurgical trauma. A cystogram may also be useful following surgical trauma. Although ascites, urinoma, and vesicocutaneous fistulae represent concerns, long-term complications of trocar injury to the dome of the bladder should be rare.

History and physical examination

Surgery and diseases that distort anatomy cause the greatest concern for possible trocar and needle damage. A previous cesarean section incision can pull the peritoneum in an anterior direction and increase the risk of trocar perforation. It may also pull the bladder peritoneum up on the uterus, which increases the risk of bladder damage while dissecting this area. Likewise, endometriosis and infection that obliterates the anterior cul-de-sac can increase such risks.

A physical examination may alert the physician to previous surgery not disclosed when the history was taken. A drawing of the abdomen in the records can be carried to the operating room to ensure greater precautions at the time of surgery

Intraoperative precautions

A full bladder can be avoided by catheterization. For short cases, an in-and-out catheterization can be employed. For longer cases, the catheter should be drained in a sterile closed system. This closed system is also used to monitor the volume and appearance of urine.

After emptying the bladder, the next step in preventing trocar damage involves visualization of the anterior compartment prior to placing the trocar. If the peritoneum of the anterior abdominal wall is distorted, the insertion site may be modified. In addition, if the bladder still appears full, kinking of the catheter may have occurred. This condition should be corrected and the bladder drained.

Intraoperative recognition and therapy

Surgeons who have recognized bladder perforation at the time of surgery have been alerted to this condition by the appearance of the bladder pushed forward by the trocar, by the appearance of bladder muscularis separated by the trocar (Fig. 9.1), or by the presence of gas in the Foley drainage bag (2). As the trocar is inserted, its tip is observed. If the trocar appears to be pushing a muscular organ forward, repositioning at this time may avoid further damage. If injury has already occurred, the damage can be assessed by a retrograde cystogram with washout (as discussed later in this chapter).

The presence of hematuria prior to other manipulation of the bladder can be investigated at this time. With

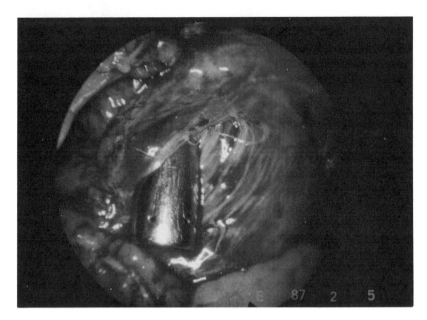

Fig. 9.1 The sleeve of the trocar is seen coming through the bladder muscularis. Methylene blue has been injected into the bladder and no evidence of a leak appeared. The trocar was removed and no leak was observed. This condition was treated with seven days of Foley drainage without subsequent problems.

the trocar kept in place, the bladder is distended with a methylene blue solution to see whether it distends on the other side of the trocar or around the trocar. This procedure also checks for intraperitoneal leak—but may miss a retroperitoneal leak. A cystoscopy would enable the surgeon to visualize the trocar if it is inserted in the bladder.

If the damage is recognized at surgery, the most direct approach is to leave the trocar in place, carry out a mini-laparotomy, and perform a purse-string (3), two-layer (4), or three-layer (5) closure. Leaving the trocar in place for the repair means that both the entrance and exit sites can be more easily identified. If the repair is performed after removal of the trocar, the intraperitoneal exit site is extended for visualization of the extraperitoneal entrance site. The entrance site is repaired from the inside of the bladder, followed by repair of the exit site. Closure is performed using chromic (4) or Vicryl (6) sutures. Permanent sutures should be avoided because of the possibility of calculus formation. The repair procedure resembles the care of laceration of the bladder when lysing dense abdominal adhesions (7).

The Foley catheter may be left in the patient for 7 to 14 days following direct repair (3). This duration can be modified depending on the degree of damage (6). A cystogram is generally performed following nonsurgical trauma but has been avoided in some patients following surgical trauma. If no leak occurs, the catheter can be removed at this time. If a leak is identified, catheter should remain in place for 14 to 30 days before repeating the cystogram (4, 8).

A second approach is based on the observation that immediate closure is needed following blunt trauma with tears averaging 5 cm, but drainage may suffice for repairs of iatrogenic damage, such as perforation at the time of transurethral surgery (9). In this approach, the trocar is removed and 400 cc of a solution colored with methylene blue is instilled into the bladder to check for an intraperitoneal leak. If a spill is found, repair or drainage can be used without a cystogram. If no intraperitoneal leak is located, a retrograde cystogram can be performed by instilling 400 cc of radiopaque dye into the bladder and then performing a flat plate of the bladder to search for a retroperitoneal leak. This process is followed by a washout film after the bladder has been lavaged with saline until clear (5, 10). If no intraperitoneal spill is found but dye is loculated in the extraperitoneal space, drainage and observation may be useful (8).

A Foley catheter is left in place for 10 to 14 days for drainage in a fashion similar to that following nonsurgical trauma (4, 5, 8, 9, 11). The patient is discharged with a leg bag and receives antispasmodics for the bladder and prophylactic antibiotics. Before the Foley catheter is removed, a cystogram is performed to demonstrate whether the bladder has healed. If the leak persists, the catheter may be left in for as long as 30 days (4).

This approach has been applied with immediate laparoscopic two-layer closure of the intraperitoneal laceration, Foley drainage for six days, and follow-up observation. A patient managed in this fashion was asymptomatic at one year of follow-up (2).

A third approach to repair may be attempted in the absence of a demonstrable leak when the surgeon is concerned about the delayed development of a fistula. This drainage-type management is based on the observation that the total extent of damage using clamps and sutures may be underestimated at the time of injury (4). In addition, the level of damage increases following perforation with prolonged manipulation of the perforating instruments prior to recognition of the injury (2). Furthermore, the patient may develop retention, due to atony or obstruction from clots, and dilation of the bladder greater than the 400 cc used for testing.

Postoperative recognition and therapy

Failure to diagnose the condition at the time of surgery can lead to significant delays in treatment, as few signs or symptoms specifically point to bladder perforation as a complication. A decreased urinary output, anuria, bloody urine, suprapubic bruising, mass in the abdominal wall or pelvis, abdominal swelling, or peritoneal signs may occur. In the absence of infected urine, peritoneal signs rarely arise.

If the patient is unable to void and catheterization reveals no urine, the instillation of 200 cc of sterile solution, followed by less solution on aspiration, should reveal the diagnosis. If an intraperitoneal leak persists, azotemia can occur with the BUN-creatinine ratio shifting to exceed 10:1 (5, 12).

A retrograde cystogram with washout is performed when a leak from the bladder is suspected (9). With a delay in diagnosis, such injuries are handled similar to other traumatic ruptures. Intraperitoneal leaks are repaired and drained (5), while extraperitoneal leaks are drained (8). The drain is left in place and a cystogram is performed prior to its removal in these cases. If the leak persists, drainage continues for as long as 30 days before the cystogram is repeated.

Complications

Complications include urinary ascites, peritonitis, urinomas, azotemia, and vesicocutaneous fistulae. Although these problems have all been observed following surgical damage to the bladder, the highest risk appears related to open surgery with an unrepaired defect in the dome of the bladder (4).

When these complications arise, they are often accompanied by a state of maximal tissue reaction. At this time, drainage is used to promote healing, encourage spontaneous closure, and minimize further complications. Although vesicocutaneous fistulae generally close spontaneously, persistent leak may require catheterization or surgical repair. Surgical repair is not considered until at least three to six months after surgery. Operating prior to this time may increase the risk of failure.

A patient has consulted the author by telephone following an apparent trocar-related intraperitoneal leak accompanied by anuria that was not noted while she was in the hospital. Following discharge, she developed *E. coli* peritonitis and was admitted to the intensive care unit. She did well after second discharge but was concerned about possible damage to her reproductive organs. At follow-up four years later, she had not become pregnant or had further surgery.

Summary

When trocar damage to the bladder is seen, immediate repair of both the intraperitoneal and extraperitoneal components through a minilaparotomy is the most direct approach to treatment. Removing the trocar and performing retrograde studies with 400 cc of methylene blue, followed by the same volume of radiopaque dye, for a cystogram may identify certain patients who do not need immediate repair. Anuria, abdominal swelling, and azotemia should alert the physician to the possibility of an unrecognized leak following surgery.

When repair is performed, a catheter is left in place for 7 to 14 days and a cystogram considered prior to removing the catheter to ensure the absence of any leak. If a retroperitoneal leak is corrected by drainage, the catheter is left for 14 days and a cystogram performed prior to its removal. If the leak persists at 7 to 14 days, drainage is continued for as long as 30 days prior to repeating the cystogram. Long-term problems should be rare, and most are correctable via drainage or observation.

REFERENCES

1. Yuzpe AA. Pneumoperitoneum needle and trocar injuries in laparoscopy. A survey on possible contributing factors and prevention. J Reprod Med 1990;35:485–490.
2. Reich H, McGlynn F. Laparoscopic repair of bladder injury. Obstet Gynecol 1990;76:909.
3. DeCherney AH. Laparoscopy with unexplained viscus penetration. In: Nichols DH, ed. Clinical problems, injuries and complications of gynecologic surgery. Baltimore: Williams & Wilkins, 1988:63.
4. Ridley JH, ed. Gynecologic surgery. Errors, safeguards, salvage. 2nd ed. Baltimore: Williams & Wilkins, 1981:35–39.
5. Peters PC. Intraperitoneal rupture of the bladder. Urol Clin N Am 1991;16:270.
6. Thompson JD. Vesicovaginal fistula following total abdominal hysterectomy. In: Nichols DH, ed. Clinical problems, injuries and complications of gynecologic surgery. Baltimore: Williams & Wilkins, 1988:169.
7. Maxson WS, Hoffman DI, Nezhat F, Adamson GD. Complications of operative laparoscopy. In: Adamson GD, Martin DC, eds. Endoscopic management of gynecologic disease. Philadelphia: Lippincott-Raven Publishers, 1996:361–383.
8. Corriere JN Jr, Sandler CM. Management of the ruptured bladder: seven years of experience with 111 cases. J Trauma 1986;26:830.
9. Corriere JN Jr, Sandler CM. Management of extraperitoneal bladder rupture. Urol Clin N Am 1991;16:275.
10. Cass AS. Diagnostic studies in bladder rupture. Urol Clin N Am 1991;16:267.
11. Robards VL Jr, Haglund RV, Lubin EW, et al. Treatment of rupture of the bladder. J Urol 1976;116:178.
12. Shah PM, Kim K, Samirez-Schon G, et al. Elevated blood urea nitrogen: an aid to the diagnosis of intraperitoneal rupture of the bladder. J Urol 1979;22:741.

Trocar Injuries to the Stomach | 10

John Tripoulas and Jamie A. Grifo

Incidence

Penetration of the stomach by the Veress needle or trocar is a rare event. One survey of 32,719 laparoscopies listed nine cases of gastric perforation for an overall incidence of 0.027% (1). In the same series, 87 total gastrointestinal perforation injuries were reported, which demonstrates that gastric perforation represents only a small proportion of the total. Nevertheless, the prevention, management, and sequelae of gastric perforation at laparoscopy are topics with which the laparoscopic surgeon should be acquainted. It is rare to find many people who have had personal experience with this complication. In addition, only case reports exist regarding management techniques and outcome. There are no studies that compare various methods for management. Consequently, any experience with this serious complication must be managed with the utmost care and with the expertise and input of a number of general and gynecological surgeons. The literature should be used as a guide.

Prevention of gastric perforation

To prevent gastric perforation by the instruments of laparoscopy, a knowledge of the conditions that predispose the patient to this injury is mandatory. The two most common conditions that lead to gastric injury are distortion of the abdominal anatomy and difficult induction of anesthesia. It is extremely unlikely that Veress needle and trocar insertion performed utilizing the proper technique in a patient who has not had prior surgery would produce gastric perforation unless one of these two conditions are met. Previous surgery with resultant adhesions and anatomical distortion, especially to the periumbilical region, predisposes the patient for laparoscopic injury. A thorough review of previous operative notes must be performed before laparoscopy is considered.

Laparoscopy is relatively contraindicated in cases of abdominal carcinomatosis, massive hemoperitoneum, pelvic or abdominal peritonitis from tuberculosis, and generalized abdominal peritonitis. It is considered a high-risk procedure in patients with previous abdominal surgery (2). Most of these contraindicated conditions predispose the abdominal cavity to anatomical distortion. One case mentioned in the literature describes a ruptured pyosalpinx and the subsequent gastric perforation upon laparoscopy (2). The omentum was adherent to the inflamed fallopian tubes and the downward traction on the omentum placed the stomach just beneath the umbilicus, resulting in a Veress needle injury.

A difficult induction of anesthesia can result in a large volume of gas being delivered to the stomach lumen. The resultant distention can position the stomach just beneath the incision site and lead to gastric perforation.

The use of general anesthesia is always accompanied by a slight risk of gastric inflation. This complication can occur due to the inadvertent placement of the endotracheal tube in the esophagus (3) or prior to intubation when manual ventilation is carried out (4). An inflated stomach is at high risk for perforation by the trocar and Veress needle. Because it may prove difficult to assess whether the stomach has been inflated, any airway management problem should be addressed by the insertion of a (large-bore) nasogastric drainage tube or an oropharyngeal tube. Most experienced laparoscopists advise that all patients undergoing general anesthesia for laparoscopy should have gastric drainage. Furthermore, Alexander and Brown (5) recommend that neither the Veress needle nor the trocar be inserted until the patient has been placed in at least 15° of a head-down Trendelenburg position. Given the evolution of office laparoscopy, it is possible that gastric perforation perpetrated by difficult induction of anesthesia may soon become an obsolete risk factor. If office laparoscopy that requires only IV (or PO) sedation becomes the standard of care, the complications associated with general anesthesia will be eliminated (6).

Techniques to prevent gastric perforation

Technical tips, some previously mentioned, to prevent gastric perforation include the following:

1. Lift the abdominal wall (some surgeons use towel clips for this step, most use a 4 by 8 cm gauze and a gloved hand).
2. The angle of the Veress needle should be such that it is aimed at a point just below the bifurcation of the aorta.
3. The nasogastric or oropharyngeal tube should be placed after induction of anesthesia.
4. Place the patient in a 15° Trendelenberg position prior to Veress needle and trocar insertion (5). (Note that many laparoscopists do not adhere to this recommendation.)
5. Ensure that adequate pneumoperitoneum is created to prevent injuries to the stomach at the time of trocar insertion—usually between 3 and 5 liters of gas may be required (7). Some laparoscopists directly insert the trocar with no Veress needle insertion (8–11).
6. Use a sharp trocar (7).
7. Avoid perpendicular insertion of the trocar without adequate elevation of the abdominal wall.
8. Control the thrust so as just to penetrate the abdominal wall and not lose control of the force after the penetration has been completed.
9. Place the index finger of the hand inserting the trocar down the shaft of the trocar to serve as a stop if the trocar slides in too rapidly.

One approach to avoiding Veress needle injuries to the stomach, bowel, and bladder is to not use the Veress needle at all. Indeed, an evolving literature is developing around the idea of directly inserting the trocar without the prior development of a pneumoperitoneum (8). Complication rates with this method are no different than with the Veress needle, and this technique has even been used on patients who have had previous surgery (9–11). One study utilized a randomized, prospective design comparing direct trocar insertion to prior insufflation with a Veress needle in patients undergoing laparoscopic tubal ligation. The investigators found that direct trocar insertion resulted in a significantly lower number of insertions and the use of a smaller volume of carbon dioxide. It also resulted in a shorter operating time. One major complication arose in each group—an inadvertent bowel perforation in the direct trocar insertion group requiring laparotomy for repair. One late major complication appeared in the Veress needle group that required hospitalization for an ileus treated conservatively with antibiotics and intravenous fluids. Each group included approximately 100 patients. Because of the size of the study and the relatively low frequency of the complications being studied, it is difficult to conclude that direct trocar insertion offers a great advantage (11). Although most authors prefer initial insufflation via the Veress needle, surgeon skill and comfort are clearly important factors that must be considered when comparing the two methods.

Finally, inserting the trocar under direct vision—particularly in patients who have had prior surgery or other conditions that predispose to distorted anatomy (e.g., pregnancy, trauma)—minimizes the potential for insertion injuries. New instruments (Visiport, Ethicon, Somerville, New Jersey) are currently available and allow for insertion under direct vision. These trocars have scopes attached to them.

Management of stomach perforation

Management of gastric injuries depends on which instrument caused the perforation. In the case of Veress needle puncture, reparative surgery is not necessary as these wounds usually seal themselves and do not leak gastric contents into the abdominal cavity. Conservative management with nasogastric suction for 24 to 48 hours, withholding fluids and food, and close observation are required. Some general surgeons advise exploration to assess the extent of damage and to perform immediate repair. Loffer and Pent (1) state, however, that a Veress needle perforation to the stomach can safely be managed by observation alone. It is wise to follow the recovery of the patient with a complication of this type with nasogastric drainage for a few days. Loffer and Pent also suggest that a Veress needle injury to the bowel or bladder can be managed in this fashion.

If the trocar is the perforating culprit, the wound must be repaired at laparotomy. The trocar should be left in place until the abdomen is opened to facilitate locating the trauma (12). Oversewing the defect is required. It is performed by first placing a continuous locked 2-0 suture through all layers of the gastric wall. Vicryl or Dexon is preferable to chromic catgut. The hemostatic stitch is very important to control extensive bleeding that may occur from the rich submucosal network of blood vessels in the stomach. Next, an outer inverting row of interrupted nonabsorbable mattress sutures of the Lembert or Halsted type is placed (13). These sutures in the outer layer should not be through and through as in the first row, but should extend only through the seromuscular coat and the submucosal layer of the stomach. The outer row of imbricating sutures provides adequate serosal approximation of the stomach wall, seals readily, and prevents leaks.

Wounds of the stomach are not drained externally because they are unlikely to leak. Nevertheless, it is important to suction and irrigate the peritoneal cavity, paying special attention to the subhepatic and subphrenic spaces and the lesser sac so that all food particles and spilled gastric juices can be removed. If heavy abdominal contamination at operation is evident, the skin and subcutaneous tissues should not be closed. Primarily, closure should be delayed.

After the operation, nasogastric tube suction should be maintained for several days until active peristalsis resumes and the danger of postoperative gastric dilatation passes. The gastric aspirate should be observed for excessive bleeding. Serial hematocrit determination to rule out hemorrhage should be obtained.

Potential complications include hemorrhage from or leakage of the suture line or abscess formation. If the hemostatic suture line is compromised in any fashion, any or all of these complications are likely to develop. A further problem related to leakage of the sutures is the development of subphrenic, subhepatic, or lesser sac abscesses secondary to the spilling of gastric contents. These abscesses are suspected in patients who have persistent pain, nausea, and fever postoperatively and who have unexplained fever for more than a few days after the operation. If this complication is suspected, ultrasound or computed tomography studies are helpful in evaluation.

Two case reports from the trauma literature may offer some insightful ways to modify surgical management of trocar injuries to the stomach in the future by using laparoscopy instead of traditional surgical techniques. One such report describes the laparoscopic repair of two 8–10mm stab wounds to the anterior wall fundus of the stomach in a hemodynamically stable patient. (This patient had been stabbed twice in the abdomen and underwent diagnostic laparoscopy to evaluate his injuries.) The gastric lacerations were closed using the Endo stapler (Ethicon, Somerville, New Jersey) and titanium staples. Next, an omental patch was pulled over the gastric staple line and secured with additional staples. The stomach was then distended with air introduced through the nasogastric tube. The absence of bubbling through the repair site indicated a secure closure. A drain was placed near the staple line (14).

A second report from the literature describes the laparoscopic repair of a stomach injury using a gasless technique. (In this report a hemodynamically stable gunshot wound patient underwent abdominal exploration using gasless laparoscopy.) This technique does not require pneumoperitoneum but instead relies on the internal support of the abdominal wall with an armature placed through a small umbilical incision. Conventional surgical instruments may be used. In this case, the stomach was retracted caudad using Babcock clamps and two small perforations on the anterior gastric fundus were repaired with 2-0 silk Lembert sutures using a standard-length needle holder. Surgical knots were tied directly through the subumbilical incision and omentum was plicated over the perforations.

Although still a hypothetical concept, laparoscopic repair of trocar injuries may soon become a reality. The above two case reports suggest the feasibility of such a procedure (15).

Summary

Fortunately, trocar and Veress needle injuries are rare events. A number of reported cases with management plans and outcomes have been presented in the literature.

Veress needle injuries to the stomach have been managed successfully by observation and nasogastric drainage as well as by laparotomy. No studies have compared the two methods. In addition, probably not all Veress needle injuries to the stomach are recognized.

Trocar injuries to the stomach, on the other hand, present a more serious complication. No prudent surgeon would follow this surgical misadventure by observation. Instead, immediate laparotomy, leaving the trocar in place, with assessment of the extent of damage and immediate repair is required. Observation of the recovering patient for bleeding and abscess formation follows. An understanding of this potential complication and its management is required for all practicing laparoscopists.

New horizons in the prevention and management of laparoscopic gastric perforation are currently evolving. These trends include the development of office laparoscopy (which does not rely on general anesthesia), the availability of new instruments that allow for trocar insertion under direct vision, and the creation of stapling devices and the gasless technique that potentially could be used to repair gastric trocar injuries without celiotomy.

REFERENCES

1. Loffer F, Pent D. Indications, contraindications and complications of laparoscopy. Obstet Gynecol Surv 1975;30:407–427.
2. Hirt PS, Morris R. Gastric bleeding secondary to laparoscopy in a patient with salpingitis. Obstet Gynecol 1982;59:655–657.
3. Reynolds RC, Pauca A. Gastric perforation, an anesthesia induced hazard in laparoscopy. Anesthesiology 1973;38:84–85.
4. Endler GC, Moghissi KS. Gastric perforation during pelvic laparoscopy. Obstet Gynecol 1876;47(suppl 41):40–42.
5. Alexander GD, Brown EM. Physiology alterations during pelvic laparoscopy. Am J Obstet Gynecol 1969;105:1078–1081.
6. Feste J. Outpatient diagnostic laparoscopy using the optical catheter. Contemp Obstet Gynecol 1995;August:54–63.
7. Pelland PC. Sterilization by laparoscopy. Clin Obstet Gynecol 1983;25:321–333.
8. Copeland C, Wing R, Hulka J. Direct trocar insertion at laparoscopy: an evaluation. Obstet Gynecol 1983;62:655.
9. Dingfelder JR. Direct laparoscope trocar insertion without prior pneumoperitoneum. J Repro Med 1978;21:45–48.

10. Sardi MH. Direct laparoscopy without prior pneumoperitoneum. J Repro Med 1986;31:684–687.
11. Borgatta L, Gruss L, Barad D, Kaali S. Direct trocar insertion versus Veress needle use for laparoscopic sterilization. J Repro Med 1990;35:891–894.
12. Gentile GP, Siegler AM. Inadvertent intestinal biopsy during laparoscopy and hysteroscopy: a report of two cases. Fertil Steril 1981;36:402–404.
13. Schwartz SI, Shires GT, Spencer FC. Principles of surgery, 6th ed. New York: McGraw-Hill, 1994;198–199.
14. Frantzides CT, Ludwig KA, Aprahamian C, Salaymeh B. Laparoscopic closure of gastric stab wounds: a case report. Surg Lap Endo 1993;3:63–66.
15. Brams DM, Cardoza M, Smith RS. Laparoscopic repair of traumatic gastric perforation using a gasless technique. J Lap Surg 1993;3:587–591.

Major Vascular Injury at Laparoscopy | 11

James M. Wheeler

Introduction

There is not an endoscopist alive who does not fear the consequences of a major vascular injury during laparoscopic surgery. Fortunately, the rare injury can be avoided by the careful performance of laparoscopy by the surgeon well versed in surgical anatomy—both normal and potentially distorted by disease.

This chapter will review the incidence of major vascular injuries, followed by demonstration of normal vascular anatomy as it relates to surface markings of the abdomen. Examples of distorted anatomy by disease and anatomic variants will be presented, followed by methods of diagnosis and treatment of major vascular injuries.

Definition and incidence

"Major" vascular injury can be defined as one that threatens the patient's life, typically immediately upon its occurrence. This definition would include injury to the great pelvic vessels, as well as the inferior and superior epigastric vessels, the superior and inferior mesenteric vessels, and large vessels supplying the abdominal or pelvic viscera. Other chapters in this text also discuss vascular injuries, so the focus herein will be on the great vessels of the abdomen and pelvis.

Major vascular injuries during laparoscopy are rare. In the 1970s, Loffer and Pent reported any vascular injury associated with bleeding in 6.4 per 1000 cases (0.6%) (1). A 1982 survey of over 125,000 laparoscopic tubal sterilizations presented an incidence of hemorrhage of 0.45 per 1000 cases (0.045%) (2). A European report of over 2700 laparoscopies for various indications presented an incidence of intraabdominal bleeding of 0.8 per 1000 cases (0.08%) (3). Most cases of intraabdominal bleeding are *not* due to injury of the great vessels, but rather, smaller vessels.

The Royal College of Obstetricians and Gynaecologists reported great vessel injury in 0.9 per 1000 cases (0.09%) (4), and a French survey presented 31 major vessel injuries in 100,000 laparoscopies for an incidence of 0.3 per 1000 cases (0.03%) (5). Many other smaller surveys or case reports document injuries of the aorta, vena cava, superior mesenteric vessels, and iliac vessels (6–12). A sign of the 1980s versus the 1970s is the appearance of case studies on major vessel injury at laparoscopy appearing in medicolegal journals (13).

To summarize, virtually every large vessel within reach of the anterior abdominal wall has been injured at laparoscopy, but fortunately on a very infrequent basis. The overall risk of major vascular injury, based on the above literature review, is less than 1 per 1000 cases (0.1%). Although this is a small risk, it certainly is not trivial. To better personalize this point, this small risk of 0.1% translates to a virtually 100% probability that the average gynecologic surgeon or one of his or her partners will experience at least one major vessel injury during their careers. Therefore, it certainly seems worthwhile to review the relevant anatomy of laparoscopic instrument insertion, and anatomic changes based on disease or normal anatomic variation.

Anatomy of laparoscopic instrument insertion

The umbilicus serves as the reference point for insertion of the laparoscopic instruments. However, the anatomic relations of the umbilicus to the great vessels can be variable between patients. In thin patients, the depths of the umbilicus can lie within 1–2 cm of the anterior surface of the aorta (14). Figure 11.1 is a transverse computed tomogram of a normal female volunteer at the L4 level (note: the left side of the figure depicts the right side of the patient). Note the plumpness of the aorta and the superior mesenteric artery that runs along over it. The

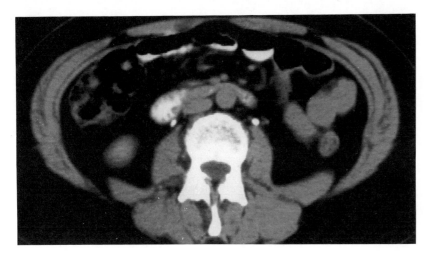

Fig. 11.1 Transverse computed tomogram of a healthy volunteer woman through L4. The left side of the image is the woman's right side. The aorta is located centrally, directly over the vertebras, and the inferior vena cava more posterolateral. The superior mesenteric artery is parallel and anterior to the aorta.

vena cava is flatter, posterior, and slightly right lateral to the aorta. It is indeed inspiring to the laparoscopist to see on this computed tomogram how the vertebral body seems to push the great vessels toward the umbilicus! Having had the opportunity to perform laparoscopy on three adolescent males to identify the location of cryptorchid testes, the author can definitely suggest extra care in the patient with an android pelvis, as the prominent sacral promontory pushes the aorta and vena cava even closer to the skin. Therefore, we usually recommend a "Z" technique, where the Veress needle and then trocar are inserted in a horizontal plane 2–4 cm through the subcutaneous or subfascial tissues prior to a more vertical insertion into the peritoneal cavity in an attempt to avoid the great vessels.

Recognizing the variations in the relations of the umbilicus to the great vessels, bony landmarks may be used to try to mentally visualize the location of the aortic/caval bifurcations. The aortic bifurcation lies over the fourth lumbar vertebral body in 75% of patients, and is within 1.25 cm above or below a line drawn between the iliac crests in 80% of women. In 9% of women, the aortic bifurcation is above L4, providing an extra degree of safety, but in 11% of women, the bifurcation is below the L4–L5 disc (15). It is recommended that an attempt be made to palpate the aortic bifurcation prior to insertion of the laparoscopic instruments. Fortunately, the vena cava, which is a more treacherous and difficult-to-repair injury, lies posterolateral to the aorta; it is infrequently injured at laparoscopy. However, one cannot palpate the vena cava through the abdominal wall.

As the laparoscopist descends into the pelvis, the external iliac vessels are lateral and superior to the uterus, and the internal iliac vessels run parallel to the ureter and the mesosalpinx (Fig. 11.2; transverse magnetic resonance image at the level of S4). Only by straying off the midline can one of these vessels be injured during instrument insertion. The external iliac vessels become quite susceptible to injury with insertion of accessory instrument sleeves lateral to the abdominis rectus muscles, *mandating* insertion only under direct visualization.

The most common vessels injured in the midline are the middle sacral vessels extending down the sacrum from the aortic bifurcation. The most common lateral vessels injured are the inferior epigastric vessels that run within 1–2 cm of the lateral edge of each rectus abdominis muscle. Again, any vessel big enough to be named can cause serious immediate bleeding or delayed intraperitoneal hemorrhage.

Figure 11.3, a sagittal magnetic resonance image of a healthy volunteer 1 cm to the right of midline, will serve to reiterate the steps suggested to avoid major injury during laparoscopic instrument insertion. After adequate anesthesia is achieved, the umbilicus is palpated to identify the aortic pulsation; the aortic arch is palpated next. Care is taken in positioning the patient in the modified dorsal lithotomy position so that her back is not extended, which would thrust the aorta even closer to the abdominal skin. The umbilical incision is made through skin only (the author prefers to use one of the deep vertical folds to avoid fat and improve cosmesis). The anterior abdominal wall is elevated, and the Veress needle (if used) is inserted *exactly* in the midline for a distance of 2–4 cm parallel to the skin, then more vertically aiming for the deep true pelvis; a uterine manipulator to deflect the genitalia downward at this point is very useful. Following achieving adequate pneumoperitoneum, the Veress needle is withdrawn and the trocar inserted along the same path using the same precautions. The laparoscope, which is connected to the light source during insufflation, is immediately inserted and inspection of the abdomen and pelvis is made for any suggestion of vascular or visceral injury. Once the umbilical insertion site seems safe, accessory trocars are inserted carefully under direct vision.

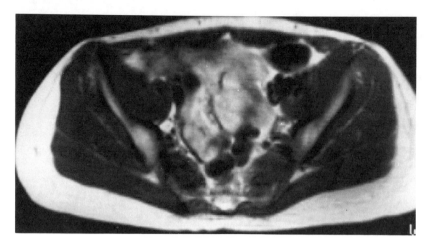

Fig. 11.2 Transverse magnetic resonance image of a volunteer woman through S4. The left side of the image is the woman's right side. The external iliac vessels lie under the lateral edge of the rectus abdominis muscles. The internal iliac vessels are more medial and inferior versus the external iliacs at this level in the pelvis.

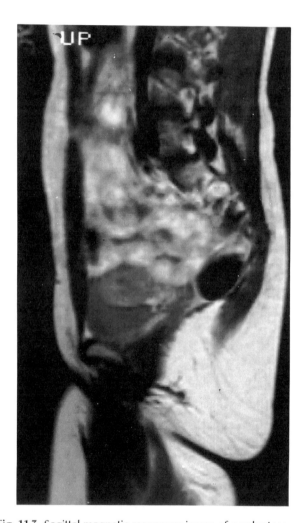

Fig. 11.3 Sagittal magnetic resonance image of a volunteer woman, 1 cm right of midline. The inferior vena cava is the larger vessel over the spine, with the left common iliac vessel seen at L5 to S1. The umbilicus is clear opposite the aortic bifurcation; this woman would have a distance of about 1.5 cm between her umbilicus and aortic arch.

Risk factors for major vascular injury at laparoscopy

As the android pelvis mentioned earlier represents, any process or anatomic variant that brings the abdominal aorta closer to the abdominal skin will increase the risk of major vessel injury; the most obvious example is rarely encountered, being an abdominal aortic aneurysm. In very thin patients, the aorta may be within 1 cm of the skin. The very obese patient is at greater risk for another reason: anatomic landmarks become more difficult to ascertain, and the laparoscopic Veress needle and trocar must be inserted in a more vertical path just to reach the peritoneal cavity.

Injury to vessels supplying the viscera will be discussed in other chapters in this book. Clearly, any process that either makes tissues less pliable (e.g., endometriosis, adhesions), or vessels more attenuated (e.g., certain vasculitides, granulomatous disease) will increase the risk for major vascular injury.

Perhaps the greatest risk factor that can be modified is the surgeon's experience. The beginning laparoscopist should be fully knowledgeable about the anatomy of the procedure and the given patient; preferably, some prior experience on an animal model is ideal and relatively available at postgraduate courses. Once learning the technique, laparoscopists must work to remain proficient: physicians performing fewer than 100 laparoscopic procedures have almost four times the complication rate of those with greater experience (14.7 versus 3.8 per 1000 cases) (16).

Diagnosing major vessel injury

Even the most careful laparoscopist may injure a vessel; prompt diagnosis and treatment is imperative to prevent the situation turning from bad to worse. If the Veress needle perforates a vessel, prompt return of blood is noted *if* it was properly inserted with the valve in the "open" position. Intraperitoneal bleeding is more easily identified by relatively sudden changes in vital signs, whereas retroperitoneal bleeding can be more occult and difficult to diagnose. If vascular injury with the Veress needle is strongly suspected, the needle is left in place to help mark the site of injury while an expeditious midline incision is made for laparotomy. A bladder catheter is placed, anesthesiology is apprised of the surgeon's concern, and a large-bore intravenous catheter is placed. A clot is sent for blood typing and screening, and colloid solutions prepared in the meantime.

A trocar injury to the great vessels is usually more dramatic and apparent, further reinforcing the supportive measures described above. With the flourishing of operative laparoscopy, major vascular injury could occur after pneumoperitoneum is achieved. If bleeding is very minimal and controlled by clamping, endoscopic repair including suturing may be considered for small vessels, but laparotomy is necessary for great vessel injury.

Repair of major vessel injury

Once laparotomy has begun, the first priority is to compress the aorta to minimize exsanguination risk; this goal is accomplished with an assistant's hand, an aortic compressor, or a vascular clamp. The field is cleared of blood in a quick hand-over-hand motion using laparotomy sponges. The vessel injury is found, and a finger placed over it for hemostasis while repair materials are gathered. Fluid resuscitation continues while the damage is sought and repaired.

Small vessels producing significant bleeding—e.g., middle sacral or inferior epigastric vessels—are ligated. The surgeon must know collateral blood supply and drainage prior to ligating a vessel. Larger vessels are repaired with 4/0 Prolene over a Dacron reinforcing bolster; larger defects may require an interposition graft. This work is best done by a trained cardiovascular surgeon, yet the laparoscopist must know the basic principles of vascular repair.

If a large artery is clamped for over 10–15 minutes, systemic anticoagulation with heparin should be considered once the repair is complete and the patient stable.

Venous injuries are more difficult to repair other than by ligation because their walls are thinner. Because of collateral venous circulation, almost all veins—even the inferior vena cava—can be ligated without significantly impeding blood return to the heart.

Once the patient reaches the recovery room, careful neurovascular assessment is done of the lower limbs in addition to usual intensive care support. Arteriography is indicated only if disruption of the suture site or leakage is clinically suspected.

After 4–6 weeks have passed since an arterial injury, Doppler flow studies would be helpful in characterizing the flow through the repaired vessel. If neural compromise occurred due to transient loss of blood supply, physical and occupational therapy should begin as soon as the patient is stabilized.

Summary

A major vascular injury at laparoscopy is a dangerous surgical complication. Thorough anatomic knowledge and understanding of the procedure will reduce the risk of such an injury. Should an injury occur, prompt diagnosis and treatment will help to limit the morbidity and mortality that can result from the rare major vessel injury at laparoscopy.

ACKNOWLEDGMENTS: The assistance of Dr. Steven Sax, Department of Radiology, The Methodist Hospital, is acknowledged for his help with computed tomograms and magnetic resonance images presented in this chapter.

REFERENCES

1. Loffer F, Pent D. Indications, contraindications and complications of laparoscopy. Obstet Gynecol Surv 1975;30:407–427.
2. Phillips JM, Hulka JF, Peterson HB. American Association of Gynecologic Laparoscopists' 1982 membership survey. J Reprod Med 1984;29:592–594.
3. Frenkel Y, Oelsner G, Ben-Baruch G, Menczer J. Major surgical complications of laparoscopy. Eur J Obstet Gynecol Reprod Biol 1981;12:107–111.
4. Chamberlain G, Brown JC, eds. Gynaecological laparoscopy: the report of the confidential inquiry into gynaecological laparoscopy. London: Royal College of Obstetricians and Gynaecologists, 1978:114.
5. Mintz M. Risks and prophylaxis in laparoscopy: a survey of 100,000 cases. J Reprod Med 1977;18:269.
6. Bartsich EG, Dillon TF. Injury of superior mesenteric vein: laparoscopic procedure with unusual complication. N Y State J Med 1981;81:933.
7. Karam K, Hajj S. Mesenteric hematoma of a Meckel's diverticulum: a rare laparoscopic complication. Am J Obstet Gynecol 1979;135:544.
8. Kurzel RB, Edinger DD Jr. Injury to the great vessels: a hazard of transabdominal endoscopy. South Med J 1983;76:656–657.
9. McDonald PT, Rich NM, Collins GJ, et al. Vascular trauma secondary to diagnostic and therapeutic procedures: laparoscopy. Am J Surg 1978;135:651–655.
10. Peterson HB, Greenspan JR, Ory HW. Death following puncture of the aorta during laparoscopic sterilization. Obstet Gynecol 1982;59:132–133.
11. Shin CS. Vascular injury secondary to laparoscopy. N Y State J Med 1982;82:935–936.
12. Erkrath KD, Weiler G, Adebahr G. Lesion of the aorta abdominalis in gynecologic laparoscopy. Geburtshilfe Frauenheilkd 1979;39:687–689.
13. Lignitz E, Puschel K, Saukko P, Koops E, Mattig W. Iatrogenic hemorrhagic complications in gynecologic laparoscopies—report of 2 cases with a fatal course. Z Rechtsmed 1985;95:297–306.
14. Hulka JF. Major vessel injury during laparoscopy. Am J Obstet Gynecol 1980:138–590.
15. Goss CM, ed. Gray's anatomy. 27th ed. Philadelphia: Lea & Febiger, 1959:684.
16. Phillips J, Keith D, Hulka J, et al. Gynecologic laparoscopy in 1975. J Reprod Med 1976;16:105.

Vascular Insult to the Intestinal Mesentery | 12

Jeffrey C. Seiler

Vascular mesenteric injuries are less frequent than other vascular injuries because of the greater mobility of the mesentery compared with the large fixed retroperitoneal vessels. This injury could potentially occur more frequently, however, as gynecologists become more aggressive in pelviscopic surgery, and as other specialties begin to use laparoscopic technology, especially in the upper abdomen.

Mesenteric injury

Mesenteric injury is more likely to occur when the mesentery and its associated vessels are in a fixed position. In the virgin abdomen without adhesions, an entry of the Veress needle or a trochar inserted at too perpendicular an angle may trap the mesenteric vessels between the posterior body wall and the penetrating instrument. In the obese patient, the surgeon may direct the trocar to a more perpendicular position or use longer instruments, both of which increase the risk of this type of trauma. Additional trocars increase the risk of injury as well. In circumstances where adhesions are present, the mesentery may assume a more fixed position. This situation often arises when the small bowel is adherent to the anterior abdominal wall, tenting the mesentery and fixing it in the path of the needle or trocar entry.

Although used less frequently now than in the past, lasers present another potential risk for mesenteric damage. Because of the hidden nature of the vessels, a laser entering the mesentery—either planned or accidental—could open up the vessel, resulting in bleeding that cannot be controlled with laser coagulation. The CO_2 laser is probably the laser type most likely to cause this trauma in nonfat areas because of its beam delivery system and poor coagulating ability (1). Fiber-directed lasers also have the potential to traumatize the mesenteric vessels. Because fat stops the CO_2 laser beam, however, the KTP, argon, and YAG lasers are more likely to produce damage deep in the mesentery.

Another potential source of injury involves adhesiolysis. Consequently, the operating surgeon should minimize grasping the mesentery as a means of traction. As vessels are usually hidden in the mesenteric fat, direct trauma may occur when they are torn.

Anatomy

The anatomy of the mesentery impedes identification and repair of trauma to a vessel. The mesentery itself ranges in length from 4 to 25 cm, with shorter segments present at the origin and termination of the structure. Its course winds from the left upper quadrant to the right lower quadrant. The blood supply originates in the superior mesenteric artery, which arises from the aorta and emerges into the mesentery between the pancreas and duodenum. Only if the trocar were directed superiorly into the upper abdomen, away from the pelvis, would trauma to this portion of the superior mesenteric artery occur. The superior mesenteric vessel courses along the more distal portion of the mesentery, supplying multiple branches to the small bowel. Before it moves into the mesentery, it gives rise to the ileocolic artery, which traverses along the base of the mesentery to the cecum; there the superior mesenteric and ileocolic arteries anastomose, forming a complete loop (Fig. 12.1).

The superior mesenteric gives off intestinal branches (averaging approximately 16 in number, but with a considerable range in frequency). These intestinal arteries divide into ascending and descending branches that anastomose with branches of the adjacent intestinal arteries, thereby forming an arcade of vessels. Secondary arcades are often noted, and as many as five arcades have been described in the midportion of the mesentery. The most distal arcade leads to the vasa recta, straight vessels to the intestines that are 1 to 5 cm in length. The abundant arcades permit significant collateral circulation, although the smaller vasa recta rarely anastomose with one

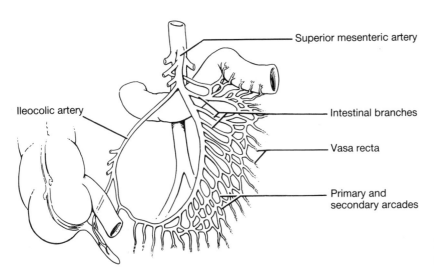

Fig. 12.1 Arterial supply of the intestinal mesentery.

Labels on figure: Superior mesenteric artery; Intestinal branches; Vasa recta; Primary and secondary arcades; Ileocolic artery

another. The venous system closely parallels the arterial system described (2).

The mesentery is composed of mostly fat. The relatively great accumulation at the base diminishes as the mesentery approaches the small bowel. Because the vasculature is hidden within this fat, laparoscopic identification of bleeders can prove difficult. Except for the vasa recti vessels adjacent to the small bowel, the vasculature of the mesentery is rarely seen through the laparoscope.

Surgical repair

Trauma to the superior mesenteric artery would create the most significant interruption of the mesenteric vasculature. Because of its importance in supplying the entire small bowel, such damage would necessitate repair by either grafting or a bypass procedure performed by a vascular surgeon.

As noted earlier, identification of the site of injury to the branches of the superior mesenteric is hindered by the fat surrounding these vessels. As the hematoma spreads into the fat, pinpointing the site of bleeding becomes even more difficult, even in the open abdomen. When trauma is identified, quick action may limit the size of the hematoma, enabling the site of damage to be more easily located. The most distal arteries (vasa recti) are the most easily seen. If hemostasis could be obtained, the lack of collateral circulation of these vessels would permit quick management of the problem. Clasping a bleeder with an atraumatic clamp can control the bleeding initially until appropriate instrumentation is available and hemostasis can be achieved. Electrocautery can be used, but bipolar should be selected to avoid transmission of the current along the vessels into the small bowel. The application of a hemoclip offers an alternative to bipolar coagulation.

As the site of trauma goes deeper into the mesentery, away from the bowel, vessel identification becomes more difficult because of the increasing fat content. If a traumatic perforation of the fat has occurred adjacent to the site of bleeding, the opening may permit easier viewing of the bleeding vessel. If the bowel is adherent (tenting the mesentery), rapid identification may be obtained. If trauma was caused by the initial entry, introduction of a secondary trocar may prove challenging because of the reduced visualization. Such trocars would be necessary for coagulation or for the application of clips.

If the hematoma identified seems small and is not enlarging, observation may be adequate. This case is most likely to occur if only venous damage has occurred. When evaluating a bleeding site, the surgeon should remain cognizant of the magnification created by the laparoscope (the bleeding may appear much worse than it is). Magnification may range from none to an eightfold increase, depending on the proximity to the site of trauma (3). Pulling the trocar back to eliminate this large magnification will keep the surgeon's vision in prospective.

In the case of an enlarging hematoma for which the source of the bleeding cannot be identified, a laparotomy should be undertaken promptly. Extensive laparoscopic manipulation coupled with a rising surgeon anxiety level may increase the bleeding and hematoma size, making subsequent identification even more difficult. A midline incision can provide rapid access to the site of trauma. Once the abdomen is open, manual exploration of the trauma site should allow adequate vessel identification, after which hemostasis should be accomplished easily. Because of the abundant arcades and extensive collateral circulation, both ends of the severed artery should be secured. Although bowel circulation is unlikely to be compromised if any vessel distal to the superior mesenteric is tied off, observation of the bowel should still be undertaken after obtaining hemostasis. If any question arises, a general surgeon should be consulted. Blunt trauma to the abdominal cavity has been associated with bowel infarction (4).

Attempts should be made to remove as much blood as possible, although most of it will diffuse through the mesentery. Drains would not provide much benefit to the procedure.

A hematoma that is missed could produce a small bowel obstruction or, if it dissects retroperitoneally, a paralytic ileus. A CAT scan would be most helpful in these circumstances. If the hematoma was not identified intraoperatively, is not enlarging, and is associated with a stable hemoglobin, observation is probably the better approach.

Precautions

In closed laparoscopy, trauma to the mesentery may be minimized by careful insertion of the needle and initial trocar, directing them toward the cul-de-sac and not into the fixed back of the patient. If the patient is obese or upper abdominal surgery is planned, a more perpendicular entry is required. The abdominal wall should then be elevated to avoid too deep penetration. If the patient has undergone prior surgery, this risk may be minimized by use of open laparoscopy or identification of nonadherent areas by inserting a spinal needle with saline and injecting to find an open space before insertion. A disposable trocar with a retractable sheath is also a safety factor that should be considered when the patient has received prior abdominal surgery. In addition to the protection bestowed by the sheath, the ease of entry of the disposable system can reduce the potential for deep penetration (5). To reduce the risk of damage from secondary trocars, insertion under direct visualization or videolaparoscopy is advised.

Open laparoscopy, which is increasing in popularity, minimizes the risk of mesenteric trauma because the mesentery is separated from the abdominal wall in virtually all cases—even where prior surgical procedures have been performed. Unfortunately, it cannot eliminate trauma to other organs adherent to the entry site as effectively.

In summary, damage to the mesenteric vessels with laparoscopy is unusual because of its mobility. If trauma occurs, however, rapid correction must be undertaken to avoid a large hematoma and difficulty in identifying the damaged vessel.

REFERENCES

1. Fisher JC. Basic laser physics and interaction of laser light with soft tissue. In: Shapshay SM, ed. Endoscopic laser surgery handbook. New York: Marcel Dekker, 1987:118.
2. Hollinshead WH. Anatomy for surgeons, vol. 2, 2nd ed. New York: Harper & Row Publishers, 1971:461–466.
3. Cook AS, Rock JA. The role of laparoscopy in the treatment of endometriosis. Fertil Steril 1991;55:4, 663.
4. Buhari SA. Isolated mesenteric vascular injury following a blunt abdominal trauma—a case report. Singapore Med J 1995;39:2, 222.
5. Corson SL, Batzer FR, Gocial B, Maislin G. Measurement of the force necessary for laparoscopic trocar entry. J. Reprod Med 1989;34:282–284.

13 | The Franklin–Kelly Technique for Insertion of the Laparoscope

Randle S. Corfman

Introduction

During the course of medical education one may be fortunate to learn a fact, a technique, or a "trick" that profoundly impacts subsequent practice. The accumulation of these tricks, when combined with a sound knowledge of basic surgical principles, is manifested as clinical savvy—that is, the "right stuff"—as the fledgling surgeon leaves the nest of formal medical education and soars on his or her own wings. It may be only then that the true wisdom from mentors of days gone by are recognized, when we thank our lucky stars that "Dr. X" crossed our paths.

It is with this idea in mind that the author plans to describe in detail a technique taught by a most admired mentor, Robert Kelly, who in turn learned the technique from Robert Franklin, a superb laparoscopic and microsurgeon. The author adopted the technique into his practice and enjoyed the privilege of sharing it with resident physicians and fellows; they, in turn, have passed their knowledge on to others. Perhaps the greatest tribute to the Franklin-Kelly technique consists of the many phone calls and notes the author has received from former students expressing their gratitude for its use.

The basic premise

The initial placement of the Veress needle and laparoscopic trocar and sheath is a "blind shot" that makes everyone in the surgeon theater take pause. This concern is particularly palpable when the patient is at risk for entry injuries—most notably in the case of an obese patient or a patient with a previous midline skin incision that approaches the inferior margin of the umbilicus.

Certainly one approach is to perform an open laparoscopy to gain entry to the peritoneal cavity. Such a procedure is not without risk, however, and the technique often makes it difficult to maintain an adequate pneumoperitoneum; this requirement itself presents a series of technical difficulties that can be difficult to overcome.

Traditional techniques for placement of the instruments involved elevation of the abdominal wall by grasping the skin inferior to the umbilicus, often with the help of an assistant, and then inserting the Veress needle. Following insufflation to gain a pneumoperitoneum, the trocar and sheath were introduced with a corkscrew motion. The laparoscope was introduced so that the surgeon could see what he or she had just passed through; the physician could then visualize the anatomy through the laparoscope and hope that it had not transgressed any unintended anatomy. Kelly pointed out that utilization of this technique could create problems if any significant adhesions were present between the bowel and the anterior wall. Passing through these structures would result in co-elevation as the surgeon elevated the skin, thereby increasing the likelihood on perforation of these structures (Fig. 13.1).

In addition, this popular technique was not easy to use in the obese patient. Lifting the anterior abdominal wall often was performed using towel clips and other such instruments—methods that struck many neophyte surgeons as slightly barbaric.

Many surgeons chose to make a semilunar incision in the inferior subumbilical margin, a practice that also made little sense to Kelly. He suggested that the objective of initial maneuvers was to gain entry into the peritoneal cavity at a site possessing the least distance from the skin to the anterior peritoneum. This distance increased as one moved inferiorly from the umbilicus (dramatically so in the obese patient), making entry more difficult.

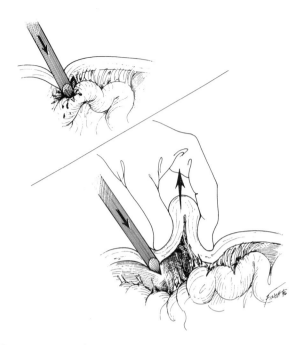

Fig. 13.1 Potential risk of bowel injury with trocar placement at laparoscopy.

The Franklin-Kelly technique

Preparation

In preparation for the Franklin-Kelly technique, the patient is placed in the low dorsal lithotomy position and the entire abdomen is prepped thoroughly with the superior margin at the level of the xiphoid. Before any incision is made, the instruments should be assembled and all systems checked out. For example, operating room personnel should ensure that the light source is in position and is operative, that the CO_2 insufflator is operative and attached to the gas tank, that the video system is ready to go, and that all members of the team are prepared.

The anesthesiologist or anesthetist is then asked to decompress the stomach by passing an orogastric or nasogastric tube. The surgeon or an assistant empties the patient's bladder, all prior to making an incision. The table is placed at a comfortable height.

Insertion of the Veress needle

The Veress needle is examined and checked to ensure that the spring mechanism is functional and that it has been assembled correctly. Occasionally the gas exit port can be hidden by the sleeve, impeding release of the gas.

The skin is infiltrated with a small amount of dilute bupivacaine. A curved clamp can be used for lateral

retraction to expose the base of the umbilicus. A No. 11 blade is used to make the skin incision, beginning at the base of the umbilicus and extending inferiorly to a distance that permits entry of the trocar and sheath (Fig. 13.2). Care must be taken to avoid overextension of the incision, an error that can lead to inadvertent leakage of gas and partial loss of a pneumoperitoneum.

The bifurcation of the great vessels lies directly beneath the umbilicus. The danger inherent in making the incision is that—particularly in the thin patient—the scalpel tip can lacerate such structures and subsequently turn a routine laparoscopy into a laparotomy and call for a vascular surgeon.

The surgeon gently lifts the anterior abdominal wall, pulling the umbilicus inferiorly so as to avoid the bifurcation of the great vessels. The Veress needle is inserted through the anterior abdominal wall, using the fingertips to identify the passage through the various tissue planes. The Veress needle is directed toward the cul-de-sac (Fig. 13.3). During this time, the gas line is not attached to the needle.

The surgeon's grip on the anterior abdominal wall is relaxed and the insufflator is attached to the Veress needle with the insufflator in the off position. Only then does the surgeon elevate the anterior abdominal wall again. As no pressure differential between the atmosphere and the peritoneal cavity exists, elevation of the anterior abdominal wall should produce a drop in the internal pressure. This drop should result in a corresponding negative pressure reading on the insufflation instrument. Failure to realize this pressure drop indicates that the tip of the Veress needle is preperitoneal, that it is within relatively dense tissue, or that it is within the lumen of the bowel. If the intraabdominal pressure fails to drop relative to the opening pressure, the surgeon should withdraw the Veress needle and redirect its entry.

Once the desired pressure drop is achieved, the insufflator is activated and CO_2 gas is released into the abdominal cavity. The grip on the anterior abdominal wall is maintained until approximately 1 liter is instilled, making it less likely to insufflate the omentum. After initial insufflation, the flow rate can be increased substantially. The abdomen is insufflated to 15 mm Hg, or until it becomes quite taut. (In the obese patient a substantially greater pressure may be required.) With this status achieved, the spinal needle test is applied.

Spinal needle test

A 22-gauge spinal needle is attached to a 10-cc syringe filled with 2 cc of saline.

The spinal needle is inserted through the incision, adjacent to the Veress needle, in the anticipated path of the trocar (Fig. 13.4). While the needle is advanced, the plunger is gently retracted; gas bubbles will return

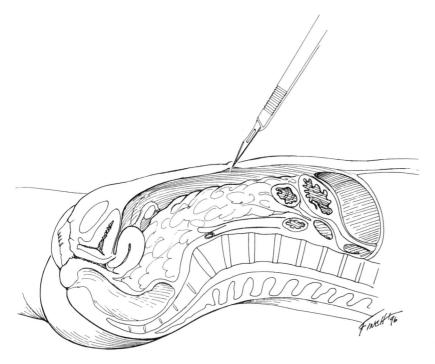

Fig. 13.2 Incision of skin vertically at umbilicus.

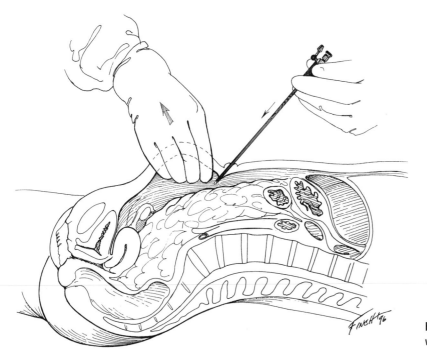

Fig. 13.3 Elevation of anterior abdominal wall with placement of Veress needle.

through the saline at the instant that the needle reaches a gas-containing space. The spinal needle is removed and the needle redirected laterally to ensure that the space near the umbilicus is free of obstruction. In the patient with a previous midline incision scar, for example, it is not uncommon to observe no return of gas in the direction of the scar. This finding would suggest that an obstruction exists (most likely bowel adherent to the anterior abdominal wall). By redirecting the spinal needle, the surgeon uses this technique to find a window through which the trocar can be safely directed (Fig. 13.5). The rationale behind this approach is that it is better to make a false passage with a small spinal needle than with a 10-mm trocar.

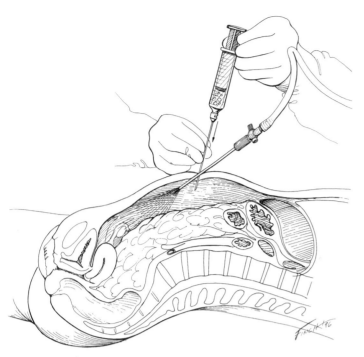

Fig. 13.4 Spinal needle test to probe space beneath umbilical incision.

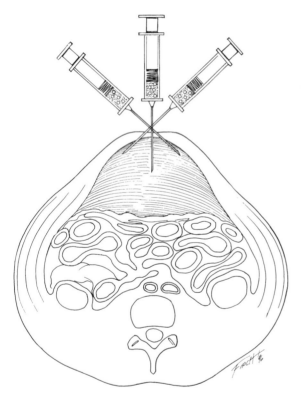

Fig. 13.5 Spinal needle probing in multiple directions.

The distance between the skin and the point of return of gas, as measured by the spinal needle, is noted. This important measurement is then used to determine the distance that the trocar and sheath can be safely advanced—that is, the safety zone.

Placement of the trocar and sheath

When the desired insufflation has been achieved, the Veress needle is removed. The trocar and sheath are examined, and the sharpness of the trocar is confirmed. To use a dull trocar is to invite trouble with trocar placement.

The trocar is grasped circumferentially with the surgeon's inferior-most hand at a distance from the trocar tip *less than* that determined to be the safety zone, as measured by the spinal needle test. For example, if the spinal needle test revealed the safety zone to be 4 cm, the trocar and sheath should be gripped 3 cm from the tip, providing a margin of safety of 1 cm.

The tip of the trocar is gently directed into the incision and cautiously advanced until it is slightly engaged through the fascia of the rectus abdominus (Fig. 13.6). It should not be directed significantly toward the underlying structures, but rather only slightly result in an indentation of the distended abdomen.

The trocar and sheath are then advanced inferiorly (Fig. 13.7), using the strength of the rectus fascia to permit entry of the instruments into the abdominal cavity. The sheath is advanced only to a distance less than that indicated as the safe area—that is, to the finger

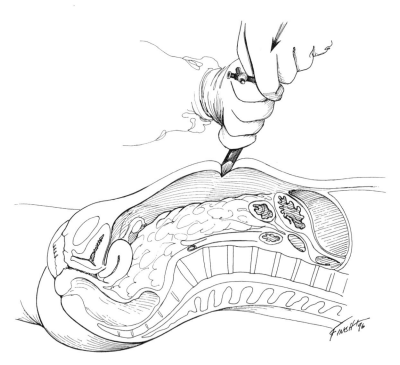

Fig. 13.6 Introduction of trocar without lifting abdominal wall. Care is taken to catch fascia with the tip.

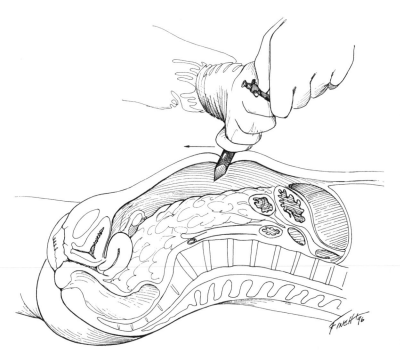

Fig. 13.7 Trocar is placed into abdominal cavity by directing pressure inferiorly.

"stop" of the surgeon's nondominant hand. In cases where the spinal needle test has, for example, indicated obstruction directly inferiorly but with a clear area to the right of the midline, the trocar and sheath are inserted in this direction.

The trocar is immediately removed and the sheath advanced. The laparoscope, which was previously attached to the light cable and video camera, is rapidly advanced into the abdominal cavity to inspect the contents. In this manner, rapid discovery of damage can be made and corrective or reparative action taken.

Summary

By using these techniques together, a number of transgressions "through the anatomy" can be avoided. Certainly no technique can prevent all unintended damage to anatomic structures, but the Franklin-Kelly technique can provide the surgeon with indicators that can modify the surgical approach to placement of laparoscopic instrumentation. In my hands this technique has proved very useful, and it is the author's hope that it will prove useful for subsequent generations of surgeons.

14 | Bladder Injuries During Laparoscopic Surgery

Stephen F. Schiff

Classification

Bladder injuries can generally be classified into four broad categories:

1. Contusion.
2. Interstitial tear.
3. Intraperitoneal rupture/laceration.
4. Extraperitoneal rupture/laceration.

The most common types of bladder trauma sustained during laparoscopic surgery are intraperitoneal or extraperitoneal injuries.

By definition, intraperitioneal injuries involve perforation or rupture of the bladder and peritoneum, with urinary drainage into the peritoneal cavity, surrounding loops of intestine, and other abdominal organs. This type of injury is often seen secondary to blunt suprapubic trauma with a full bladder where the dome literally "blows out" along with the overlying peritoneal reflection. In extraperitoneal injuries, the peritoneum remains intact and urinary leakage from the damaged bladder is generally limited to the space of Retzius and the true pelvis.

Mechanism of injury

During laparoscopic surgery the most likely mechanism of injury would be as follows:

1. Penetrating trauma from trocar or other operating instruments causing a puncture or laceration.
2. Thermal trauma from laser or cautery instruments.
3. Crushing trauma from clamps or other operating instruments.

Bladder lacerations or perforations are usually related in scope to the instrument used in creating the injury. The magnitude of the damage is often readily apparent upon visual inspection. However, with thermal injuries, looks can be deceiving. A zone of devitalized tissue surrounds the actual point of thermal damage that may not survive after repair unless it is debrided beforehand. This condition is quite similar to the "blast effect" on surrounding tissue seen with bullet injuries.

Perhaps the simplest way to reduce the likelihood of bladder injury during laparoscopic surgery is to keep the bladder drained with a Foley catheter during surgery. There is no doubt that a distended bladder is more likely to be injured than one that is kept flaccid and empty.

Diagnosis

The challenge in bladder injuries during laparoscopic surgery is twofold: (1) considering the possibility that an injury has occurred; and (2) making the diagnosis accurately and in a timely fashion.

During surgery, the patient may actually be of some assistance in alerting the surgeon that a bladder injury has occurred. With regional anesthesia if an intraperitoneal perforation has been made and urinary ascites causes diminished diaphragmatic excursion, patients may complain of respiratory difficulty. However, the surgeon should not rely on patients complaints of suprapubic pain or fullness.

If a Foley catheter is used (it is recommended for all laparoscopic surgery), there may be a drop in urinary output and/or the urine may become bloody. Of course, serious injury may occur without any of the above-mentioned signs or symptoms.

Laparoscopically, the surgeon may observe or suspect a bladder injury. Urine may be seen in the pelvis, usually secondary to an extraperitoneal perforation or laceration. If an injury is suspected but no definite urine is seen, $5\,cm^3$ of IV indigo carmine or methylene blue can be administered and one can watch the bladder laparoscopically for leakage. Remember that much of the bladder is hidden within the true pelvis and injuries of the lateral and posterior wall may be missed visually. Therefore, if bladder damage is still suspected, a gravity cystogram should be performed immediately. A 50/50 mixture of standard contrast medium and normal saline is made. Approximately $250\,cm^3$ is infused into the bladder by gravity drainage and a film obtained. If a rupture is seen, the catheter is placed to gravity drainage immediately. If not, another $150\,cm^3$ is infused and anteroposterior, oblique, and lateral films are obtained. The bladder is drained and a drainage film is then taken. Small bladder perforations may only be seen on the lateral, oblique, or drain-out films.

Radiographically, intraperitoneal injuries will allow contrast to fill the cul-de-sac, outline loops of bowel, and extend along the pericolic gutter. Extraperitoneal injuries will show areas of extravasated contrast within the perivesical space. Sometimes contrast may be seen extending retroperitoneally or along the inguinal canal. If a pelvic hematoma is present, the bladder may appear compressed.

Perhaps the most dangerous bladder injury is the one that is missed at the time of surgery. Certain signs and symptoms should alert the surgeon to the possibility of bladder injury.

Suprapubic pain and fullness with or without diminished urine output may suggest bladder injury. The definitive diagnosis can be made by cystography as described above.

If an intraperitoneal bladder injury has been missed, a dramatic increase in the blood urea nitrogen (BUN) may occur due to urinary contact with the peritoneum. Once again, the definitive diagnosis is made by cystography.

Thermal injuries to the bladder may not manifest themselves initially. Sudden hematuria well into the postoperative period may be a sign of thermal damage. A true perforation may not yet be present and therefore a negative cystogram may be misleading. Cystoscopy should be performed to identify any areas of devitalized tissue.

Management

There is general consensus that all intraperitoneal bladder injuries should be repaired by open surgery at the time the diagnosis is made.

A midline suprapubic incision is made to allow adequate exposure to the abdomen and pelvis. Once the urine is evacuated, the peritoneal and bladder perforations/lacerations are identified. The peritoneal laceration is closed in a single layer with 3-0 chromic catgut. The bladder injury is debrided back to viable tissue. A large-bore suprapubic tube (24–26 French) is brought out through a separate stab wound in the bladder and

secured to the bladder with a 2-0 chromic catgut "Z" stitch. The bladder laceration itself is closed watertight in three layers using 2-0 chromic catgut; the mucosa and muscularis in running locking stitches; and the adventitial tissue with interrupted stitches. The suprapubic tube is brought out the abdominal wall through a separate stab wound—not at one end of the incision. The peritoneal cavity is *not* drained, although the space of Retzius is. The abdominal incision is closed in the standard manner.

It is a matter of style as to which catheter—urethral or suprapubic—is removed first. Once the urine clears of blood, one catheter is removed and the pelvic drain is removed once drainage subsides. A gravity cystogram is performed on day 7–10. If no extravasation is noted at that time, the catheter is removed.

Extraperitoneal injuries are somewhat more controversial in their management. Most small rents can be managed nonoperatively with large-bore Foley catheter drainage for 10 days. Usually, the bladder will heal and extravasated urine and blood will resorb. The patient should have uninfected urine, and appropriate catheter care should be employed. If the patient is to be explored for other reasons, the bladder may be repaired via a cystotomy with the laceration closed from the inside with 2-0 chromic catgut. The cystotomy closure, suprapubic tube placement, and pelvic drainage are as previously described. The cystogram should be performed at 10 days. If no extravasation is noted then, the Foley catheter is removed.

Patients with known infected urine should be explored and drained even with extraperitoneal lacerations, due to the very high likelihood of developing infected urinomas or hematomas.

Complications

As mentioned previously, the biggest trap is not thinking of the diagnosis. Often, bladder injuries can be treated nonoperatively with excellent results. Delay in diagnosis only increases the risk of developing infected hematomas and urinomas. If these complications occur, especially in patients being treated with catheter drainage, they must be drained surgically and appropriate antibiotic coverage instituted. Infected urine with intraperitoneal injuries can lead to peritonitis and sepsis; surgical repair of these injuries should be performed at the time of diagnosis.

Conclusion

Management of bladder injuries is generally quite straightforward. Nevertheless, early consultation with urological colleagues can help ensure an excellent outcome when these injuries do occur.

Suggested reading

Cass AS. Diagnostic studies in bladder rupture: indications and techniques. Urol Clin North Am 1989;16:267–273.

Corrier JN. Trauma to the lower urinary tract. In: Gillenwater JY, Grayhack JT, Howards SS, Duckett JW, eds. Adult and pediatric urology. 2nd ed. Chicago: Year Book Medical Publishers, 1987:499–505.

Corrier JN, Sandler CM. Management of the ruptured bladder: 7 years of experience with 111 cases. J Trauma 1986;26:830–833.

Corrier JN, Sandler CM. Mechanisms of injury, patterns of extravasation and management of extraperitoneal bladder rupture due to blunt trauma. J Urol 1988;139:43–44.

Corrier JN, Sandler CM. Management of extraperitoneal bladder rupture. Urol Clin North Am 1989;16:275–277.

Peters PC. Intraperitoneal rupture of the bladder. Urol Clin North Am 1989;16:279–282.

Complications of Laparoscopic Burch Colposuspension

15

Edward M. Beadle, James B. Presthus, and Chau-Su Ou

Introduction

The Burch colposuspension, first reported by John Burch in 1961, has become the "gold standard" for genuine urinary stress incontinence (1). Compared with other surgical procedures, the Burch colposuspension has shown more consistent success and better long-term cure rates (2). As laparoscopic instrumentation and techniques improved, this open procedure became amenable to conversion. Vancaillie and Schuessler reported the first laparoscopic suture procedure in 1991 (3). Ou *et al.* followed shortly with a surgical mesh and staple modification of this procedure (4). In addition, a preperitoneal approach was reported in 1993. These variations of the original open procedure are being evaluated in controlled trials and will be judged accordingly over time.

No published series to date have reported complication rates of these techniques. The authors presented data at the 23rd AAGL-World Congress of Endoscopy in 1994 (Table 15.1). These data reflect the initial 165 patients in the mesh and staple series and show the common minor and major complications. They were later expanded with three additional series presented at the 24th AAGL-World Congress of Endoscopy in 1995 (Table 15.2). Although each author used a different modification of the Burch procedure, the rates of complications that they found are very similar.

Intraoperative complications

The laparoscopic Burch is an elective operation. A thorough explanation of the surgery to the patient is mandatory. Informed consent requires that patients understand all potential risks, complications, failures, and alternative treatments. Patients should have realistic expectations regarding the outcome of surgery. In particular, they should understand that complications such as urinary retention, detrusor instability, and recurrence of stress incontinence cannot be totally avoided. It is also important that the patient recognizes that laparoscopy is merely a means of access. If that access proves unsatisfactory because of technical difficulties or complications, then the surgery may need to be converted to a traditional open procedure.

The laparoscopic Burch procedure should be performed only by surgeons experienced in advanced laparoscopy. The key to the procedure involves correct placement of suture or mesh to support the urethrovesical junction with a broad hammock of paravaginal fascia (5). The goal of the surgery is to arrest the hypermobility of the urethra and allow intra-abdominal pressure transmission to compress the urethra and maintain continence. In addition, the normal posterior rotational descent of the bladder is preserved, as is the integrity of the urethra (6).

Access to the space of Retzius can be accomplished by either a transperitoneal or preperitoneal approach. The transperitoneal approach begins as a standard intra-abdominal laparoscopy, and all potential complications inherent to conventional laparoscopy can occur. With this approach, the entire pelvis and abdomen may be explored. Combined procedures—such as laparoscopically assisted vaginal hysterectomy, oophorectomy, or culdoplasty—require the transperitoneal technique.

The preperitoneal or extraperitoneal approach typically involves the use of commercial balloon dissectors. In addition, the dissection can be performed bluntly using standard trocars. The approach involves an open laparoscopic technique at a subumbilical site. To minimize the risk of subcutaneous emphysema, insufflation pressure should be less than 8 to 10 mm Hg. Assisting trocars are placed under direct vision lateral to the epigastric vessels.

Surgeons experienced with the preperitoneal approach cite as its advantages faster dissection, decreased chance of bladder injuries, and the option of regional anesthesia.

Table 15.1. Complications of laparoscopic Burch procedure.

Stapling Technique—21/165 Patients	
UTI	5
Detrusor instability	4
Hematuria	2
Subcutaneous hematoma	2
Pain	1
Bladder injury	3
Hernia (trocar)	2
Enterocele	1
Rectocele	1

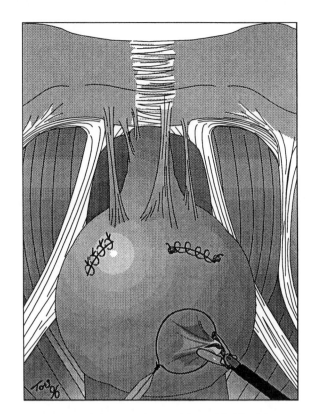

Fig. 15.1 Three techniques for repairing a bladder injury. (© Ethicon Endo-Surgery.)

Potential disadvantages are bleeding, tearing into the peritoneum resulting in a pneumoperitoneum that may restrict the surgeon's view, subcutaneous emphysema, and the inability to explore the pelvis and perform other intra-abdominal procedures.

Trocar placement for the laparoscopic Burch procedure is usually more cephalad and lateral, which allows triangulation for suturing or adequate distance in which to use a stapling device. Direct visualization of the inferior epigastric vessels is essential to minimize transection and bothersome bleeding from the insertion of accessory trocars.

Although trocar site herniation may occur at any site, it is most common with trocars greater than 10 mm. Trocar movement, removal, and replacement may cause fascial tears as large as 2 or 3 cm. Partial and complete small bowel obstruction secondary to herniation through these fascial defects has been reported (7). Numerous fascial closure devices are available to simplify closing these trocar sites. We recommend suture closure of fascia for any trocar site exceeding 5 mm.

Urinary tract infections secondary to catheterization can be minimized with administration of prophylactic antibiotics. As with most advanced laparoscopic procedures, wound or surgical site infections are rare.

Access to the space of Retzius from the abdominal cavity requires exiting anterior to the bladder and medial to the umbilical ligaments. Bladder injury is one of the more common complications noted during the early learning curve for the laparoscopic approach. The bladder may be filled with 250 to 400 cc of methylene blue-stained saline to outline the bladder's superior margin and avert any inadvertent cystotomy. A bladder injury may result from the initial peritoneal incision and

Table 15.2. Major complications of laparoscopic Burch colposuspension.

	Percent			
	Ou *et al.* n = 165	Liu n = 186	Ross n = 148	Lyons n = 179
Bladder injury	1.8	2.1	1.4	2.2
Hemorrhage	1.2	0.5	1.4	0.0
Urinary retention	1.2	2.1	N/A	1.1
Detrusor instability	2.4	2.1	2.0	24.8
Ureteral obstruction	0.0	0.5	0	1.1

dissection within the retropubic space or during exposure of the paravaginal fascia. To facilitate retraction of the bladder and identification of the proper site for sutures or staples, the operator can use his or her finger in the vagina to elevate the paravaginal fascia.

A perforation of the bladder less than 5 mm in length should heal spontaneously with continuous drainage for seven to ten days. In contrast, larger defects require closure. Repair of the defect can be accomplished by using either intraperitoneal or extraperitoneal suturing techniques with absorbable suture material. A simple method of performing a running closure is available with the use of the Lapro-Ty (Ethicon Inc., Somerville, New Jersey) system. Absorbable clips rather than conventional knots are used to anchor the ends of the suture line. Perforations on the dome of the bladder may be closed by using a pretied loop suture. These techniques are illustrated in Fig. 15.1. After repairing the bladder, continuous drainage is recommended for seven to ten days. The bladder heals rapidly, and this complication should not require abandonment of the laparoscopic approach.

Dissection in the space of Retzius is almost bloodless if carried out in the proper plane. In most cases, excessive bleeding indicates the dissection is too close to the bladder. The correct dissection should lie within the loose areolar tissue anterior to the bladder. Hemorrhage may occur from injury to the obturator or inferior epigastric vessels (8, 9). For example, injury to the venous plexus located along the attachment of the lateral vagina fornices may lead to troublesome bleeding. Bipolar coagulation will control most bleeding. Laparoscopic clips, hemostatic agents, or the argon beam coagulator can be used if the bleeding persists or appears close to vital structures.

Suture or mesh attachment to the paravaginal fascia should be made 1.5 to 2.0 cm lateral to the urethrovaginal junction to avoid the neurovascular supply to the urethra. Urethral injuries may occur from injudicious dissection. In addition, inaccurate suturing or stapling can cause injury. A large Foley catheter with a 25-cc bulb may be placed before beginning the procedure to aid in identifying the urethra and the bladder neck.

Early postoperative complications

Return of normal voiding function varies considerably. Transient voiding difficulties have a reported incidence as high as 25% (10–12). Urinary retention may be related to partial outflow obstruction, postoperative edema, or narcotic use. Patients who have a history of such problems are at higher risk. If a posterior colporrhaphy has been performed in combination with the Burch, spontaneous voiding is often delayed secondary to irritation of the levator muscles and inability to completely relax the pelvic floor. This problem will usually resolve itself in time. Patient reassurance along with either continuous or intermittent self-catheterization is recommended. Only rarely is medical therapy an improvement over expectant management.

A small percentage of patients will have a more prolonged delay of spontaneous voiding (12). This effect may be the result of overelevation of the bladder neck that produces kinking or compression of the urethra. It is important to understand that no absolute position of the urethra is associated with continence—the amount of urethral mobility affects development of this condition. Therefore adequate support of the urethra—not excessive elevation—is the surgical goal. It is not necessary to tightly approximate paravaginal fascia to Cooper's ligament. At the end of the procedure, a 1-cm space should remain between the urethra and the symphysis (Fig. 15.2).

Detrusor instability is a recognized complication of the Burch procedure (11, 13). Patients should be aware

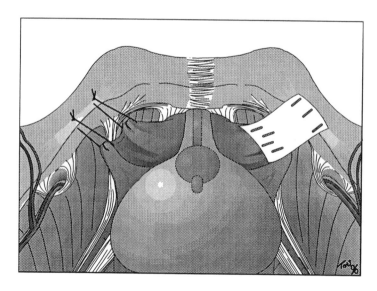

Fig. 15.2 Comparison of traditional suture and mesh technique. (© Ethicon Endo-Surgery.)

that they may have postoperative incontinence secondary to detrusor instability even though the stress component has been corrected.

Preoperative urodynamic studies have shown a 15% to 30% concurrence of detrusor instability with genuine urinary stress incontinence. As shown in Table 15.2, a postoperative incidence of 2% to 28% is associated with the laparoscopic Burch. The exact pathophysiology is unknown, but some cases may be related to overcorrection and partial outflow obstruction. Patients may be treated with drug therapy, bladder training, and behavior modification.

Ureteral injury is rare, but a few cases have been reported (9, 14). Obstruction may occur due to kinking of the ureter from the acute elevation of the anterior vaginal wall. Suture ligation or cautery injury arise only rarely because of the inferior insertion of the ureters into the bladder trigone. The common symptoms associated with ureteral injury include flank pain, fever, and anuria, which usually appear in the first 48 to 72 hours. An intravenous pyelogram may show hydronephrosis and the site of obstruction. Therapeutic options include cystoscopic antegrade stent placement, percutaneous nephrostomy with or without retrograde stent placement, and reoperation to alleviate the obstruction (15, 16).

If sutures or staples are placed into Cooper's ligament, groin pain may occur. Expectant management and analgesics are the traditional means of treatment. If symptoms persist, reoperation to remove the offending suture or staple should be delayed if possible. This waiting period allows adequate time for scarring and fixation so that the outcome of the surgery is not jeopardized.

Late postoperative complications

The most challenging late postoperative complication is the development of genital prolapse. Incidence of uterine descent and the formation of an enterocele and/or rectocele was reported to range from 5% to 20% in a large series of open Burch procedure cases (8, 10, 12). Wiskind reported that 26% (35 of 131 patients) required another procedure for associated prolapse (17). The same intrinsic weakness of the pelvic floor that leads to urinary stress incontinence predisposes these women to prolapse problems later in life. In addition, the vaginal axis may be altered by pulling the vagina anteriorly, thereby exposing the vaginal apex and posterior vaginal wall to the direct vector of intra-abdominal pressure.

It is imperative to identify all sites of prolapse preoperatively and correct these defects during the initial operation. Concurrent laparoscopic culdoplasty—i.e., uterosacral ligament fixation and Moschowitz stitches—can effectively close a deep cul-de-sac and reduce the incidence of this complication. When performing a culdoplasty, the ureters must be identified. If necessary, a relaxing incision can be made in the peritoneum to ensure that the ureters are not pulled in and obstructed.

Bladder calculi may occur from either permanent stitch or staple placement into the bladder. Careful dissection and proper stitch or staple placement should prevent this complication. In addition, cystoscopic evaluation of the bladder prior to completion of the case may identify errant sutures or staples. Simple removal and replacement are all that is necessary at the time of surgery. Late identification of a suture or staple in the bladder may be managed cystoscopically.

As an alternative to the traditional suture technique, the laparoscopic hernia stapler or tacker and surgical mesh may be used. The first operation to use a laparoscopic hernia stapler and Prolene mesh was performed by Ou in July 1991. Concerns have been voiced about these materials, however, and questions remain as to whether unique complications may arise from their use.

The use of synthetic mesh and staples is not new to surgery. Mesh has been used for the repair of hernia defects for many years (18). Different materials have been used, with the most popular and widely used being polypropylene mesh (Prolene and Marlex). This monofilament plastic, which offers minimal elasticity or stretch capacity, is nonallergenic, nononcogenic, resistant to infection, and resistant to rejection. Most importantly, the mesh is a weave in which interstices between the fibers allow immediate fibroplastic ingrowth. As a consequence, it provides a framework promoting the formation of scar tissue. The result is a very strong fascia or tendon-like structure consisting of mesh encased in fibrous tissue. The mesh itself will support up to 250 lb/in^2, and the tissue ingrowth can only increase this level of support.

In his original paper, Burch used absorbable suture material to perform his operation (1). Many surgeons today continue to use absorbable suture material. Obviously, the suture does not maintain the support; rather, the scarring associated with healing provides the foundation for long-term success. Many authors have commented on ways to increase the scarring by removing fat from the space of Retzius, using reactive suture material or other agents, and even encouraging bleeding. (18). It seems logical that the use of mesh would provide a reasonable alternative.

Stapling devices are accepted and dependable surgical tools that have been used extensively in chest and abdominal surgery. Titanium staples are nonreactive and will not disrupt any future radiological studies the patient may have. When fired, the staple forms a box with no sharp points exposed.

One concern about the use of mesh and staples has focused on the fear of erosion or migration. This potential complication is not unique to these materials. Any permanent suture may become a nidus of infection and cause erosion or rejection. In more than four years and over 500 Burch procedures performed by the authors, we have not encountered this complication. Likewise, a review of all medical device complications related to the use of hernia staplers and polypropylene mesh reported to the FDA for the years 1900–1995 did not reveal any reports commenting on erosion or migration.

In cases where mesh has eroded, such as suburethral sling procedures, the mesh and urethra have opposed one another. The mesh pulls up into the urethra and the urethra is pushed into the mesh by abdominal pressure. This tension and the potential for contamination of the mesh by opening the vagina explain why this effect is a significant complication associated with pubovaginal slings. In the laparoscopic Burch procedure, the mesh and staples suspend the vagina. These materials pull away from the vagina and the vagina is pushed away from the mesh and staples by abdominal pressure.

Finally, the return of incontinence following a Burch colposuspension can be considered a complication. It is extremely distressing for both the patient and the doctor. This condition may result from improper patient selection or technical failure.

The first operation to correct urinary stress incontinence offers the best chance of success. Reoperations are generally more difficult and less successful. Therefore, choosing the right surgical candidate and the correct procedure initially is of paramount importance. The ideal candidate for a Burch procedure will demonstrate genuine urinary stress incontinence, a hypermobile urethra, adequate vaginal capacity and mobility, and no evidence of intrinsic sphincteric dysfunction. Patients not meeting these criteria may be better served by a sling procedure or other treatment modality.

Technical failure can result from misplacement of sutures, inadequate fixation of paravaginal tissue to Cooper's ligament, or sutures pulling out of tissue (19). As a result, careful dissection to identify urethra, bladder neck, bladder, and paravaginal fascia is extremely important. Attachments should be secure and properly positioned. When sutures or mesh are properly anchored to paravaginal fascia, the operator should be able to feel the anterior vaginal wall lift when traction is applied to the suspending material. It is better to suture into the vagina than to have a meager bite of fascia. The vagina will reepithelialize over the sutures.

Conclusion

The surgical treatment of urinary stress incontinence is a challenging, frustrating, and rewarding pursuit. Patients are eternally grateful when an uncomplicated long-term cure is achieved. Complications and failures will occasionally occur, however, and are an irrefutable fact of surgery. It is the surgeon's responsibility to be aware of and recognize these potential complications and pitfalls. He or she must know how to avoid complications if possible and manage them when required. For their part, patients must understand that success cannot be guaranteed and that new problems or worsening of their condition may occur.

The complications related to a laparoscopic procedure are the same as those seen from a traditional approach, with the exception of those related to the use of trocars. Bleeding, infection, injury to other organs, voiding dysfunctions, genital prolapse, and failures can occur regardless of the technique. The advantages of laparoscopy are better visualization, reduced hospitalization time, less pain, and faster recovery. Future clinical studies will demonstrate if the long-term success and complication rates are better, worse, or no different compared with those of open surgery.

REFERENCES

1. Burch JC. Cooper's ligament urethrovesical suspension for stress incontinence. Am J Obstet Gynecol 1968;100:764.
2. Bergman A, Elia G. Three surgical procedures for genuine urinary stress incontinence: five-year follow-up of a prospective randomized study. Am J Obstet Gynecol 1995;175:66–71.
3. Vancaillie TG, Schuessler W. Laparoscopic bladder neck suspension. J Laparoendoscopic Surg 1991;1:169–173.
4. Ou CS, Beadle EM, Presthus JB. Laparoscopic bladder neck suspension using hernia mesh and surgical staples. J Laparoendoscopic Surg 1993;36:563–566.
5. DeLancey JOL. Structural support of the urethra as it relates to stress incontinence: the hammock hypothesis. Am J Obstet Gynecol 1994;170:1713–1723.
6. Hurt WG. Retropubic urethropexy or colposuspension. In: Hurt WG, ed. Urogynecologic surgerg. Gaithersburg, Md.: Aspen, 1992:81–95.
7. Kador N, Reich H, Liu CY, et al. Incisional hernias after major laparoscopic gynecologic procedures. Am J Obstet Gynecol 1993;168:1493–1495.
8. Korda A, Ferry J, Hunter P. Colposuspension for the treatment of female urinary incontinence. Aust NZ J Obstet Gynecol 1989;29:146–149.
9. Maulik TG. Kinked ureter with unilateral obstructive uropathy complicating Burch colposuspension. J Urol 1983;130:135–136.
10. Ericksen BC, Hagen B, Eik-Nes SH, et al. Long term effectiveness of the Burch colposuspension in female urinary stress incontinence. Acta Obstet Gynecol Scand 1990;69:45–50.
11. Vierhout ME, Mulder AFP. Denovo detrusor instability after Burch colposuspension. Acta Obstet Gynecol Scand 1992;71:414–416.
12. Wiskind AK, Stanton SL. The Burch colposuspension for genuine stress incontinence. In: Thompson JD, Rock JA, eds. TeLinde Operative Gynecology, vol I. Philadelphia: Lippincott, 1993:1–13.
13. Galloway NTM, Davies N, Stephanson TP. The complications of colposuspension. Br J Urol 1987;60:122–124.
14. Drutz HP, Baker KR, Lemieux MC. Retropubic colpourethropexy with transabdominal anterior and/or posterior repair for the treatment of genuine stress incontinence and genital prolapse. Int Urogynecol J 1991;2:201–204.
15. Ferriani RA, Silva de Sa MF, deMoura MD, et al. Ureteral blockage as a complication of Burch colposuspension. Report of six cases. Gynecol Obstet Invest 1990;29:239–240.
16. Kohorn EI. The surgery of stress urinary incontinence. Obstet Clin North Am 1989;16:841–852.
17. Wiskind AK, Creighton SM, Stanton SL. The incidence of genital prolapse after the Burch colposuspension. Am J Obstet Gynecol 1992;167:399–403.
18. Capozzi JA, Beckenfield JA, Cherry JK. Repair of inguinal hernia in the adult with prolene mesh. Surg Gynecol Obstet 1988;168:1–5.
19. Tanagho EA. Colpocystourethropexy: the way we do it. J Urol 1976;116:751–753.

16 | Ureteral Injury Associated with Transection of the Uterosacral Ligaments

David A. Grainger

Introduction

Minimally invasive surgery continues to expand in terms of both indications and scope of procedures. With this growth and the fact that more difficult cases are performed laparoscopically comes increasing reports of injuries to the urinary tract. The magnitude of this type of injury sustained at laparoscopy is still not well known.

Anatomically, many laparoscopic procedures, including the laparoscopic uterine nerve ablation (LUNA), closely approximate the ureter. The goals of this chapter will be to discuss the anatomy of the pelvic ureter, the innervation of the pelvic organs, and the merits and risks of the LUNA procedure. In addition, a review of the published reports of ureteral injury at laparoscopy will be presented, along with the recommended mode of diagnosis and treatment. Lastly, methods of reducing the chance of ureteral injury during extensive pelviscopic procedures will be described.

Anatomy

The ureter enters the pelvis at the pelvic brim, crossing over the common iliac artery and vein. It courses caudad, crossing under the uterine artery and entering the cardinal ligament at the level of the cervix. Next, the ureter pierces the cardinal ligament, coming anteriorly and medially to enter the trigone of the bladder. At the level of the cervix, the ureter appears 1 to 1.5 cm lateral to the uterosacral ligament. Adventitia connect the ureter to the medial peritoneum. Although the blood supply to the ureter has a multiplicity of sources, skeletonizing large segments of the ureter may result in ureteral stricture (2).

Pelvic surgeons operate closest to the ureter at the level of the infundibulopelvic ligament, the uterine artery, and the cervix. It is important to realize that the normal anatomical relationships in these three areas may be altered by common disease processes, such as leiomyoma or endometriosis. For instance, in patients with cul-de-sac endometriosis, the ureter may be much closer to the uterosacral ligament than the normal 1.5 cm, and thus more susceptible to injury (3). In the cul-de-sac, after the ureter has entered the cardinal ligament, it can no longer be visualized transperitoneally—increasing the likelihood of injury during laparoscopy.

Great variation is observed in the nervous innervation of the uterine corpus and cervix. In general, three sources supply extrinsic nerves to the uterus. First, motor fibers arising in the upper sympathetic ganglia eventually coalesce to form the inferior hypogastric plexus (at the sacral promontory), diverging over the lateral surface of the pelvis to re-form as the cervical ganglion of Frankenhauser. Fibers from this plexus pass along the uterosacral ligaments to the smooth muscle of the uterus. Second, sensory fibers arise in the eleventh and twelfth sympathetic ganglia, and follow a course similar to that described above. Third, both motor and sensory fibers to the lower uterine segment and cervix arise in the first through fourth sacral nerves, eventually forming ganglia lateral to the cervix.

Operations to denervate the pelvis can be complicated by the diversity of afferent sensory fibers between individual patients. This complexity may partly explain the varied results obtained with the LUNA procedure.

Laparoscopic uterine nerve ablation

In 1955, Doyle described a procedure that involved resecting the afferent pain fibers in the area of the uterosacral ligaments via culdotomy or laparotomy (4). This procedure was later modified and performed laparoscopically, where it has gained popularity in the treatment of patients with central pelvic pain. Published studies report success rates of 60% when this laparoscopic uterine nerve ablation (LUNA) procedure is employed to treat patients with chronic pelvic pain unresponsive to medical management (5–7). Although no complications were reported in one group of 54 women, long-term follow-up revealed a significant recurrence of symptoms (7).

These studies raise several issues regarding LUNA that need clarification. First, the studies did not include a control group (i.e., laparoscopy, but no LUNA); as a result, the known placebo effect of laparoscopy could not be evaluated. Second, the anatomic distribution of sensory nerves to the pelvic organs is variably included in the uterosacral ligament. Because it would be unlikely for any patient to have all sensory fibers contained in the uterosacral ligament, even a complete transection of this ligament would not be expected to sever all of the afferent sensory fibers from the uterus. Based on these observations, routine use of the LUNA procedure is difficult to justify on scientific grounds, as its efficacy may not exceed that of a placebo.

If the procedure is performed as described by Lichten (7) (Fig. 16.1), two complications are possible: (1) bleeding from the artery at the base of the uterosacral ligament, and (2) ureteral injury, either directly or secondarily. Attempts to control bleeding via electrocautery—unipolar or bipolar—may result in thermal damage to the ureter. In the presence of endometriosis and nodularity of the uterosacral ligament, the ureter may be severed inadvertently as part of the dissection of the cul-de-sac. Regardless of the procedure being performed, special attention must be given to the location of the ureter, and every attempt made to avoid injury to this structure.

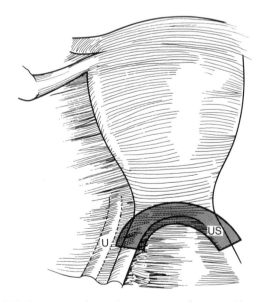

Fig. 16.1 Laparoscopic uterine (uterosacral) nerve ablation. The cross-hatched area represents the location of transection/vaporization.

Ureteral injury: prevention

Several methods for protecting the ureter from injury have been described in the literature, whether the procedure is being performed laparoscopically or at laparotomy. The first approach involves a sharp dissection of the ureter away from the operative field. For the LUNA procedure, particularly in the absence of cul-de-sac obliteration, this technique is not only feasible but also relatively easy to accomplish (8). The ureter is identified as it approaches the uterosacral ligament, and a peritoneal incision made between the ureter and the ligament. The ureter can thus be mobilized laterally. This procedure becomes more difficult, however, in the presence of the scarring and inflammation that accompany endometriosis. In addition, because it is tedious at laparotomy to dissect the ureter out of the cardinal ligament (i.e., to expose its course to bladder entry), it is therefore unrealistic to perform this task at routine laparoscopy. Fortunately, this step is rarely necessary.

The second method described focuses on "hydrodissection" (9). An incision is made superior to the ureter, and 150 to 200 cc of lactated Ringer's solution is infused into the retroperitoneal space. This method, although reported to lateralize the ureter onto the psoas muscle, may be more useful in localizing the ureter rather than protecting it. In a series of 19 patients undergoing laparotomy for benign disease, we performed hydrodissection and evaluated the retroperitoneal space directly (10). In none of the cases was the ureter located on the psoas muscle. With lactated Ringer's solution, transperitoneal visualization often proved difficult. When the hydrodissection media was changed to contain indigo carmine, however, the ureter could more easily be identified throughout its pelvic course. Subsequently, these observations have been extended to laparoscopy with equal success in localizing the ureter.

Note that the ureter may be traced in this fashion only to its penetration of the cardinal ligament at the level of the cervix. Use of a combination of hydrodissection and blunt dissection may result in a more lateral displacement of the ureter. This technique, which is similar to the more routine retroperitoneal dissection at laparotomy, requires a larger incision in the lateral peritoneum.

Ureteral injuries: collected literature

In 1990, we published a paper reporting on five ureteral injuries occurring at laparoscopy, and reviewing the eight previously reported cases (1). One of these cases resulted from a LUNA procedure; in fact, the patient had undergone the same procedure for pelvic pain one year prior to the injury. It is difficult to rationalize the indications for a repeat procedure, given the questions about its efficacy. In this case, the anatomy of the ureter was most likely altered from the previous uterosacral ligament transection, drawing the ureter medially. The second procedure resulted in transection of the ureter 2 cm from the ureterovesicle junction, and required a laparotomy with transverse uretero-ureterostomy.

Most laparoscopic ureteral injuries present one to five days postoperatively with increasing abdominal pain, fever, leukocytosis, and either urinary ascites or urinoma formation. The patient presenting with these symptoms should have evaluation of the urinary tract with an intravenous pyelogram (IVP); if injury to the urinary tract is found, the initial therapy should involve attempts at either retrograde or antegrade stenting. These injuries are not trivial, and require aggressive intervention to preserve renal function of the affected side. Two of the 13 patients described in the literature that we reviewed ultimately underwent a nephrectomy.

Recently, Gomel reported a ureteral injury that occurred during a pelviscopic procedure but that was recognized at the time of the initial operation (11). This injury was stented, and the serosal edges of the ureter reapproximated laparoscopically. If any questions arise about the integrity of the urinary system at laparoscopy, the intravenous injection of indigo carmine will permit appropriate evaluation.

Recent reviews of gynecologic surgery indicate a similar incidence of ureteral injury (0.4%) for major pelvic surgical procedures, whether performed at laparoscopy or laparotomy (12, 13). Laparoscopic assisted vaginal hysterectomy has also been associated with ureteral injury, seemingly due to distortion of or extensive dissection of the cardinal ligaments (14, 15). Injuries resulting in uretero-tubal fistula formation after cauterization of endometriosis have also been reported (16).

Summary

The incidence of ureteral injury at laparoscopy is unknown. Clearly, the more severe the pelvic disease, the more likely that an injury to some pelvic organ may occur as a result of the surgical procedure. In the case of injuries to the urinary tract, prompt recognition and treatment will most likely result in a favorable outcome for the patient. If the diagnosis is not suspected and treatment delayed, a significant risk of compromised renal function on the affected side is incurred.

To avoid this complication, every effort should be made to identify the ureter during laparoscopy, including sharp dissection with direct retroperitoneal visualization or injection of indigo carmine retroperitoneally with transperitoneal visualization of the ureter.

In addition, advocates of the LUNA procedure for the treatment of chronic pelvic pain must be forthcoming with an appropriately controlled study evaluating the placebo effect of laparoscopy. If the procedure is not efficacious, even the rare risk of ureteral injury occurring as a result of the operation should restrict its use in modern gynecological practice.

REFERENCES

1. Grainger DA, Soderstrom RM, Schiff SF, Glickman M, DeCherney AH, Diamond MP. Ureteral injury at laparoscopy: insights into diagnosis, management, and prevention. Obstet Gynecol 1990;75:839–843.
2. Houtrey CE. Surgical anatomy. In: Buschsbaum HJ, Schmidt JD, eds. Gynecologic and obstetric urology. Philadelphia: W.B. Saunders, 1982:26–31.
3. Maxson WS, Hill GA, Herbert CM, et al. Ureteral abnormalities in women with endometriosis. Fertil Steril 1986;46:1159–1161.
4. Doyle JB. Paracervical uterine denervation by transection of the cervical plexus for the relief of dysmenorrhea. Am J Obstet Gynecol 1955;70:1–16.
5. Daniell JF. The role of lasers in infertility surgery. Fertil Steril 1984;42:815–823.
6. Lichten EM, Bombard J. Surgical treatment of primary dysmenorrhea with laparoscopic uterine nerve ablation. J Reprod Med 1987;32:37–41.
7. Lichten EM. Three years experience with LUNA. Am J Gyn Health 1989;5:9.
8. Redwine DB. Laparoscopic excision of endometriosis by sharp dissection. Presented at American Association of Gynecologic Laparoscopists, Orlando, Fla., Nov 1990.
9. Nezhat C, Nezhat FR. Safe laser endoscopic excision or vaporization of peritoneal endometriosis. Fertil Steril 1989;52:149–151.
10. Grainger DA, Miller K, Feuille E, Delmore JE, Horbelt DV, Webster BW. Hydrodissection as a means of protecting the ureter: evaluation by retroperitoneal dissection at laparotomy. Oral presentation, American Fertility Society, Orlando, Fla., Oct 21–24, 1991.
11. Gomel V, James C. Intraoperative management of ureteral injury during operative laparoscopy. Fertil Steril 1991;55:416–419.
12. Goodno JA, Powers TW, Harris VD. Ureteral injuries in gynecologic surgery: a ten year review in a community hospital. Am J Obstet Gynecol 1995;172:1817–1822.
13. Saidi MH, Sadler RK, Vancaillie TG, Akright BD, Farhart SA, White AJ. Diagnosis and management of serious urinary complications after major operative laparoscopy. Obstet Gynecol 196;87:272–276.
14. Woodland MB. Ureter injury during laparoscopically assisted vaginal hysterectomy with endoscopic linear stapler. Am J Obstet Gynecol 1992;167:756–757.
15. Kadar N, Lemmerling L. Urinary tract injuries during laparoscopically assisted hysterectomy: causes and prevention. Am J Obstet Gynecol 1994;170:47–48.
16. Steckel J, Badillo F, Waldbaum RS. Uretero-fallopian tube fistula secondary to laparoscopic fulguration of endometriosis. J Urol 1993;149:1128–1129.

Ureteral Complications of Laparoscopic Surgery in Gynecology | 17

Salim Bassil, Michelle Nisolle, Mireille Smets, and Jacques Donnez

Surgical procedures of the female genital tract are known to be associated with ureteral injury. In particular, many laparoscopic procedures of this type closely approximate the ureter. Since laparoscopy has been used in gynecology, ureteral injury has been estimated to occur in 0.5% to 2% of pelvic operations (1, 2, 3). The development of new instruments and the involvement of laparoscopy in more complicated surgical procedures may increase this incidence. In this chapter we will discuss the occurrence of ureteral injury and the recommendations for its prevention and management.

Diagnosis

Although only 18 cases of ureteral injury in laparoscopy-related procedures have been reported in the literature (Table 17.1), extreme care must be taken when dissecting within the pelvis (3). In only two cases described in the literature was the diagnosis made intraoperatively (4, 5). Usually, the patient tends to present 48 hours to 7 days postoperatively, with symptoms of abdominal pain, peritonitis, leukocytosis, and fever being noted. Flank tenderness or hematuria are rarely described. In some cases, an evaluation of abdominal fluid drainage with measurement of urea and creatinine may aid in diagnosis. In a few rare cases, the diagnosis was made two to three weeks after endoscopic surgery (Fig. 17.1). The presence of ascites and/or a pelvic mass is indicated by sonography, and the diagnosis is confirmed by intravenous pyelography (Fig. 17.2).

Management

The repair of ureteral injuries must be undertaken with the collaboration of a urological surgeon. Percutaneous or cystoscopic techniques can probably be used to manage most such injuries (3). Exploratory laparoscopy and/or laparotomy can be employed for surgical repair in cases requiring end-to-end reanastomosis, reimplantation of the ureter to the bladder, transureteral ureterostomy, and similar procedures.

In our department (6), three patients avoided laparotomy for ureteral repair. Nevertheless, one patient underwent management in another hospital. In this case, the surgeon did not try to stent the ureter and performed a uretero-ureterostomy. The insertion of a ureteral stent allowed drainage of urine, resolution of the pelvic urinoma, and spontaneous healing of the injured site (Fig. 17.3). The placement of such ureteral stents may be accomplished in a retrograde manner. If technically possible, this method of treatment is preferable in managing such types of ureteral injuries.

Prevention

The ureter enters the pelvis at the pelvic brim, crossing over the common iliac artery and vein. It then courses posteriorly, crossing under the uterine artery and matching the level of the cervix. At this point, the ureter is 1 to 1.5 cm lateral and anterior to the uterosacral ligament. Unfortunately, direct visualization of the ureter can prove difficult via pelviscopy. Although the ureter may be visualized through the peritoneum in the upper pelvis, it cannot be identified reliably in the area of the uterosacral ligaments. Identification is particularly difficult when endometriosis or pelvic adhesions are present. In addition, some procedures such as laparoscopic hysterectomy, lymphadenectomy and laparoscopic uterine nerve ablation (LUNA) increase the risk of ureteral injuries (2). Although specific guidelines are not available to prevent this serious complication, the following general points should be considered.

Table 17.1. Summary of 18 cases of ureteral injury resulting from laparoscopy that are reported in the literature.

Case Number	Time of Presentation	Indication for Initial Procedure	Treatment Modality	Method of Diagnosis	Treatment
1 (6)	7 days	endometriosis (LUNA)	CO_2 laser/unipolar cautery	IVP-CT scan	retrograde stent (double J)
2 (6)	7 days	salpingoovariolysis	CO_2 laser/bipolar cautery	IVP	retrograde stent (double J)
3 (6)	7 days	laparoscopic hysterectomy	bipolar cautery	IVP	retrograde stent (double J)
4 (3)	48 h	endometriosis	unipolar cautery	IVP	end-to-end anastomosis
5 (3)	48 h	adhesions/ endometriosis	unipolar cautery	IVP	transverse uretero-ureterostor
6 (3)	24 h	uterosacral ligament transection	unipolar cautery	repeat laparoscopy	transverse uretero-ureterostor
7 (3)	36 h	adhesions	bipolar cautery	repeat laparoscopy	end-to-end anastomosis
8 (3)	48 h	endometriosis	CO_2 laser/bipolar	IVP	percutaneous stent
9 (7)	5 days	endometriosis	unipolar cautery	IVP	transverse uretero-ureterostor
10 (8)	2 weeks	sterilization	bipolar cautery	IVP	Boari flap
11 (9)	unknown	endometriosis	unipolar cautery	IVP	unknown
12 (10)	3 weeks	sterilization	cautery (not specified)	laparotomy	ileal interposition
13 (11)	3 weeks	diagnostic laparoscopy	trocar injury (J)	IVP	end-to-end anastomosis
14 (12)	5 days	adhesions	cautery (not specified)	IVP	stent at laparotomy
15 (13)	4 days	sterilization	bipolar cautery	IVP, repeat	retrograde stent
16 (14)	5 days	sterilization	bipolar cautery	IVP	transverse uretero-ureterostor
17 (4)	preoperatively	radical LAVH	scissors section	urine spillage	transverse uretero-ureterostor
18*	3 weeks	laparoscopic adnexectomy	bipolar cautery	IVP	transverse uretero-ureterostor

LUNA = laser uterine nerve ablation.
LAVH = laparoscopy-assisted vaginal hysterectomy.
IVP = intravenous pyelography.
*Personal data.

The operator must understand the anatomy of the pelvic ureter and appreciate its proximity to the cervix in cases of endometriosis or when performing LUNA or other risky procedures. Sometimes dissection of the ureter may help avoid complications. In addition, some authors have advocated using hydrodissection or hydroprotection to protect retroperitoneal structures (15, 16). This technique involves making a small incision on the lateral parietal peritoneum and inflating fluid into the retroperitoneal space. Hydroprotection is particularly helpful when a laser is used in the procedure. In cases of laparoscopic hysterectomy (LH), ureteral and/or bladder damage occurs at a rate of 2% (17). The technique of laparoscopic supracervical hysterectomy (LASH) appears to reduce the risk of such damage (5).

Electrocauterization must always be performed with strict visual control of the structures lying under and around the field of application. Bipolar coagulation is preferred to monopolar coagulation (18). It is sometimes erroneously assumed that bipolar coagulation is "completely safe"; in fact, it is safe only when the bipolar forceps are correctly positioned a sufficient distance from the ureter and used for a well-calculated coagulating time (3, 13). A longer coagulation induces a diffusion of thermal energy and the current may damage the vascular supply around the coagulated tissue, leading to delayed tissue necrosis (19, 20).

To prevent such problems, the surgeon must check the energy unit (i.e., isolation, return electrode, power setting), and ensure that it functions correctly. In many

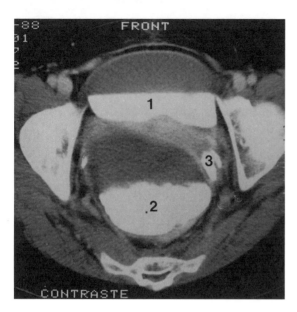

Fig. 17.1 CT scan: the bladder is filled with contrast medium (1). Note the spillage of the contrast medium from a ureteral fistula (3) into the retroperitoneal space (2).

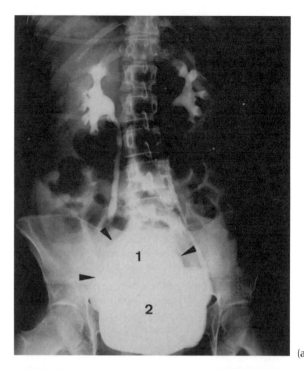

(a)

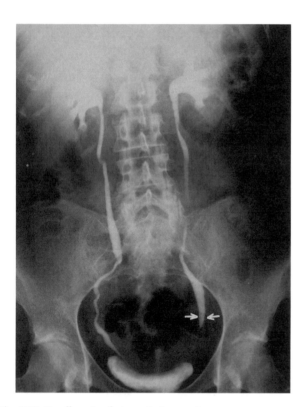

Fig. 17.2 Small ureteral stenosis (arrows).

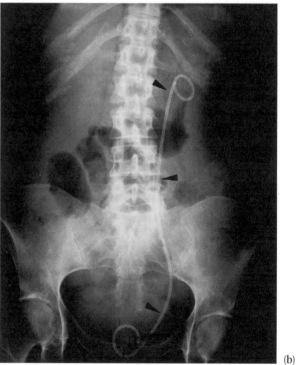

(b)

Fig. 17.3 (a) Extravasation of contrast medium in a right urinoma (1). The arrows show its limit behind the bladder (2). (b) A double-J stent was placed for three months (arrows).

instances, burn injuries result from faults in the electro-coagulation equipment and its use. Faulty insulation of the cautery device may also cause burns (21). The use of a hyperfrequenced electrocautery unit with a low peak voltage of 600 V and a maximum output of 100 W is preferred to other high-energy (3000–8000 V), spark-gap-type generators (22, 23).

Conclusion

The indications for laparoscopic surgery have expanded greatly during the past decade, prompting a reappraisal of the risks involved in operating by endoscopy. These risks, in addition to the risk of general anesthesia, have been increased by the introduction of new operative devices and instruments.

Ureteral complications have a specific etiology that is usually preventable or treatable if recognized in time. Often, they consist of thermal injuries and are only diagnosed postoperatively. This delay in diagnosis represents a major problem because it worsens the patient's prognosis and increases morbidity. The incidence of ureteral injuries is unknown.

Injuries of a ureteral nature often require repair by laparotomy. The likelihood of laparotomy appears to be directly related to the degree of complexity of the laparoscopic surgical procedure and to the experience of the surgeon. Understanding these complications and how to assess them is the only way to avoid them in the future. Consequently, besides the anatomical knowledge required in surgical training, a minimum of technical knowledge of the new instrumentation (e.g., laser, electrosurgery, automated stapling devices) is recommended.

REFERENCES

1. Gomel V, James C. Intraoperative management of ureteral injury during operative laparoscopy. Fertil Steril 1991;55:416–419.
2. Woodland MB. Ureter injury during laparoscopy-assisted vaginal hysterectomy with the endoscopic linear stapler. Am J Obstet Gynecol 1992;17:756–779.
3. Grainger DA, Soderstrom RM, Schiff SF, Glickman MG, De Cherney AH, Diamond MP. Ureteral injuries at laparoscopy: insights into diagnosis, management and prevention. Obstet Gynecol 1990;75:839–843.
4. Lee CL, Huang KG, Lai YM, Lai CH, Soong YK. Ureteral injury during laparoscopically assisted radical vaginal hysterectomy. Hum Reprod 1995;10:2047–2049.
5. Donnez J, Bassil S, Smets M, Nisolle M. LASH: laparoscopic supracervical (subtotal) hysterectomy. In: Cusumano P, Deprest J, eds. Advanced gynecologic laparoscopy. New York, London: Parthenon Publishing Group, 1996:79–83.
6. Donnez J, Bassil S, Anaf V, Smets M, Nisolle M. Ureteral and bladder injury during laparoscopic surgery. In: Donnez J, Nisolle M, eds. An atlas of laser operative laparoscopy and hysteroscopy. New York, London: Parthenon Publishing Group, 1994:273–243.
7. Cheng YS. Ureteral injury resulting from laparoscopic fulguration of endometriotic implant. Am J Obstet Gynecol 1976;8:1145–1146.
8. Stengel JN, Felderman ES, Zamora D. Ureteral injury: complication of laparoscopic sterilization. Urology 1974;4:341–342.
9. Daly JW, Higgins KA. Injury to the ureter during gynecologic surgical procedures. Gynecol Obstet 1988;16:19–22.
10. Irvin TT, Gligher JC, Scott JS. Injury to the ureter during laparoscopic tubal sterilization. Arch Surg 1975;110:1501–1503.
11. Schapira M, Dizerensch H, Essinger A, Wauters JP, Loup P, Von Niederhausern W. Urinary ascites after gynecological laparoscopy. Lancet 1987;1:871–872.
12. Winslow PH, Kreger R, Ebbesson B, Oster E. Conservative management of electrical burn injury of ureter secondary to laparoscopy. Urology 1986;27:60–62.
13. Bauman H, Jaeger P, Huch A. Ureteral injury after laparoscopic tubal sterilization by bipolar electrocoagulation. Obstet Gynecol 1988;71:483–485.
14. teBrevil W, Boeminghaus F. Harnleitorlasion bei laparoskopistcher lubensterilisation. Geburts Frauenheilkd 1977;27:572–576.
15. Donnez J, Nisolle M. Instrumentation and operational instructions. In: Donnez J, Nisolle M, eds. An atlas of laser operative laparoscopy and hysteroscopy. New York, London: Parthenon Publishing Group, 1994:21–24.
16. Nezhat C, Nezhat FR. Safe laser endoscopic excision or vaporization of peritoneal endometriosis. Fertil Steril 1989;52:149–151.
17. Cusumano P, Deprest J, Hardy A, Van Herendal B, Verly M. Multicentric registration on laparoscopic hysterectomy: a one year experience. Proceedings of the first European Congress of Gynecologic Endoscopy. Clermont-Ferrand, France, Sept 1992:46.
18. Seiler JC, Gidwana G, Ballard L. Laparoscopic cauterization of endometriosis for fertility. A controlled study. Fertil Steril 1986;46:1098–1100.
19. Schwimmer WB. Electrosurgical burn injuries during laparoscopy sterilization. Treatment and prevention. Obstet Gynecol 1974;44:526–530.
20. Jaffe RH, Willis D, Bachem A. The effect of electric currents on the arteries. A histologic study. Arch Pathol 1929;7:244–252.
21. Irvin TT, Goligher JC, Scott JS. Injury to the ureter during laparoscopic tubal sterilization. Arch Surg 1975;110:1501–1503.
22. Levinson CJ, Schwartz SF, Saltzstein CE. Complication of laparoscopic tubal sterilization: small bowel perforation. Obstet Gynecol 1973;41:253–256.
23. Corson SL, Bolognese RJ. Electrosurgical hazards in laparoscopy. JAMA 1974;927:1261.

Complications of Sharp and Blunt Adhesiolysis

18

David B. Redwine

Frequency of complications related to laparoscopic adhesiolysis

Pelvic adhesions can be a consequence of previous surgery or pelvic pathology. Resting silently somewhere in the abdominal cavity, such adhesions create concern during placement of laparoscopic trocars and can complicate laparoscopic surgery. Despite these concerns, complications related to endoscopic adhesiolysis remain rare. A search of the medical literature published since 1966 did not reveal any article specifically detailing such complications. Although several authors (1–4) discuss laparoscopic adhesiolysis, none mentions any complications related to the procedure.

The computerized database of the Endometriosis Institute of Oregon was searched for complications related to laparoscopic adhesiolysis performed at the Endometriosis Treatment Program at St. Charles Medical Center (Bend, Oregon). A total of 1467 laparoscopies were undertaken for treatment of endometriosis and other pathology between July 1978 and January 1996. Of this total, 1122 patients (76.5%) had a history of previous surgery by laparoscopy or laparotomy, which confers some risk of pelvic or abdominal adhesions. Adhesiolysis was performed on the total patient group when necessary using blunt dissection, sharp dissection, and electrosurgery. Twenty patients experienced significant complications during laparoscopy involving adhesiolysis, for a crude rate of 1.4% (Table 18.1)

Because not all 1467 patients listed in the Oregon database had adhesions at the time of their laparoscopy, it is more revealing to survey patients with pelvic or abdominal adhesions at laparoscopy. The revised American Fertility Society classification system for endometriosis is heavily weighted toward adhesions. To achieve Stage III or Stage IV, a patient usually must have significant pelvic adhesions. When only patients with Stages III and IV endometriosis or those patients with lower stages of endometriosis and associated pelvic or abdominal adhesions ($N = 546$) are considered, the complication rate reflects 20 cases out of a total of 546 (3.7%). (Six patients underwent laparoscopically assisted vaginal hysterectomy.)

Of these 20 patients, three required second operations and two required transfusion; one patient required both reoperation and transfusion. Not all of the complications observed were necessarily due to adhesiolysis, however. In addition, no complication attributable to unintended monopolar electrosurgical damage occurred in any patient.

Despite the high incidence of previous surgery among these patients, a laparoscopic trocar perforated the bowel of only one patient, with this mishap occurring after needle insufflation. In this patient with multiple previous laparotomies, laparotomy was performed by a general surgeon for intestinal repair, and the bowel was perforated during entry as well. This finding indicates that laparotomy offers no guarantee against intestinal perforation in patients with previous surgery.

The author has avoided the use of needle insufflation of the abdomen since 1990. Direct blind insertion of a 10-mm reusable umbilical trocar in more than 840 patients has resulted in no unintended injury in any patient. Several factors contribute to this record. First, the abdominal wall is elevated before trocar insertion, minimizing the chance that the trocar may pin the bowel against the vertebrae or lacerate major vessels. Second, the reusable trocar becomes somewhat dull with use, and a dull trocar is less likely to cause injury than a sharp trocar. Finally, in selected patients with previous laparotomy, an intrasheath blunt peritoneal entry was often possible, which increases safety [Fig. 18.1(A)].

Techniques of adhesiolysis

Adhesiolysis seems to be a conceptually simple process: two surfaces are stuck together and they are separated mechanically. This procedure can be performed with

Table 18.1. Complications associated with laparoscopy in patients with stage III or stage IV endometriosis or pelvic or abdominal adhesions.

Surgery Type	Number of Patients						
	Total Patients	Bleeding*	Transfusion	Reoperation	DVT**	Ileus	Infectious***
Hysterectomy	6	0	0	0	0	1	5
Excision of endometriosis	14	4	2	3	1	1	5

*Includes cases with low (<25%) postoperative hematocrit.
** DVT suspected clinically.
*** Includes patients with postoperative abscess (2) and postoperative fever suspected to be bacterial in origin.

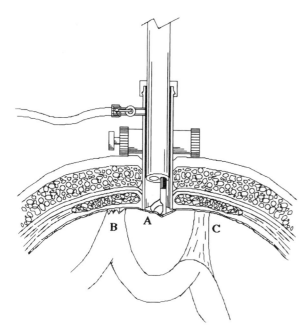

Fig. 18.1 Blunt entry into the peritoneum using intrasheath laparoscopic surgery. The 10-mm umbilical trocar has been inserted only partly through the abdominal wall. Using 3-mm scissors down the operating channel of a 10-mm operating laparoscope, the final layers of the abdominal wall are bluntly or sharply incised under direct vision (A). This step duplicates abdominal entry at open laparotomy and may help avoid inadvertent intestinal injury in patients with previous surgery. Dense, confluent adhesions binding a bowel loop to the anterior abdominal wall should usually be lysed by blunt or sharp dissection working immediately next to the parietal wall or retroperitoneally. Isolated adhesion curtains (C) can be transected near the parietal wall by any method, although it is important to watch for bleeding vessels that may retract into the cut tissue.

laser, scissors, electrosurgery, or blunt dissection (if the adhesions are filmy). Bands of adhesions can be cut or excised. No evidence suggests that any method is superior with respect to decreasing adhesion reformation, increasing fertility, or decreasing pain. Excising bands of adhesions will at least eliminate them, making surgery somewhat easier. Evidence in animal models suggests that scissors produce less tissue reaction than the CO_2 laser or electrosurgery (5, 6) and therefore might theoretically be the best tool for adhesiolysis. When using electrosurgery, higher current densities should generally be used when lysing adhesions that do not incorporate bowel, as lower power densities can result in coagulation and more widespread thermal damage. No matter what method of adhesiolysis is used, however, countertraction and tension on the adhesions must be maintained at all times.

Because the bowel wall may be indistinctly fused to the peritoneum [Fig. 18.1(B)], loops of intestine adherent to the abdominal wall should usually be separated by blunt or sharp dissection. A retroperitoneal technique that allows a small portion of peritoneum to remain attached to the bowel wall is safest, although retroperitoneal dissection can quickly lead far beyond the point of adherence. The resulting denudation of parietal wall may serve as a nidus of even more aggressive adhesion reformation. Strings or curtains of adhesions binding bowel loops to the anterior abdominal wall [Fig. 18.1(C)] can be transected near the abdominal wall by any method without fear of damage to the bowel.

Adhesiolysis must take into account the fact that curtains of adhesions or adherent omentum may contain rather sizable blood vessels. Retraction of a blood vessel into a clump of adhesions or omentum can lead to persistent hemorrhage, while attempts to coagulate the bleeder may damage the bowel. When such bleeding occurs, it is important to isolate the bleeder so that specific control has less chance to damage adjacent vital structures. While virtually all such bleeding may be prevented or controlled via a combination of bipolar or monopolar electrocoagulation, sutures are sometimes useful. Large veins have a low venous pressure and may be tamponaded by the pressure of the pneumoperitoneum. In such a case, the surgeon should examine the pelvis while evacuating the pneumoperitoneum.

Potential injuries

Although complications due to adhesiolysis are rare, understandable concerns arise over the possibility of blunt or sharp injury to the bowel. While preoperative ultrasound can frequently indicate the presence of adhesions to the anterior abdominal wall (7), it has not been shown to help in actual performance of surgery.

One potential bowel injury is a serosal tear with possible extension into the superficial muscularis. Because the colon has four layers (serosa, outer and inner muscularis, mucosa), a considerable safety margin exists, and any such injury would be expected to remain asymptomatic and need no suture.

Full-thickness penetrations of the colon by sharp or blunt dissection carry a greater risk. If such perforation occurs in the midst of a difficult adhesiolysis, most surgeons would take it as a sign that surgery is not going well laparoscopically and proceed to a laparotomy assisted by a general surgeon. If little other work must be done after colonic perforation occurs, experienced laparoscopists may elect to repair the bowel endoscopically with a double-layer closure, followed by copious irrigation of the pelvis. Bowel wall integrity can be assessed by filling the pelvis with irrigation fluid and injecting air through a sigmoidoscope. Prophylactic antibiotics should be administered, and the patient monitored for postoperative infection. Intraoperative surgical consultation is prudent as well.

A small colonic perforation is unlikely to result in fecal spillage, so a colostomy need not be an automatic initial response to such an injury. A colostomy entails two surgeries—one to create it and one to reverse it later. Such a procedure preempts the high likelihood that the patient will do well with primary repair of the bowel wall. If careful postoperative monitoring indicates that intraperitoneal infection is likely, laparotomy can then be undertaken and a colostomy performed if necessary.

Less of a safety exists with the much thinner wall of the small bowel, and consequently repair with interrupted 3-0 silk suture is recommended if any question of mucosal injury arises. If the bowel lumen is entered, repair is mandatory. This process is best accomplished with two layers. Although the contents of the large bowel are septic, small bowel contents are less so. Irrigation and evacuation of spillage from the small bowel is important, and a short course of prophylactic antibiotics may be wise.

Two clinical conditions associated with adhesions demand special consideration: Stage IV endometriosis with obliteration of the cul-de-sac, and the adherent ovary.

Stage IV endometriosis and obliteration of the cul-de-sac

Obliteration of the cul-de-sac with endometriosis usually signifies the presence of invasive disease of the uterosacral ligaments, cul-de-sac, and a rectal nodule in the wall of the bowel (Fig. 18.2). Complete surgical treatment of the disease will usually require en bloc resection (8) of these areas as well as some type of bowel surgery. Because the obliterated cul-de-sac exhibits yellowish or whitish scarring, some clinicians might not associate it with active endometriosis, merely noting "intense scarring of the cul-de-sac" but not recognizing its origin. Some surgeons may be aware of this manifestation of active endometriosis but understandably hesitate to tackle what can be the most difficult surgery in the gynecologic repertoire. Frequently the surgeon may separate the bowel from the cervix and then stop. While this technique may restore a semblance of normal anatomy, it leaves the endometriosis behind, which may be symptomatic whether the cul-de-sac is obliterated or not.

Adherent ovary

An adherent ovary consists of the ovarian remnant syndrome or persistent endometriosis waiting to happen. When the ovary is sharply or bluntly dissected off the pelvic side wall or off the bowel, some of the ovarian cortex or stroma may remain attached to the opposing peritoneal surface. With the passage of time and chronic stimulation by pituitary gonadotropins, the remnant may become cystic and cause pain. To avoid this complica-

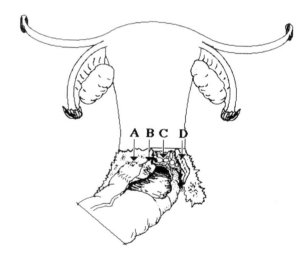

Fig. 18.2 Obliteration of the cul-de-sac (A) associated with invasive, nodular endometriosis of the anterior rectal wall (B), adjacent to the fatty tissue of the rectovaginal septum (C). The right anterior rectal wall has been removed for the sake of clarity. The right uterosacral ligament (D) is also involved by invasive endometriosis. Superficial laser vaporization or electrocoagulation may not burn deeply enough to destroy all disease.

tion, the ovary can be mobilized by dissecting behind the peritoneum, thus lifting the ovary off of the pelvic side wall (that is, the peritoneum is lifted off the side wall with the ovary still attached). When the ovary is adherent in association with endometriosis, the peritoneum in the area of the attachment frequently harbors endometriosis; thus this technique will provide complete surgical treatment of endometriosis as well. Once the peritoneum and ovary have been completely mobilized, it becomes a relatively simple task to remove the attached peritoneum from the surface of the ovary, ensuring complete removal of peritoneal disease.

Why perform adhesiolysis?

Adhesions may (9) or may not (10) cause pain. Although uncontrolled studies found that early second-look laparoscopy for adhesiolysis may improve the rate of intrauterine pregnancy (11, 12), a randomized controlled trial of patients who underwent terminal salpingostomy or salpingo-ovariolysis demonstrated that second-look laparoscopic adhesiolysis at one year did not improve intrauterine pregnancy rates or decrease rates of ectopic pregnancy (13). Adhesions are softer and easier to lyse within a few weeks of pelvic surgery (1, 2, 14). Even with laparoscopic adhesiolysis, adhesions will usually tend to re-form (15), and the more severe the adhesions, the more likely they are to reappear. For this reason, adhesion re-formation is more difficult to treat. De novo adhesion formation may be less likely to occur after laparoscopic surgery than after laparotomy (15, 16).

The low rate of complications due to trocar insertion in patients who have undergone previous operations and exhibit pelvic or abdominal adhesiolysis indicates that laparoscopic adhesiolysis is usually a safe procedure. Although adhesions are not always symptomatic, adhesiolysis may prove necessary simply to enable the surgeon to view pelvic and abdominal contents. As carefully performed adhesiolysis does not pose an undue risk to the patient, adhesiolysis should usually be attempted, both to enhance other surgical goals and to reduce the ultimate adhesion burden. The surgeon should use his or her own judgment to decide whether and how vigorously adhesiolysis should be attempted.

REFERENCES

1. Jansen RPS. Early laparoscopy after pelvic operations to prevent adhesions: safety and efficacy. Fertil Steril 1988;49:26–31.
2. Trimbos-Kemper TCM, Timbos JB, van Hall EV. Adhesion formation after tubal surgery: results of the eighth-day laparoscopy in 188 patients. Fertil Steril 1985;83:395–400.
3. Barbot J, Parent B, Dubuisson JB, Aubriot FX. A clinical study of the CO₂ laser and electrosurgery for adhesiolysis in 172 cases followed by early second-look laparoscopy. Fertil Steril 1987;48:140–142.
4. Luber K, Beeson CC, Kennedy JF, Villanueva B, Young PE. Results of microsurgical treatment of tubal infertility and early second-look laparoscopy in the post-pelvic inflammatory disease patient: implications for in vitro fertilization. Am J Obstet Gynecol 1986;154:1264–1268.
5. Filmar S, Jetha N, McComb P, Gomel V. A comparative histologic study on the healing process after tissue transection. I. Carbon dioxide laser and electromicrosurgery. Am J Obstet Gynecol 1989;160:1062–1067.
6. Filmar S, Jetha N, McComb P, Gomel V. A comparative histologic study on the healing process after tissue transection. II. Carbon dioxide laser and surgical microscissors. Am J Obstet Gynecol 1989;160:1068–1072.
7. Caprini JA, Arcelus JA, Swanson J, Coats R, Hoffman K, Brosnan JJ, Blattner S. The ultrasonic localization of abdominal wall adhesions. Surg Endosc 1995;9:283–285.
8. Redwine DB. Laparoscopic en bloc resection for treatment of the obliterated cul de sac in endometriosis. J Reprod Med 1992;37:695–698.
9. Freys SM, Fuchs KH, Heimbucher J, Thiede A. Laparoscopic adhesiolysis. Surg Endosc 1994;8:1202–1207.
10. Rapkin AJ. Adhesions and pelvic pain: a retrospective study. Obstet Gynecol 1986;68:13–15.
11. Surrey MW, Friedman S. Second look laparoscopy after reconstructive pelvic surgery for infertility. J Reprod Med 1982;27:658–660.
12. Daniell JF, Pittaway DE. Short-interval second-look laparoscopy after infertility surgery: a preliminary report. J Reprod Med 1983;28:281–283.
13. Tulandi T, Falcone T, Kafka I. Second-look operative laparoscopy 1 year following reproductive surgery. Fertil Steril 1989;52:421–424.
14. DeCherney AH, Mezer HC. The nature of post-tuboplasty pelvic adhesions as determined by early and late laparoscopy. Fertil Steril 1984;41:643–646.
15. Operative Laparoscopy Study Group. Postoperative adhesion development after operative laparoscopy: evaluation at early second-look procedures. Fertil Steril 1991;55:700–704.
16. Nezhat CR, Nezhat FR, Metzger DA, Luciano AA. Adhesion reformation after reproductive surgery by videolaseroscopy. Fertil Steril 1990;53:1008–1011.

Difficulties in Adhesion Prevention | 19

Bertil Larsson

Formation of adhesions

The mechanism of action behind the formation of adhesions is not fully understood. It appears, however, that peritoneal adhesions will develop only in peritoneum damaged by either surgical trauma or inflammatory disease.

Fibrin matrix seems to play an essential part in both adhesion formation and the healing process by inducing fibroblast activity. Thus, to prevent postoperative adhesions, a reasonable precaution would involve either avoiding fibrin or reducing its volume. As one recent experimental study implied, "Fibrinolytic inhibition postoperatively increases adhesion formation, whereas fibrinolytic stimulation decreases the formation of adhesions. Thus, fibrinolysis seeems to play a pivotal role in the early formation of adhesions" (1).

Prevention of adhesion formation

The most effective way of preventing postoperative re-formation of adhesions after adhesiolysis and formation of de novo adhesions is to avoid any trauma to the abdominal serosa. Even a slight trauma to the serosa, observed only as petechiae, undoubtly carries some risk of postoperative adhesion formation.

Laparoscopic surgery offers an advantage in its avoidance of operating towels, which may traumatize the peritoneum and induce postoperative adhesion formation. Laparoscopic procedures may also be associated with a lower risk of postoperative adhesions when less traumatizing instruments are used and when the amount of necrotic tissues in cautery incisions is minimized.

In case of inflammatory diseases (e.g., PID, appendicitis, diverticulitis), effective treatment with antibiotics is mandatory. When choosing an antibiotic, the surgeon should bear in mind that not only *Chlamydia* but also microorganisms such as *E. coli* and enterococces are very common in these conditions, especially in PID (salpingi-tis). In cases of ongoing inflammatory disease in the abdominal cavity, it is essential not to traumatize the tissue during laparoscopy or laparotomy. Preferably the tissue should not be touched by any surgical instruments or by the surgeon's fingers. Conversely, abdominal lavage with Ringer-acetate to remove excess of fibrin would be recommended. Performing surgery in infected tissue always carries a very obvious risk of postoperative adhesions.

Adhesion formation following fertility-related microsurgery

Less traumatic, microsurgical techniques used in operations for fertility include a number of specific steps (2, 3, 4). Through experimental studies in rats and pigs and in clinical series, the author has evaluated the significance of less traumatic and bloodless techniques in operations for fertility, as described by Swolin in his thesis in 1967. In addition to the gentle surgical procedure, Swolin advocated high doses of cortisone, administered intraabdominally at the end of the operation and in successively decreasing oral doses for two weeks postoperatively. Although the use of cortisone has been questioned by a number of colleagues in many countries, it has been widely used in Sweden without any registered side effects (4).

In separate studies we have registered the benefits of the following steps:

- Keeping the serosa constantly irrigated (5).
- Removing adhesions by use of microelectrodes.
- Avoiding trauma to the serosa by use of nonwoven operating towels (6).
- Avoiding necrotic residues by use of adequate suturing technique.
- Minimizing the number and size of the sutures.

In experimental studies we have shown that blood and fibrinogen per se do not induce any adhesions (7);

conversely, fibrin has been shown to induce adhesion formation (8). Reconstructive surgery—even of huge sactosalpinges—has resulted in a promising number of intrauterine pregnancies when the gentle microsurgical technique is combined with high-dose cortisone (4, 9).

The aim of the operation for fertility is to make it possible for the patient to become pregnant. The results of the treatment could consequently be given in numbers of full-term pregnancies. Such an evaluation must take a number of other factors in the fertilization procedure into account. Thus, the results of tubo-ovarian microsurgery might preferably be given in reduction of adhesion scores when considering specifically the effect of preventing re-formation of adhesions and formation of de novo adhesions.

By use of the microsurgical technique, we have observed a reduction of the adhesion scores by at least 50% in tubo-ovarian reconstructive surgery (10). Although it is not possible to completely avoid any trauma to the serosa when performing adhesiolysis in all cases, however, and adjuvant therapy is mandatory when such damage occurs.

Working together with a group of gynecologists from the Scandinavian countries and Finland, a team headed by the author has performed a number of prospective, randomized, multicenter clinical studies on other agents reported to reduce postoperative adhesion formation. All surgeons involved in the studies were highly experienced in the less traumatic microsurgical technique and the scoring system used throughout the multicenter studies.

In two separate series, we concluded that Hyskon (32% dextran 70, Pharmacia, Uppsala, Sweden) (11) and Solu-Medrone (Upjohn, Göteborg, Sweden) (unpublished data) did not significantly reduce the reformation of pelvic adhesions, when randomly applied in abdominal cavity at the end of the microsurgical laparotomy. Saline was administered in the control patients.

In the Hyskon study, 105 patients from five centers underwent surgical treatment to repair tubal and/or peritoneal damage. A reduction in the extent of the intraabdominal adhesions (statistically highly significant) was revealed in both the group that received Hyskon and the saline control group when a second laparoscopy was performed approximately 10 weeks postoperatively. The extent of adhesions in the Hyskon group was, however, not lesser than in the saline group. The pregnancy rates in the two groups were also similar.

In terms of de novo adhesions, however, we observed a significant reduction of adhesions on the oviducts in the cortisone-treated group when compared with the control group. In conclusion, our experiences do not indicate any benefit from the use of either dextran or corticosteroids in preventing postoperative adhesions.

In another multicenter study, also headed by the author, an adjuvant in the form of a locally applied Interceed barrier proved to have a significant effect in preventing re-formation of abdominal adhesions in reconstructive, less traumatic tubo-ovarian surgery (10). This series included 66 patients suffering from infertility caused, at least in part, by bilateral tubal disease with bilateral adhesions attached to ovaries, fallopian tubes, and fimbriae. Adnexa randomly covered with Interceed demonstrated significantly lower adhesion scores than the control adnexa, translating into an improvement of 39% compared with microsurgery alone in reducing adhesion re-formation scores. When combined with microsurgical techniques, Interceed reduced adhesion re-formation scores by 70%. The number of ovaries, fallopian tubes, and fimbriae without any adhesions at the time of second-look laparoscopy was significantly increased (by approximately twofold) when organs were covered with Interceed.

The beneficial effect observed separately on the ovaries was also proved in an international multicenter study (12). Fifty-five patients with bilateral ovarian disease (adhesions, cysts, and/or endometriosis) were treated at initial laparotomy. At the end of the operation, one ovary was randomly assigned to be wrapped with Interceed; the other ovary was left uncovered as a control. Second-look laparoscopy was performed 10 to 98 days later to evaluate the incidence, extent, and serverity of adhesions. Treatment with Interceed eliminated the incidence of adhesions in nearly twice as many ovaries compared with the ovaries left uncovered with Interceed. This finding translates into an 86% improvement over controls alone in preventing adhesion development. Moreover, the differential score for the severity of adhesions showed that the ovaries treated with Interceed had a significantly larger reduction in the severity of adhesions compared with controls.

Some patients suffer from infertility because of fibroids. In an ongoing clinical study, my preliminary data indicate that Interceed also has a beneficial effect in such women. In the study, the barrier is placed over the enucleation area. Especially after removal of large myomata, extensive tension might exist between the two edges of the myometrial incision. This characteristic makes it almost impossible to approximate the edges by use of very thin sutures, as is generally advocated in operations for fertility, which most often incise the myometrium. Our current routine procedure includes 3-0 sutures in the uterine wall after enucleation with Interceed administered as adjuvant therapy to cover the "sutured region." This procedure has been used in 10 cases to date, and second-look laparoscopy performed approximately ten weeks later has revealed no postoperative adhesions. Interceed is very easy to apply at any region of the abdominal cavity not only at laparotomies, but also in laparoscopic surgery.

REFERENCES

1. Holmdahl L. Fibrinolysis and adhesions. Thesis, University of Gothenburg, Göteborg, Sweden, 1994.
2. Swolin K. 50 Fertilitätsoperationen. Teil I. Literatur und methodik. Acta Obstet Gynecol Scand 1967;46:234–250.
3. Swolin K. 50 Fertilitätsoperationen. Teil II. Material und resultaten. Acta Obstet Gynecol Scand 1967;46:251–267.
4. Larsson B. Late results of salpingostomy combined with salpingolysis and ovariolysis by electromicrosurgery in 54 women. Fertil Steril 1982;37:156–161.
5. Larsson B, Perbeck L. The possible advantage of the uterine and intestinal serosa irrigated with saline in operations for fertility—an experimental study in rats. Acta Chir Scand 1986;530(suppl): 15–18.
6. Swolin K, Bends A, Larsson B, Tronstad SE, Bengtsson R, Hamberger L, Svanberg S. Traumatization of the abdominal serosa. A comparison between non-woven and cotton abdominal swabs. Acta Chir Scand 1974;140:203–204.
7. Nisell H, Larsson B. Role of blood and fibrinogen in developement of intraperitonal adhesions in rats. Fertil Steril 1978;30:470–473.
8. Fianu S, Larsson B, Jonasson A, Hedström CG, Thorgirsson T. Mechanism of action of a fibrin sealant in transabdominal urethrocystoperxy: experimental study in monkeys. Fibrin sealant in operative med. In: Schlaug G, ed. Gynecology and obstetrics–urology, vol 3. Heidelberg: Springer-Verlag, 1986.
9. Rosenborg L, Tronstad SE, Sponland G, Larsson B. Results of electromicrosurgery in 78 women for correction of infertility. A two-center comparative study. Infertility 1982;5: 25–41.
10. Larsson B, et al. Nordic Adhesion Prevention Study Group. The efficacy of Interceed (TC7) for prevention of reformation of postoperative adhesions on ovaries, fallopian tubes, and fimbriae in microsurgical operations for fertility: a multicenter study. Fertil Steril 1995;63:709–714.
11. Larsson B, Lalos O, Marsk L, Tronstad SE, Pehrson S, Bygdeman M, Joelsson I. Effect of intraperitoneal instillation of 32% dextran 70 on postoperative adhesion formation after tubal surgery. Acta Obstet Gynecol Scand 1985;64:437–441.
12. Franklin R, Malinak L, Larsson B, Jansen R, Rosenberg S, Webster B, Diamond M. Reduction of ovarian adhesions by the use of Interceed. Obstet Gynecol 1995;86:335–340.

20 | Electrocoagulation Injuries During Laparoscopic Sterilization Procedures

Richard M. Soderstrom

History

To understand the frequency and risks of electrosurgical injuries during laparoscopic sterilization, a review of history is needed. In the United States, laparoscopic sterilization procedures blossomed in 1969 when the American College of Obstetricians and Gynecologists lifted restrictions on voluntary sterilization, placing the decision in the hands of the patient and her physician. Although a ligature technique was developed for laparoscopy, it was cumbersome, and electrosurgery seemed a more expedient method to occlude the fallopian tube. At that time, most operating theaters supplied the surgeon with a large electrical generator based on the *spark gap* principle that could generate a peak voltage output of 8000 V. Since a volt is a measure of pressure forcing electrons through small electrodes into tissue, visible sparking was common. At 8000 V, under proper atmospheric conditions, electrical current may jump 1 cm. If the wattage (a measure of power) is high enough, an arc of electrical current can cause a substantial burn to nearby tissue.

During the early 1970s, a retrospective survey by the American Association of Gynecologic Laparoscopists (AAGL) uncovered a rough estimate of bowel injury incidence at 1 per 1000 sterilization procedures. Anecdotal stories of abdominal wall burns at the laparoscope trocar site encouraged instrument manufacturers to supply insulated trocar sleeves. During this time, the vast majority of sterilization procedures were unipolar techniques; some burned the tube, some burned and cut the tube, and a few burned and resected a small specimen from the tube. The frequency of bowel injury was the same regardless of technique.

By the mid-1970s, solid-state generators with lower voltage became popular for electrosurgical sterilization procedures and abdominal wall injuries ceased to occur.

With these generators, it was shown that nonconductive trocar sleeves not only were unnecessary but could also promote a capacitance effect in the metal laparoscope shell; an electrical charge, via capacitance, could injure the bowel should any portion of the laparoscope touch the bowel.

Prompted by the 1976 Health Devices Act, a committee of laparoscopists and industry representatives set out to establish standards for safe laparoscopes and accessory equipment including electrogenerators. During the three years of deliberation, industry experts determined that low-voltage generators with a low peak voltage of 600 V and a maximum of 100 W output would be adequate for laparoscopy, eliminating the theoretical risk of sparking or arcing causing accidental bowel injury. This limit on electrical power and pressure protects against abdominal wall burns and prompted the U.S. Food and Drug Administration (FDA) to endorse the committee's recommendation that only conductive sleeves for trocars above 6 mm in diameter be available. It was shown that should an active electrode touch the metal trocar sleeve or a capacitance effect occur with such a low voltage, the low density of current, in touch with the abdominal wall, would leak harmlessly back to ground without a noticeable increase in contact temperature.

In 1972, Rioux introduced the first bipolar forceps for sterilization. This concept removes the need for electrons to seek a pathway to ground, a requirement of unipolar electrosurgery. This bipolar design, however, limits the power output available to the grasping forceps. The nuances of electrophysics are such that what you see may not reflect the amount of coagulation at the core of the tubal lumen. However, with bipolar electrocoagulation it is safe to make the following statement: to burn a structure, the operator must actively grasp it and apply direct energy—sparking or arcing cannot occur.

The first bipolar forceps was marketed in the United States in 1974. By 1976, several designs were available; by 1980, bipolar methods of sterilization were favored by two-thirds of the gynecologists surveyed by the AAGL. In 1981, the Centers for Disease Control (CDC) published their opinions as to the cause of three deaths following unrecognized bowel injuries during laparoscopic sterilization. They blamed the unipolar methods used and, in concert, the AAGL recommended that "other methods of sterilization be used."

Although abdominal wall burns were eliminated, especially with bipolar methods using the low-voltage, solid-stage generators, bowel injuries continued. Penfield reviewed 10,000 cases of "open" laparoscopy and found six bowel injury cases, none associated with the use of electrosurgery (1).

In 1985, a pathology study of traumatic and electrical bowel injuries inflicted on New Zealand rabbits demonstrated distinct histologic markers created by thermal versus traumatic injury (2). Because electrosurgery seals blood vessels, thermal injuries are characterized by coagulation necrosis and a notable absence of white blood cell infiltration due to the lack of blood supply in the edge of the perforation. Traumatic injuries showed the reverse: hypervascularity with profound white blood cell infiltration and architectural disruption without coagulation necrosis (Table 20.1).

In 1990, DiGiovanni *et al.*, immediately following sterilization, tried to inflict thermal damage to bowel by touching the "hot" fallopian tube to the bowel and could not show a histologic change in the bowel (3). They also touched the bowel with electrodes immediately after they had coagulated the tube and could find no injury. To date, the author has reviewed 54 cases of bowel injury following laparoscopic procedures where electrosurgery was used. Only three were caused by electrocoagulation; the rest were secondary to trocar or needle insertion trauma, usually beyond the control of the laparoscopists.

Today, we can state: electrical injuries do not occur to the bowel unless the bowel is grasped or touched by an electrode during activation with electroenergy. The arcing and sparking theories of the 1970s are obsolete, and the move to bipolar forceps has not reduced the incidence of bowel injury. What were *thought* to be unipolar electrical accidents to the bowel were, for the most part, due to inadvertent and unrecognized trauma from trocar or needle insertion.

Should a bowel perforation occur and a high suspicion of a unipolar burn ensue, a wide resection is recommended, as it may take several days before the extent of tissue damage becomes visually apparent. The pathologist who examines the resected tissue should be aware of the histologic differences between electrosurgery and traumatic injury before he or she records the final diagnosis.

Table 20.1. Histology of bowel injuries.

Features of puncture injuries
Limited, noncoagulative-type necrosis, more severe in the muscle coat than the mucosa

Rapid and abundant capillary ingrowth with rapid white cell infiltration

Rapid fibrin deposition at the injury site followed by fibroblastic proliferation

Features of electrical injuries
Absence of capillary ingrowth or fibroblastic muscle coat reconstruction

Absence of white cell infiltration except in focal areas at the viable borders of injury

An area of coagulation necrosis

Electrical hazards unique to sterilization

Regardless of the electrical method used, a panoramic view of the field of operation should always be obtained before activating the generator. Whether one uses a double-puncture or single-puncture technique, pull back the laparoscope from the operating field to appreciate the wide-angle view. This necessity is particularly obvious when using an electrode through an operating laparoscope. The blind spot created by the presence of the electrode shrinks as the laparoscope is withdrawn from the object to be coagulated.

When using unipolar energy, 50 W of power is sufficient. In theory, the tube should be grasped, coagulated, and then regrasped moving *toward* the uterine fundus because as tissue is heated and desiccated, the electrical flow is impeded and the electrons will try to seek an alternative pathway. Should one move distal on the tube when applying a second or third burn, the energy might seek a route out through the fimbria. If the fimbria barely touches the bowel, the current density may be high enough to cause a burn. Here, bipolar forceps eliminates such a risk, but the reduced power output may hinder the laparoscopist's ability to completely occlude the tube. The visual end point used with unipolar methods is not adequate with bipolar methods. Research has shown that an undamped or nonmodulated waveform, commonly called a "cutting" waveform, should be used to allow the energy transmitted through the bipolar forceps to penetrate deep into the endosalpinx. With the undamped waveform, at least 25 W of power are needed. An inline, current flowmeter reassures the surgeon that all tissue has been coagulated. Most of the bipolar generators sold in the 1990s include such a flowmeter.

Over the years, authors have questioned the presence of a "poststerilization syndrome" that allegedly manifests itself with dysfunctional uterine bleeding. The theory behind this phenomenon proposes that the electrosurgery energy destroys some of the necessary blood supply to the adjacent ovary causing hormonal imbalance. Epidemiologists have not been able to substantiate such a claim.

In summary, the electrical methods of laparoscopic sterilization—be they unipolar or bipolar—have minimal hazards. They do require some understanding of electrophysics, but no more than is expected of laparoscopists who use lasers. The theoretical hazards of electrosurgical methods of sterilization felt to be present in the 1970s and early 1980s do not exist. In the 1990s, better education in the basic science of electrosurgery and proper laparoscopic techniques will broaden the surgeons' choices and those of their patients.

REFERENCES

1. Penfield AJ. How to prevent complications of open laparoscopy. J Reprod Med 1985;30:660–663.
2. Levy BS, Soderstrom RM, Dail DH. Bowel injuries during laparoscopy: gross anatomy and histology. J Reprod Med 1985;30:168–179.
3. DiGiovanni M, Vasilenko P, Belsky D. Laparoscopic tubal sterilization: the potential for thermal bowel injury. J Reprod Med 1990;35:951–954.

Complications of Laparoscopic Suturing and Clip Applications

21

Magdy Milad

Introduction

Although operative laparoscopy was introduced more than 50 years ago, only recently has endoscopic suturing been possible. Prior to its development, intra-abdominal hemorrhage was controlled with electrocoagulation. The possibility of thermal damage extending beyond immediate visibility precluded its application in areas in which adjacent viscera are at risk. In an attempt to avoid such injury, suturing techniques used at laparotomy were applied to endoscopic procedures. It rapidly became clear that specialized instrumentation would be required to ensure widespread acceptance of laparoscopic suturing. The rapidity with which these instruments are evolving is remarkable; their appropriate use, however, remains predicated on technical skill and sound judgment. As with all surgical procedures, laparoscopic suturing is associated with possible complications—some inherent to general suturing and others only applicable to laparoscopic suturing. In this chapter, we will review the advantages and disadvantages of suture materials, discuss knotting techniques and placement problems, and consider knot security. Additionally, we will discuss clip applications and their potential difficulties as well as stapleoscopy.

Suture material

Endoscopic surgeons should apply the same principles at laparoscopy as they would at laparotomy. The same criteria hold true for selection of suture material. The ideal suture should be easy to handle, maintain good knot security, and have a minimal tissue reaction and lasting tensile strength.

When selecting a suture it must be taken into account that once the wound has healed to maximum strength, sutures are no longer needed. Multifilament suture should be avoided in potentially contaminated tissues as it may serve as a nidus for infection. Always use the smallest possible size appropriate for tissue.

Suture material can be divided into three categories: absorbable, slowly absorbable, and nonabsorbable (1). Absorbable suture material is degraded by either hydrolysis or proteolysis and can stimulate a variable inflammatory response, depending on the suture selection. Plain catgut, for example, is derived from the mucosa of sheep intestine or the serosa of beef intestine. As a naturally occurring substance, it acts to stimulate an intense inflammatory reaction. This material undergoes rapid degradation, maintaining tensile strength for only four to five days. Treating plain gut with chromium salts delays absorption, while increasing tensile strength. Materials that do not rely upon cellular processes for absorption tend to be less inflammatory yet retain their tensile strength (e.g., Dexon and Vicryl). Although it provides easy handling, use of synthetic polyfilament suture can lead to tissue damage as the braided material passes through the tissues. Additionally, braided suture does not "slip" well, providing a challenge to the endoscopic surgeon when attempting to tighten the knot in a less than accessible area. Recently an absorbable monofilament has been developed (Monocryl) that may offer tensile strength as well as less inflammation; this material may avoid the disadvantages associated with braided suture.

Nonabsorbable sutures are produced from both natural materials (silk) and synthetic materials. In the latter category, nylon has high elasticity and is primarily used for skin closure. Polyester is a braided material that is coated with polybutilate (Ethibond). Such products provide excellent tensile strength with minimal tissue reactions. Finally, polypropylene (Prolene) is a monofilament that is essentially inert to tissues—a valuable asset in treating contaminated wounds and for vascular repairs.

The surgical needle

The main consideration in choosing a surgical needle is the need to reduce tissue trauma. Needles used at laparotomy minimize this type of injury and provide excellent strength and stability within the needle holder. The optimal selection of a needle used at laparoscopy should take advantage of these needle refinements made for use at laparotomy. Some needles designed for endoscopic suturing lack the time-honored characteristics of a conventional sharp needle with swaged-on suture (Fig. 21.1). As a result, they may produce greater tissue trauma and encounter resistance to penetration.

When selecting suture material, the needle style must be considered. Straight needles offer the obvious advantage of ease of entry into the abdomen through the 5-mm accessory sheath. Straight needles have limited application in the pelvis, however, as adjacent tissue is at risk for injury during placement. Juxtapositional structures may incur multiple needle piercings, resulting in a "tenderizing" effect. Although curved needles more than a 3/8 circle afford greater ease of application, they can be difficult to bring through the accessory sheath. One option is to employ a 5-mm laparoscope in a lateral port and bring the needle through the 10-mm sheath under direct visualization. Another option would be to manually reduce the curve of the needle, thereby permitting placement through the sheath. A "ski" or half-curved needle is also manufactured for this purpose, providing greater intra-abdominal entry, maneuverability, and needle control.

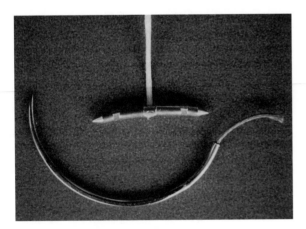

Fig. 21.1 A disposable endoscopic suturing device uses a needle (above) that lacks many of the time-honored characteristics of a conventional laparotomy needle (below). The needle has a blunt tip and a rough surface and drops the suture along the needle. Refinements to the device will improve its versatility and application.

The surgical knot

Although more than 1000 knots have been described, only a few are currently in use to secure sutures. The completed knot must be firm enough to eliminate slippage and small enough to reduce excessive tissue reaction. Excessive torsion may break suture and cut tissue. Although knot tying is a most basic principle for the surgeon at laparotomy, transferring this technique to endoscopy is less than intuitive. The combination of remote tissue manipulation with fixed entry points and a magnified view can significantly increase the difficulty level.

Historically, the pretied knot was employed to avoid intraoperative endoscopic knot tying. One of the earliest described is the Roeder loop slipknot. In the pretied form, the endoscopic loop is versatile in controlling hemostasis, tissue extirpation, and tissue approximation. The pretied loop slipknot is loaded backward into an applicator tube. The ligature is then placed into a 5-mm accessory sheath and introduced into the abdomen. The loop is placed over the tissue to be ligated, and the knot is tightened by pulling on the free end of the suture while pushing the plastic guide. In isolating the pedicle, it is important that the loop not be initially too small. Placement of the loop must take place under direct visualization so as to avoid unwanted tissue or structures.

A common mistake is to tighten the loop while the knot rests on adjacent tissue and draw it up inadvertently. In tightening the loop, one must apply steady continuous pressure—not tighten and release in multiple succession. Such "jerking" movements tend to weaken the knot (2). In the experience of the author and others, the Roeder loop used in the endoscopic loop displays a tendency to slip (3). One easy modification to prevent this problem involves the placement of a half-hitch following the application of the loop to the tissue. Alternatively, the surgeon can use knots that are less prone to slippage, due to their inherent design, such as the Duncan loop (Fig. 21.2). In using these alternative knots, an extracorporeal slipknot must be prepared.

Extracorporeal knot tying is commonly used in two settings: when the suture material or the pretied endoscopic loop knot itself is unacceptable for the application intended, and when the suture must be placed with a needle. An endoscopic suture for this purpose is available commercially (Endoknot, Ethicon, Cincinnati, Ohio) made of chromic, monofilament, or braided suture (Surgiwip, United States Surgical Corporation, Norwalk, Connecticut) attached to a straight needle that is 3 cm in length. To complete the suture apparatus, a plastic push rod is included. The suture is first grasped near the needle with a 3-mm needle holder and introduced through a trocar sleeve into the peritoneal cavity. A 5-mm needle holder is used to regrasp the needle, and the tissue is approximated. The needle is then brought through the

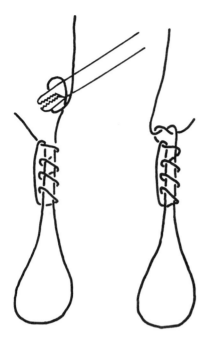

Fig. 21.2 The Duncan slipknot is more secure than the Roeder knot. (Reproduced with permission from Maerrero MA, Corfman RS. Laparoscopic use of sutures. Clin Obstet Gynecol 1991;35:387.)

original sleeve, employing the 3-mm needle holder. Next, an extracorporeal knot such as the Roeder loop or Duncan loop knot is tied and finally pushed down with the applicator. Extracorporeal knot tying can be performed with any suture material provided it is of significant length (>100 cm). Roeder or Duncan loop knots require patience and practice to be tied correctly. A more intuitive technique is the extracorporeal sliding knot used at laparotomy for less than accessible areas. The extracorporeal sliding square knot provides excellent strength as compared with the Roeder knot (4).

A reusable instrument is commonly used to "push" an extracorporeal knot back through the trocar sleeve. Several prototypes have been described, including one by McComb (personal communication), and another by Clarke (Marlow Surgical Technologies, Willoughby, Ohio). Concomitant tension must be employed on both ends of the suture while pushing the knot down on to the tissue—necessitating the aid of an assistant.

In tying the extracorporeal knot, the surgeon must be acutely aware of undue upward traction exerted on the tissue to be ligated. It is helpful for the assistant to watch the monitor as the surgeon focuses solely on tying the knot. The assistant can then warn the surgeon before an inadvertent injury takes place.

Intracorporeal suturing is more challenging. Two methods of intra-abdominal suturing are available. In the first technique, after introducing a suture with a swaged needle into the abdominal cavity, the suture is placed through the tissue using laparoscopic needle holders. A tissue grasper and needle holder can then be used to place a square knot. This type of suturing is cumbersome and requires a great deal of patience and efficiency. Recently, a second technique has been described that has proved more successful. A swaged needle attached to a long suture is introduced through a laparoscopic sleeve and the tissue sutured. A laparoscopic needle holder is introduced through the same sleeve, and the needle is grasped at right angles to the needle shaft. The needle holder is rotated several times, thereby winding the two strands of suture in the abdomen. Another needle holder, introduced through a separate port, is used to regrasp the needle, and it is passed through the loop formed closest to the tissue. By simply retracting the long end of the suture, the knot is formed and tightened. Care must be taken to avoid laceration of intra-abdominal structures by the needle, particularly during the winding phase.

As was mentioned earlier, laparoscopic intracorporeal knot tying can be technically challenging. Magnification coupled with the two-dimensional nature of videoendoscopy can lead to inefficiency and a lack of coordination. By necessity, the surgeon stands to one side of the patient—a position that can lead to disorientation in manipulating the instruments. In addition, reaching over the patient can result in early fatigue. It is important to reduce strain whenever possible. Consequently, the operating table should be placed below the surgeon's waist level. The surgeon's arm should rest comfortably on either side. Ideally, the scope should be in line with the surgeon's eyes and monitor. With the surgeon's instruments placed equidistant on either side, a perfect triangle is created.

The importance of accessory sheath selection cannot be overemphasized. Although ball-valve sheaths are designed to maintain pneumoperitoneum following removal of an instrument, they tend to catch the needle upon withdrawal. The 5-mm sheath that contains a "trap door" valve permits manual opening and closing of the valve and is an excellent choice for suturing.

If a ball-valve sheath is initially placed and a simple sheath is later desired, a long, blunt probe can be used to facilitate the exchange. The blunt probe is placed in the ball-valve sheath, and the sheath is then pulled out over the probe. This step is followed by placement of the replacement sheath over the probe and removal of the probe.

Clip appliers and surgical staplers

Recently made available to the laparoscopic surgeon are endoscopic multifire clip appliers (Ligaclip, Ethicon, and Endoclip, USSC) and linear stapler and cutter (Endopath, Ethicon, and Multifire ENDOGIA, USSC) (5). Both clips and staples are made of titanium, which has low reactivity.

Simple in design, the endoscopic clip offers three sizes based on length when closed: small (3.8 mm), medium (6.0 mm), and large (9–10 mm). Each applier contains 20 clips. The clip is passed through a 10-mm sheath, reloaded with one trigger, and fired with the pistol grip on the handle. Care must be taken so as not to maintain pressure on the reloading trigger while firing. Maintenance of this pressure permits the loaded staple to approximate but also fires a second, unapproximated staple into the abdominal cavity. To ensure proper clip placement, the surgeon can visually confirm a clip in the jaws of the applicator. One should never remove the applier with an open clip in the jaw, as the open clip could drop into the body cavity. Instead, squeeze the handle and remove the instrument with the jaws closed.

Another potential complication associated with clips involves pedicle procurement. The surgeon must carefully estimate the amount of tissue to be incorporated, so as not to take "too big a bite." The same concern applies to stapleoscopy. Staple appliers and cutters are available in 30 and 35 mm lengths and are produced in two sizes based on the height of the staple; 3.5-mm staples can ligate tissues less than 1.5 mm in width, and 2.5–2.75-mm staples will ligate tissue less than 1 mm in width. The latter type of staple is primarily used for vascular procurement. The applier is passed through a 12-mm sheath. Once the tissue is placed between the jaws of the cartridge and anvil, the approximating lever is closed. The resulting atraumatic clamp can be opened and readjusted. When the surgeon is confident of the tissue to be stapled, the pistol grip is fired. The two edges are stapled and separated. A safety interlock prevents firing if the cartridge is empty.

The endoscopic surgeon has several options when excess bleeding occurs along the cut edges. Over time, endogenous mechanisms of hemostasis may intervene naturally. Pressure using a suction aspirator or blunt probe has also been successful, but one cannot be impatient when employing this method. The author prefers to count five minutes by the clock to aid in this regard. One can also apply a clip if isolated bleeding is present. Use of electrocoagulation must be judicious, as excessive des-iccation of the tissue can cause retraction of the vessel with subsequent loss of the function of the preexisting staples. Caution is also encouraged when using a laser to control bleeding along staple lines. Although staples and clips do have a matted finish, one would expect some reflection given the risk of visceral injury present.

Summary

Intra-abdominal suture, clip, and staple applications afford the endoscopic surgeon a wide variety of techniques to achieve hemostasis. Often, these methods can be used to deal with complications incurred during a procedure. On the other hand, complications or difficulties may arise during the preventive or salvage maneuver, exacerbating an already difficult situation. In such cases it may be prudent to simply apply pressure with an atraumatic, self-retaining grasping forceps so as to allow oneself the luxury of reflection. This waiting period often permits development of a fine plan for dealing with the situation while providing the endogenous hemostatic mechanisms the opportunity to contribute. Finally, sometimes a decision must be made to proceed to laparotomy to deal effectively and decisively with the situation at hand. While this situation certainly arises in cases of major hemorrhage, it can be incurred with less significant bleeding. One must be vigilant to avoid "denial," whereby a problem, although suspected, is dismissed prematurely.

REFERENCES

1. Sanz KE. Sutures: a primer on structure and function. Contemp Ob/Gyn 1990;35:99.
2. Hay DL, Levine RL, von Fraunhofer JA, Masterson BJ. Chronic gut pelviscopic loop ligature: effect on the number of pulls on the tensile strength. J Reprod Med 1990;35:260.
3. Marrero MA, Corfman RS. Laparoscopic use of sutures. Clin Obstet Gynecol 1991;35:387.
4. Dorsey JH, Sharp HT, Clovan JD, Holtz PM. Laparoscopic knot strength: a comparison with conventional knots. Obstet Gynecol 1995;86:636–640.
5. Grainger DA, Meyer WR, DeCherney AH, Diamond MP. Laparoscopic clips evaluation of absorbable and titanium with regard to hemostasis and tissue reactivity. J Reprod Med 1991;36:493.

Hemorrhage from the Ovary or Fallopian Tube | 22

Peter F. McComb and Christina Williams

Laparoscopic reconstructive tubal surgery carries a risk of bleeding from these structures as a direct result of dissection or as an inadvertent incidental injury to the adnexa.

It is difficult to assess the frequency of hemorrhage for several reasons:

- Only cases where a hemorrhage of substantial volume has occurred due to accidental injury to the pelvic vessels tend to be reported (1–4).
- Only if hemorrhage leads to a laparotomy or blood transfusion is it classified as a "complication" in surgical records.
- The rate of bleeding at laparoscopy is not easily estimated, especially if the patient is in the Trendelenburg position.
- A variable amount of bleeding is expected to occur in many laparoscopic procedures.

Vascular supply to the ovary and tube

The arterial supply to the oviduct is dual, with variable contributions from both the ovarian and uterine arteries. The lateral ampulla and fimbria, which are supplied by both arteries, are the most profusely vascularized segments of the tube. This region also represents the site of entry and exit of the ovarian vessels to and from the hilum of the ovary.

Venous drainage follows a similar distribution, with a rich anastomotic arch noted between the ovarian hilum and mesosalpinx. Varicosities are frequently observed in the mesoovarium.

Predisposing circumstances for vascular injury

Although it is possible for coarse manipulation of normal adnexae at laparoscopy to cause vascular injury and hemorrhage, most hemorrhage occurs because of a distortion of the anatomical relationship between the tube, ovary, broad ligament, and pelvic side wall.

Many conditions that require endoscopic reconstructive surgery—for example, adhesive disease or endometriosis—are associated with a loss of the normal anatomy and may serve as a source of increased vascularity (5). Some congenital defects of the oviduct, such as certain forms of fimbrial phimosis and distal tubal obstruction, are particularly prone to hemorrhage at the time of endoscopic correction.

Ovarian cyst formation related to ovulation (such as a vascular corpus luteum cyst) can increase the risk of bleeding at the time of adnexal manipulation. A dramatic example is the extremely vascular ovary that is hyperstimulated by induction of ovulation.

Predisposition to hemorrhage may occur when a torsion of the adnexum has occurred. In such a case, the ischemic necrosis of the vessel wall results in loss of vascular integrity.

Endoscopic surgery carries a risk of vascular injury at the time of introduction of instruments through the abdominal wall (1, 2). Large studies have documented a vascular complication rate between 3 and 7 per 10,000 cases; mortality rates range from 10% to 53% (1, 2, 6). This risk increases when the patient is thin or obese. Most reported vascular injuries are related to the iliac veins and arteries during adhesiolysis or tubal ligation.

Hemorrhage from the adnexae can be either immediate or delayed. The pneumoperitoneum induces pressures of 10 to 12 mm Hg. Releasing the pressure at the end of the procedure terminates the tamponade effect on "occult venous injury." Injury may then appear in the immediate postoperative period in the form of a hemoperitoneum requiring reexploration. To check for this condition, the pneumperitoneum is released; after several minutes, it is reestablished, and the operative field inspected.

Causes of vascular injury

A distinction can be made between arterial and venous trauma. Manipulation of tissues with probes or graspers may lead to tearing of the wall of a vein. This condition is typified by blunt dissection of an ovary from the pelvic side wall. In such a case, scarring fuses the ovarian cortex to the tissues of the ovarian fossa. The fibrosis is stronger than a vein wall; the vein itself is torn and pronounced hemorrhage may ensue (the proximity of the ureter hinders efforts to control bleeding).

Sharp dissection techniques are more likely to injure an artery or arteriole. Such damage occurs irrespective of whether electrical, laser, or mechanical (scissors) incisions are employed.

Electrical and laser incisions induce a shoulder of thermal damage that coagulates small vessels adjacent to the cut. The hemostatic effect usually remains limited to vessels less than 1 mm in diameter. Use of electrical or laser energy does not preclude bleeding from larger veins or arteries, however. Sharp incision with scissors will cause more bleeding, but less damage to tissues adjacent to the incision. For this reason interstitial injection of vasopressor solution is advocated by some surgeons.

Procedure-specific vascular injuries

Oviductal banding

The applicator metal grasping prongs that elevate the oviduct in preparation for applying the Silastic ring can penetrate the mesosalpinx and injure an artery or vein (7). Because the vessels lie free and unsupported between the leaves of peritoneum, this perforation can produce a broad ligament hematoma. Scrutiny of the mesosalpinx at the outset and selection of an avascular window preclude this injury.

Ectopic pregnancy–salpingostomy

The standard laparoscopic approach to ectopic pregnancy has been to incise the antimesenteric border of the fallopian tube over the site of the gestational tissue. Interstitial injection of vasopressor solution helps to counteract the increased vascularity of the tissues. The vascular vasopressor supply in the distal ampulla is profuse, being supplied by both uterine and ovarian arteries. If hemorrhage occurs from the implantation site of the ectopic pregnancy, after the gestational tissue has been removed, further infiltration of the mesosalpinx both proximally and distally may be necessary.

If the ectopic pregnancy is well implanted and therefore well vascularized, a 5-0 polypropylene suture can be sewn through the mesosalpinx to restrict the vascular supply to the implantation site. This technique was effective in a recent isthmic ectopic pregnancy with a human chorionic gonadotropin level of 108,631 I.U./mL. In placing the suture, care must be taken to avoid the vessels within the mesosalpinx.

Salpingoovariolysis–peritubal and periovarian adhesions

The potential for bleeding during salpingoovariolysis is directly proportional to the cohesiveness and density of the adhesions, and the proximity to adjacent structures. Specifically, bowel mesentery and omental vessels are very easily injured and do not benefit from any intrinsic tamponade effect because of their loose peritoneal covering. Instead, preliminary coagulation and/or fine suturing is required.

Careful dissection via sharp scissors can divide adnexal adhesions in layers by defining the avascular windows between the blades of curved scissors. This technique minimizes the amount of coagulation needed for hemostasis and the extent of subsequent tissue damage.

Accidental injury of the iliac veins during lysis of adnexal adhesions has been documented in the literature (1, 2, 6). Extreme care must be used when the anatomy is grossly distorted and when thermal energy is used (as in electrosurgery or lasers used for adhesiolysis).

Hydrosalpinx–terminal salpingostomy

The blood supply to the hydrosalpinx is attenuated because of fibrosis subsequent to inflammation. If the hydrosalpinx is free, the terminal occlusion may be incised with scissors with little subsequent bleeding (Fig. 22.1).

Two instances predispose the patient to hemorrhage in such cases: (1) the presence of neovascularization between the hydrosalpinx and the ovary, and (2) inadvertent incision of the mesosalpinx (Fig. 22.2).

Neovascularization represents a response to inflammatory devascularization of the tube. The new vessels arise from the ovary and supply the occluded end of the oviduct. Often the occluded ostium is adherent to the surface of the ovary. Unless the pathogenesis of the creation of these vessels is appreciated, the endoscopist will not expect the vessels to be in this location. Bleeding can be brisk and inaccessible if these vessels are incised.

Incision of the mesosalpinx can cause either overt bleeding or hematoma formation (surprisingly quickly). Fusion of the hydrosalpinx to the ovarian surface or broad ligament makes it difficult to differentiate the tubal wall from the mesosalpinx; only when arterial bleeding occurs does it become apparent that the mesosalpinx has been penetrated.

Another situation in which the mesosalpinx may be inadvertently incised arises when the distending dye solution leaks from the hydrosalpinx into the mesosalpinx. From personal experience (unfortunately), one author (McComb) has noted that the newly distended mesosalpinx may resemble the classical retort configuration of

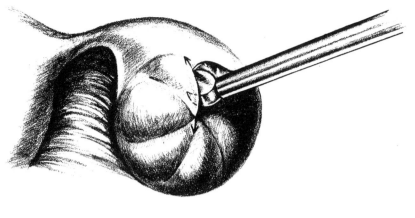

Fig. 22.1 Neosalpingostomy by laparoscopy: the relatively bloodless incision of the radial fusion scars of the terminus of the hydrosalpinx with scissors.

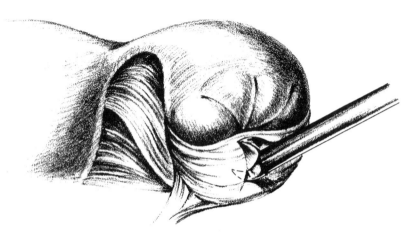

Fig. 22.2 Neosalpingostomy by laparoscopy: pertubation dye solution has leaked from the hydrosalpinx into the mesosalpinx to distend the mesosalpinx. The surgeon believes the mesosalpinx to be the terminus of the hydrosalpinx, incises the mesosalpinx, and hemorrhage occurs.

a hydrosalpinx (see Fig. 22.2). Only upon reviewing the video recording of the procedure was the earlier leakage of the dye into the mesosalpinx seen to occur.

Tubal reanastomosis

The advent of laparoscopic techniques to handle light-weight sutures (7-0) now permits tubal anastomosis. At the time of transection of the oviductal stumps, the vessels that course parallel to the tube are susceptible to damage. Elevation of the tube within the curved blades of the scissors allows close inspection of the limit of the myosalpinx and can minimize the risk of this injury.

Ovarian cystectomy

As the cyst lining is dissected or stripped from the ovarian tissue, areas of fibrosis are often encountered that require sharp dissection. At the level of the hilum of the ovary, the major ovarian vessels disperse to supply the ovarian tissue. Hemorrhage may occur if these vessels are damaged. To minimize this risk, the surgeon should maintain surveillance of the external surface of the ovary so as to avoid incision of the hilum.

In the case of an endometrioma, the ovary may be densely adherent to other pelvic structures—for example,

the rectum, ureter, or ovarian fossa. Loss of recognizable anatomy at the time of laparoscopic cystectomy can lead to inadvertent fenestration of the capsule and incision of the extraovarian pelvic vessels. To avoid this event, the surgeon must select, judiciously, the cases for this type of surgery, be prepared to discontinue the endoscopic procedure, and at all times remain aware of the level of dissection within the ovarian tissue.

Plication of the ovarian ligament to the round ligament

This endoscopic procedure entails passing a suture from the round ligament beneath the oviductal isthmus, through the ovarian ligament or ovary, and back to the round ligament. This technique rotates and elevates the ovarian tissue away from denuded pelvic peritoneal surfaces and avoids subsequent adhesion formation. If the needle is passed through the mesosalpinx too close to the isthmus, the vessels immediately beneath the tube may sustain damage.

Stabilization of adnexal torsion

Once the torsion has been diagnosed and untwisted, the lateral aspect of the mesoovarium is sutured (beneath the fimbria) to the pelvic side wall. This method realigns the axis of adnexal rotation and positions the oviduct and ovary so as to prevent recurrence of the torsion. The tortuous veins of the mesoovarium are avoided by scrutinizing the tissue as it is stretched over the point of the needle. Once the mesoovarium is secured, the side wall is stitched with multiple shallow bites of peritoneum (as opposed to deep bites) to preclude vascular injury to the iliac vessels or the infundibulopelvic ligament.

Ovarian transposition

Transposition of the ovary and tube to an extrapelvic location to preserve ovarian function during radiotherapy for Hodgkin's disease or cervical/rectal carcinoma has been performed laparoscopically. This procedure requires extensive electrocoagulation and transection of the ovarian ligament and mesosalpinx to mobilize the ovary, which is then sutured in the paracolic gutter. Given the proximity of the iliac vessels and the tension imposed upon newly coagulated tissues, this procedure carries a potential for hemorrhage that can require prompt laparotomy.

Salpingectomy–salpingoophorectomy

Endoscopic removal of the oviduct or ovary to treat ectopic pregnancy or severe inflammatory changes (such as an ovarian remnant) requires the use of suture loops, electrocoagulation, and stapling devices. Of necessity, large vascular pedicles are developed; these pedicles are associated with a subsequent risk of immediate or delayed bleeding if the vessels are not properly secured.

Management of hemorrhage

Laparoscopically induced bleeding may be life-threatening (2). The surgeon may not appreciate the extent of blood loss, especially if blood is able to flow to the upper abdomen because the patient is in the Trendelenburg position. Immediate laparotomy with resuscitative measures should not be delayed.

As soon as hemorrhage is detected, the surgeon must state the urgency of the situation. The nursing and anesthesia staff may not appreciate this urgency, and therefore not respond rapidly with assistance. Video camera monitoring is usually very helpful, but occasionally the images produced can be underestimated or misunderstood. A droplet of blood on the tip of the endoscope can obscure the optical channel as effectively as a liter of blood in the pelvis. If any question arises about the source of bleeding, degree of hemorrhage, or ability to control it, then an immediate laparotomy (without evacuation of the pneumoperitoneum) is mandatory. It is not necessary to reposition the patient from the leg/foot stirrups.

When the source of hemorrhage is evident, the bleed-ing considered controllable, and the blood loss not rapid, attempts at achieving hemostasis at laparoscopy may be reasonable.

The surgeon should immediately obtain a suction-irrigator, bipolar electrocoagulating forceps (the Kleppinger designs are most versatile), vasopressor solution, and grasping forceps. Suction and irrigation are essential to permit identification of the source of bleeding. The bipolar forceps are usually effective when an arterial or venous bleeder can be isolated from surrounding structures—for example, in the case of arterial bleeding encountered from omental adhesions or inadvertent incision of the mesosalpinx.

Grasping forceps are used to apply pressure to bleeding tissues to gain time for the source of bleeding to be identified. Vasopressor solution is ideal for control of diffuse bleeding that is either encountered (e.g., in ovarian cystectomy with bleeding from the ovarian hilum) or anticipated (e.g., in ectopic pregnancy or terminal salpingostomy).

In addition, suture with lightweight material can achieve hemostasis, particularly when the bleeding originates from tissue that cannot be coagulated without potential compromise to fertility or to vital structures. This condition is exemplified by bleeding near the ureter or bladder, bowel, ovary, or oviduct. The advent of instrumentation (the suture knot pusher) to handle fine suture has enhanced the ability to treat hemorrhage rapidly at laparoscopy without damage to surrounding tissues.

Other methods available include stapling devices or suture loops. Although these techniques are rarely needed in bleeding that is encountered during fertility-enhancing procedures, it is important for the surgeon and the operating room staff to be familiar with them because they can achieve hemostasis of a rapid bleeder within a very short period of time.

Conclusion

Hemorrhage from the oviduct and ovary at laparoscopy ranges from innocuous to life-threatening. If the surgeon has any question as to the source, volume of bleeding, or ability to achieve hemostasis at laparoscopy, then laparotomy is essential. Otherwise a variety of measures may be employed to halt the hemorrhage. Interstitial injection of vasopressor solution and fine suturing are the least damaging of these options.

REFERENCES

1. Hanney RM, Alle KM, Cregan PC. Major vascular injury and laparoscopy. Aust N Z J Surg 1995;65:533–535.
2. Nordestgaard MD, Kenton C, Bodily MD, Osborne RW, Buttorff JD. Major vascular injuries during laparoscopic procedures. Am J Surg 1995;159:543–545.

3. Yupze AA. Pneumoperitoneum needle and trocar injuries in laparoscopy. A survey on possible contributing factors and prevention. J Reprod Med 1990;35:485–490.
4. Peterson HB, Hulka JF, Phillips JM. American Association of Gynecologic Laparoscopists' 1988 membership survey on operative laparoscopy. J Reprod Med 1990;35:587–589.
5. Magos AL, Baumann R, Turnbull AC. Managing gynaecological emergencies with laparoscopy. Br Med J 1989;299:371–374.
6. Chapron C, Querleau D, Mage G, Madelenat P, Dubuisson JB, Audebert A, Erny R, Bruhat MA. Complications of gynaecologic laparoscopy. Multicentric study of 7604 laparoscopies. J Gynecol Obstet Biol Reprod 1992;21:207–213.
7. Franks AL, Kendrick JS, Peterson HB, Unintended laparotomy associated with laparoscopic tubal sterilization. Am J Obstet Gynecol 1987;157:1102–1105.

23 | Tubal Bleeding After Salpingostomy for Ectopic Pregnancy

Michael P. Diamond and Charla M. Blacker

Use of linear salpingostomy to treat ectopic pregnancy

For patients wishing to preserve their fertility, ectopic pregnancies can be efficiently treated by conservative surgery. Most commonly, the procedure consists of a linear salpingostomy incision on the antimesenteric border of the fallopian tube; it is performed at both laparotomy and laparoscopy. In recent years, this procedure has gained in popularity because multiple series have shown that the subsequent pregnancy rate after salpingostomy does not differ from that after salpingectomy, and because the repeat ectopic pregnancy rate is no higher than after more radical therapy. In fact, in patients treated by linear salpingostomy for ectopic pregnancy, the repeat ectopic pregnancies occur with equal frequency in the ipsilateral and contralateral fallopian tube. This finding suggests that the prior ectopic pregnancy is not the major factor contributing to repeat eccyesis, but that a bilateral condition (either congenital or developmental) predisposes such patients to an increased risk of ectopic pregnancy.

Although linear salpingostomy for the treatment of ectopic pregnancy can be performed in any portion of the fallopian tube, it has most commonly been described for treatment of ampullar ectopic pregnancies. When this procedure is performed in the ampullar aspect of the tube, the risk of subsequent tubal occlusion or fistula formation is low. In contrast, salpingostomy in the isthmic portion of the fallopian tube frequently results in occlusion or fistula formation at the site of the salpingostomy incision.

Outcomes for these procedures may be related to structural differences of the tube in these locations. In the isthmus, the serosa of the tube is more intimately attached to the underlying muscularis; incision over an isthmic ectopic pregnancy almost always results in entry into the tubal lumen. Conversely, the serosa of the ampullar segment is much more loosely applied to the muscularis, allowing expansion of the ectopic pregnancy into the potential space between the serosa and muscularis, rather than within the lumen of the tube. Thus, treatment of ampullary ectopic pregnancies is less likely to involve the tubal lumen itself. This statement does not imply that a connection could not exist between the ampullar ectopic bed and the tubal lumen; the latter does not, however, always suffer extensive violation in these procedures.

Complications during linear salpingostomy

Two major problems arise during conservative surgery for ectopic gestation: bleeding at the salpingostomy incision site and bleeding from the implantation site. Careful planning and forethought can decrease the incidence of such troublesome bleeding, however.

Bleeding from a salpingostomy incision

In an attempt to minimize the likelihood of bleeding from a salpingostomy incision, many physicians inject a dilute pitressin solution into either the antimesenteric border in the fallopian tube or the mesosalpinx (and sometimes into both). The pitressin solution typically consists of 1 ampule of pitressin (20 I.U.) in 100 mL of normal saline.

Mesosalpingeal injection of pitressin is thought to cause contraction of the vessels supplying the fallopian tube, thereby reducing the pulse pressure at the incision and implantation sites. The injection must be performed carefully, as damage to the mesosalpingeal vessels can result in bleeding into the broad ligament. Antimesenteric injection is usually performed over the entire serosal surface of the ectopic gestation. If it is administered at laparoscopy, either a second puncture probe or use of a spinal needle that is placed through the anterior abdominal wall may be employed. When using a spinal needle, the needle should be advanced at the correct angle immediately over the fallopian tube, as correction becomes more difficult once the needle penetrates the abdominal wall.

To minimize difficulties with needle placement, the abdominal wall over the ectopic should be palpated to identify the site and angle of inclination for needle placement. If a large pneumoperitoneum is present, partial evacuation will decrease the distance that the needle must traverse to reach the fallopian tube. Use of a grasping instrument will facilitate manipulation of the tube and allow better control of this portion of the procedure.

While proponents of pitressin use claim that it minimizes bleeding during the course of the procedure, opponents remain concerned about the possibility of delayed bleeding postoperatively. In fact, the latter has been a relatively infrequently described occurrence.

In theory, the salpingostomy incision should be made with an instrument that allows coagulation of the serosal blood vessels, such as a laser, harmonic scalpel, or some form of electrosurgery such as a needle electrode. (If an electrosurgical option is selected, care should be taken to avoid creating a situation in which capacitance coupling occurs.) At this time, none of these modalities has proved more efficacious than the others. Thus, the choice of cutting modality should be based on availability and surgeon preference.

Should bleeding result from a salpingostomy incision, surgical management will vary based on the clinical circumstances and the desires of the patient. As a last resort, salpingectomy can be performed via either laparoscopy or laparotomy. In most cases where a conservative procedure has been attempted, the surgeon will usually prefer to avoid this more radical procedure.

In many cases, bleeding arises from the serosal margin of the fallopian tube. With irrigation, such bleeding sites can often be identified, allowing point coagulation. If the procedure is being performed laparoscopically, microbipolar instrumentation represents a good choice to obtain hemostasis. Use of a carbon dioxide (CO_2), argon, or KTP laser for control of bleeding is usually not helpful (unless only a very minimal amount of oozing is observed). When available, the argon beam coagulator can also be employed to achieve hemostasis.

In situations where the operating room is not prepared for use of electrocautery, bleeding may be minimized by grasping the tube at the bleeding site with atraumatic forceps while appropriate preparations for the use of electrocautery are made. Additionally, many surgeons are becoming increasingly facile at laparoscopic suturing. If the source of bleeding can be identified, this technique represents another option.

Bleeding from the implantation site

A second source of bleeding identified at salpingostomy comes from within the implantation site. Often, this type of bleeding results from overaggressive debridement of the ectopic bed. A general principle in trying to remove products of conception from the ectopic bed is to remove all tissue that comes easily but not any additional tissue. After removing tissue that is easily extracted, the site frequently appears to have residual tissue at its base. Thus, the decision as to how much tissue to remove is very difficult. If the surgeon is not sufficiently aggressive, persistent ectopic pregnancies may be more likely to occur; on the other hand, if the surgeon is overly aggressive, the likelihood of developing bleeding from the base increases.

The laparoscopic irrigator can be a valuable tool for thorough, but less traumatic removal of the ectopic pregnancy. It is gently inserted between the ectopic sac and the tubal wall; using hydropressure, the ectopic can then be lifted from its bed without grasping the tissue. After irrigating, any new tissue that is easily extracted can be removed, although tissue that offers resistance to easy removal by grasping should not be debrided.

Bleeding within the implantation site is often difficult to identify. One approach is the use of irrigation to visualize the ectopic bed, with subsequent point coagulation of the bleeding site. The irrigation fluid serves to remove coagulum from the bleeding vessel (increasing the accuracy of cautery) and minimizes damage to the fallopian tube itself by cooling tissues peripheral to the site of electrocoagulation. If bleeding from the bed of the ectopic cannot be identified during irrigation, the surgeon is then forced to be less specific in attempting to control the hemorrhage. In many cases, the source of the bleeding appears at the proximal or distal angle of the salpingostomy incision. This region of the tube can be grasped with an micropolar forceps and coagulated. A second option would be to extend the linear salpingostomy incision, thus providing greater visualization, with the hope of then being able to identify the site of bleeding. A third option is to grasp the tube in its entirety with a unipolar or bipolar coagulation instrument and to coagulate the entire tube in a fashion similar to performance of the tubal ligation. Although this technique is very likely to be successful, it will almost assuredly result in tubal obstruction. A fourth option is performance of partial salpingectomy. This procedure can be undertaken through cauterization of the tube on either side of the ectopic bed and excision of this portion of the tube; alternatively, the surgeon can use pretied suture ligatures, surgical staples, or devices that simultaneously staple and cut.

The specific determination of how to proceed will depend in large part on the experience of the surgeon and the operating personnel available to assist. In situations where difficulty is encountered, the surgeon must realize that attempts at tubal conservation must be modified by concern for the patient's well being and a more extensive procedure performed as needed. Similarly, if the procedure is being performed laparoscopically and difficulty is encountered that precludes laparoscopy, conversion of the procedure to laparotomy is entirely appropriate.

Ectopic Pregnancy: Persistent Trophoblastic Tissue

24

Steven J. Ory

Introduction

Kelly *et al.* first described persistent ectopic pregnancy or persistent trophoblastic disease after conservative treatment of tubal pregnancy, a unique complication of conservative treatment of ectopic pregnancy, in 1979 (1). As conservative procedures for ectopic pregnancy have become more extensively utilized, awareness of this potentially serious complication of ectopic pregnancy has increased over the past decade. Patients with persistent ectopic pregnancy incur a risk of tubal rupture and hemorrhage similar to that associated with patients initially presenting with suspected ectopic pregnancy. The incidence of persistent trophoblast after conservative laparoscopic treatment of ectopic pregnancy has ranged from 3% to 21% in unpublished reports (Table 24.1) (7). A laparoscopic approach may confer higher risk than laparotomy, although both risks are underreported in the literature.

Pathophysiology

Three mechanisms have been proposed to explain the pathophysiology of persistent ectopic pregnancy. Budowick *et al.* have suggested that the growing ectopic gestation rapidly penetrates the wall of the fallopian tube as well as spreading along the luminal surface (9). They suggest that this phenomenon occurs relatively early in the development of a tubal pregnancy, and subsequent trophoblastic proliferation occurs in an extratubal location. Because conservative surgical treatment involves removing all visible ectopic tissue from the tubal lumen, additional trophoblastic tissue behind the lumen in the muscularis layer may not be visible at the time of surgery and could be left in situ. This problem may be compounded at laparoscopy when it is not possible to palpate the fallopian tube and otherwise identify additional trophoblastic tissue.

Pauerstein *et al.* observed that extraluminal trophoblastic spread was not the predominant mode of dissemination, but was noted to occur in only one-third of carefully studied fallopian tubes (10). They suggested that segmental resection might become the conservative treatment of choice for ectopic pregnancy, and that it would probably be necessary to individualize the treatment plan depending upon whether trophoblastic spread was intraluminal or extraluminal.

Stock presented an alternative hypothesis following his review of eight cases of persistent tubal pregnancy (11). He performed a histopathologic examination of five fallopian tubes removed after initial treatment failure (two patients underwent laparoscopic salpingostomy, two patients received salpingotomy at laparotomy, and one patient underwent salpingostomy at laparotomy) and three cases of fimbrial expression. In addition, he examined three fallopian tubes that were removed at the time of the primary procedure for uncontrolled bleeding following unsuccessful salpingotomy. Stock noted that the remaining trophoblastic tissue was medial to the initial incision in four of five patients with persistent trophoblasts and two of the three salpingectomies performed for uncontrolled bleeding. None was associated with invasive growth of the trophoblast to the muscularis, and all residual trophoblastic tissue was intraluminal. He concluded that the syndrome of persistent trophoblasts is a consequence of incomplete evacuation of the chorionic villi.

Cataldo has suggested an additional means of dissemination. He described a case of a patient who had a uterine fundal serosal implant 45 days after laparoscopic treatment for tubal pregnancy. Three other cases have been described in which persistent trophoblastic tissue was found outside the tube. Cataldo suggested a possible mechanism involving reimplantation of viable trophoblastic cells shed from the fimbriated end of the tube. Alternatively, viable cells could be disseminated during operative manipulation of the ectopic pregnancy with postoperative proliferation (12). Cartwright has

Table 24.1. Incidence of persistent trophoblastic disease.

	Total (no.)	Persistent	
		No.	%
Pouly et al. (2)	317	11	4.0
Brumsted et al. (3)	25	1	4.0
Silva (4)	8	1	12.5
Vermesh et al. (5)	30	1	3.0
Henderson et al. (6)	15	3	21.0
Seifer et al. (7)	81	10	12.0
Lundodff et al. (8)	52	5	9.6
Total	528	32	6.0

described viable implants occurring on omental surfaces (13). This phenomenon is probably more common than is clinically suspected and is usually self-limited unless tubal rupture or hemorrhage by another mechanism occurs.

Clinical features

Patients with persistent ectopic pregnancies most often present with symptoms similar to those occurring at initial presentation, with pain being the most common symptom. More recently, patients have been detected before they developed symptoms through persistent or rising human chorionic gonadotropin (hCG) levels. Persistent ectopic pregnancy occurs most often after treatment of ampullary tubal pregnancies. The mean number of days between initial operation and reoperation is 26 days, with a range of 18 to 42 days (14). In approximately 90% of cases, trophoblastic tissue is present at the time of reoperation. Persistent trophoblastic tissue has been found after histologic confirmation of removal at the initial procedure. Fimbrial expression has been associated with an increased risk of persistent ectopic pregnancy (14).

Several risk factors for persistent ectopic pregnancy have been described. Seifer et al. performed a multivariate, stepwise, logistic regression analysis on 11 women with persistent ectopic pregnancy and reported that affected patients were more likely to have a shorter duration of amenorrhea (less than 42 days from last menstrual period) and a fallopian tube diameter of 2.0 cm or smaller at the time of initial presentation (7). Both observations suggest that early intervention was associated with higher risk of persistent disease. Paradoxically, Lundoff et al. noted that patients with preoperative hCG levels exceeding 3000 IU/L (International Reference Preparation) and those with levels exceeding 1000 IU/L on the second postoperative day were more likely to

experience persistence (8). Vermesh et al. noted that the declines in serum hCG and progesterone were similar in patients with resolving ectopic and persistent ectopics three and six days postoperatively (15). Patients with persistent ectopic pregnancy, however, were more likely to have higher hCG levels and progesterone levels six days postoperatively. As a result, Vermesh's group recommended that hCG levels be obtained six days following surgery and at three-day intervals thereafter.

hCG levels

Several studies have demonstrated a two-component disappearance rate for hCG following termination of pregnancy (16, 17). hCG has a half-life of 5 to 9 hours during the initial fast phase and 22 to 32 hours during the second, slower phase. It may remain detectable for as long as 60 days after termination of a normal, first-trimester pregnancy (18). hCG disappearance curves are remarkably similar for spontaneous abortions, elective abortions, and following treatment of ectopic pregnancy with salpingectomy or conservative tubal procedures (16–18). The interval to complete disappearance of hCG is most closely correlated with initial hCG levels. Kamrava et al. evaluated hCG levels following salpingectomy in conservative surgery and noted that serum clearance of hCG could continue for at least 24 days (17). One patient in their study who had a persistent elevation of hCG at 24 days following fimbrial expression ultimately experienced a successful resolution without intervention. Kamrava's group was unable to determine the interval to complete resolution, but it is probable that this patient had a protracted resolution phase or a "plateauing" of her hCG levels. The researchers also confirmed that the initial hCG level was the most significant factor in determining the length of time until hCG levels became undetectable.

DiMarchi et al. reported a patient that had detectable hCG levels for 60 days following conservative surgery (19). The patient ultimately experienced a spontaneous resolution. Vermesh et al. demonstrated that a precipitous drop in hCG levels during the first six days following surgery is not a reliable criterion for excluding the possibility of persistence (15). They suggested that the diagnosis of persistent ectopic pregnancy could be suspected if hCG levels did not decrease to 10% of their initial value within 12 days after surgery. In addition, they noted that a serum progesterone level greater than 1.5 ng/mL for 9 days following surgery was highly suggestive of persistent tubal pregnancy.

Hagstrom reviewed 158 patients with unruptured tubal pregnancies. The serum progesterone and hCG levels for each patient were obtained twice preoperatively. Fourteen patients required reoperation for persistent trophoblasts. Eleven of the 14 complicated patients had preoperative progesterone levels greater than 35 nmol/L and 12 of the 14 (86%) had daily hCG increases greater than 100 mIU/mL, compared with 31% of the patients who did not experience persistent trophoblasts. Patients with a progesterone level exceeding 35 nmol/L and a one-day hCG increase exceeding 100 mIU/mL experienced a 61% risk for repeat operation for persistent trophoblasts. Those patients with progesterone levels below 35 nmol/L and a one-day hCG increase of less than 100 mIU/mL were associated with a 2% risk.

Treatment options

As with all complications of surgery, prevention of persistent tubal pregnancy is preferable to treatment. Patients should be advised of this potential complication of conservative surgery for ectopic pregnancy preoperatively if they consent to a conservative procedure. Risk of persistent tubal pregnancy may be reduced by making a diligent effort to remove all trophoblastic tissue at the time of the initial surgery, carefully inspecting the tube, vigorously irrigating the tubal lumen, and achieving complete hemostasis. It may be prudent to extend the linear salpingostomy incision medially if persistent bleeding occurs as this location is often noted to be a site of persistence.

Following initial surgery, monitoring of hCG levels is important to detect persistence. Various recommendations for the frequency of hCG determinations have been made. Vermesh *et al.* suggest obtaining an initial hCG measurement six days postoperatively, and at three-day intervals thereafter (15)—a sampling frequency that would permit early diagnosis and intervention. They also feel that a serum progesterone determination on day nine is helpful in making the diagnosis. No intervention is necessary as long as the hCG levels do not increase and the patient remains asymptomatic. Most patients with persistent elevations will experience spontaneous resolution without additional therapy.

When the diagnosis of persistent ectopic pregnancy is established by increasing hCG levels, the occurrence of hemorrhage, or recurrent pain, treatment options include systemic methotrexate therapy or reoperation, including salpingectomy or a second attempt at conservative surgery. Because of the possibility of extraluminal trophoblastic disease, the latter surgery may be fraught with the same potential for recurrence as existed initially. Salpingectomy offers the opportunity for definitive treatment, but deprives the patient of any fertility-sparing advantages. Although limited data are available, methotrexate may represent the treatment of choice for persistent ectopic pregnancy. It appears to be safe, effective, and well tolerated (20–27).

Several regimens have been described for treatment of ectopic pregnancy with methotrexate. The regimen of 1 mg/kg methotrexate every other day for four doses followed by 0.1 mg/kg citrovorum factor every other day for four days on alternating days has been used most extensively as primary treatment for ectopic pregnancy, but is also reported to be effective for persistent ectopic pregnancy.

Patsner and Kenigsberg used 0.4 mg/kg oral methotrexate per day (25 mg/day) for five days to successfully treat a patient with persistent ectopic pregnancy on an outpatient basis (23). Therapy was well tolerated and no change in the complete blood count or liver function test was noted. Rose and Cohen used 100 mg/m² IV methotrexate as a bolus administered over one hour, followed by 200 mg/m² administered as a 12-hour infusion (24). This treatment was followed by 10 mg/m² citrovorum factor every 12 hours for four doses. Three patients were successfully treated with this regimen. The authors cited the advantage of being able to complete therapy within three days.

Stovall *et al.* described successful resolution in 29 of 30 patients receiving a single dose of methotrexate as *primary* treatment for ectopic pregnancy (25). They administered a single dose of 50 mg/m² IM methotrexate without citrovorum rescue. This regimen offers several advantages, including ease of administration, treatment on an outpatient basis, and minimal toxicity with a lower dose. Although none of the regimens utilizing methotrexate for treatment of ectopic pregnancy has been sanctioned by the U.S. Food and Drug Administration (FDA), a significant volume of clinical experience supports the use of methotrexate for primary treatment and a more limited experience offers reassurance about its safety and efficacy for persistent disease.

Hoppe *et al.* treated 19 consecutive patients with expected persistent ectopic pregnancy following conservative surgery with a single intramuscular injection of methotrexate (50 mg/m²) (26). Nineteen patients experienced complete resolution of their elevated hCG levels without additional surgery. Typically transient increased levels of hCG were observed during the first three days of therapy, followed by consistent declines. Two patients were hospitalized for observation and analgesia, and one patient appeared to have a self-limited intra-abdominal hemorrhage and received a blood transfusion.

Bengtsson treated 15 patients with evidence of persistent trophoblast after conservative laparoscopic surgery with oral methotrexate (10–20 mg per day for 4–5 days) (27). Ten patients also received folinic acid and 15 mg of methotrexate. Treatment was successful in 14 of 15 cases, and the mean interval for decline of hCG measurements to undetectable levels was 24 days.

Little is known about the reproductive performance of patients following treatment for persistent ectopic pregnancy. Seifer reviewed the records of 50 patients treated at three medical centers over a six- to seven-year interval. All patients were followed for a minimum of one year. The patients were treated with repeat salpingostomy or salpingectomy (34 patients) or methotrexate therapy (16 patients). Thirty-two patients attempted conception following treatment, and 19 achieved clinical pregnancies. Patients with normal contralateral fallopian tubes at initial surgery were more likely to have a successful clinical pregnancy. Patients treated with surgery had a shorter interval to subsequent conception than patients who received methotrexate (28).

REFERENCES

1. Kelly RW, Martin SA, Strickler RC. Delayed hemorrhage in conservative surgery for ectopic pregnancy. Am J Obstet Gynecol 1979;133:225–226.
2. Pouly JL, Mahnes H, Mage G, Canis M, Bruhat MA. Conservative laparoscopic treatment of 321 ectopic pregnancies. Fertil Steril 1986;46:1093–1097.
3. Brumsted J, Kessler C, Gibson C, Nakajima S, Riddick DH, Gibson M. A comparison of laparoscopy for the treatment of ectopic pregnancy. Obstet Gynecol 1988;71:889–892.
4. Silva PD. A laparoscopic approach can be applied to most cases of ectopic pregnancy. Obstet Gynecol 1988;72:944–947.
5. Vermesh M, Silva PD, Rosen GF, Stein AL, Fossum GT, Sauer MV. Management of unruptured ectopic gestation by linear salpingostomy: a prospective, randomized, clinical trail of laparoscopy versus laparotomy. Obstet Gynecol 1989;73:400–404.
6. Henderson SR. Ectopic tubal pregnancy treated by operative laparoscopy. Am J Obstet Gynecol 1989;160:1462–1469.
7. Seifer DB, Gutmann JN, Doyle MB, Jones EE, Diamond MP, DeCherney AH. Persistent ectopic pregnancy following laparoscopic linear salpingostomy. Obstet Gyneco 1990;76:1121–1125.
8. Lundorff P, Hahlin M, Sjoblom P, Lindblom B. Persistent trophoblast after conservative treatment of tubal pregnancy: prediction and detection. Obstet Gynecol 1991;77:129–133.
9. Budowick M, Johnson TRB Jr, Genadry R, Parmley TH, Woodruff JD. The histopathology of the developing tubal ectopic pregnancy. Obstet Gynecol 1980;34:169–171.
10. Pauerstein CJ, Croxatto HB, Eddy CA, Ramzy I, Walters MD. Anatomy and pathology of tubal pregnancy. Am J Obstet Gynecol 1986;67:301–309.
11. Stock RJ. Persistent tubal pregnancy. Obstet Gynecol 1991;77:267–270.
12. Cataldo NA, Nicholson M, Bihrle D. Uterine serosal trophoblastic implant after linear salpingostomy for ectopic pregnancy at laparotomy. Obstet Gynecol 1990;76:523–525.
13. Cartwright PS. Peritoneal trophoblastic implants after surgical management of tubal pregnancy. J Reprod Med 1991;36:523–524.
14. Bell OR, Awadalla SG, Mattox JH. Persistent ectopic syndrome: a case report and literature review. Obstet Gyecol 1987;69:521–523.
15. Vermesh M, Silva PD, Sauer MV, Vargyas JM, Loo RA. Persistent tubal gestation: patterns of circulating β-human chorionic gonadotropin and progesterone and management options. Fertil Steril 1988;50:584–588.
16. Rizkallah T, Gurpide E, Van d Wiele RL. Metabolism of hCG in man. J Clin Endocrinol Metab 1969;29:92–100.
17. Kamrava MM, Taymor ML, Berger MJ, Thompson IE, Seibel MM. Disappearance of human chorionic gonadotropin following removal of ectopic pregnancy. Obstet Gynecol 1983;62:486–488.
18. Steier JA, Bergsjo P, Myking OL. Human chorionic gonadotropin in maternal plasma after induced abortion, spontaneous abortion, and removed ectopic pregnancy. Obstet Gynecol 1984;64:391–394.
19. DiMarchi JM, Kosasa TS, Kobara TY, Hale RW. Persistent ectopic pregnancy. Obstet Gynecol 1987;70:555–558.
20. Hagström HG, Hahlin M, Bennegard-Edén B, Sjöblom P, Thorburn J, Lindblom B. Prediction of persistent ectopic pregnancy after laparoscopic salpingostomy. Obstet Gynecol 1994;84:797–802.
21. Cowan BD, McGehee RP, Bates GW. Treatment of persistent ectopic pregnancy with methotrexate and leukovorum rescue: a case report. Obstet Gynecol 1986;67:50–1S.
22. Higgins KA, Schwartz MB. Treatment of persistent trophoblastic tissue with salpingostomy with methotrexate. Fertil Steril 1986;45:427–428.
23. Patsner B, Kenigsberg D. Successful treatment of persistent ectopic pregnancy with oral methotrexate therapy. Obstet Gynecol 1988;50:982–983.
24. Rose PG, Cohen SM. Methotrexate therapy for persistent ectopic pregnancy after conservative laparoscopic management. Obstet Gynecol 1990;76:947–949.
25. Stovall TG, Ling FW, Gray LA. Single-dose methotrexate for treatment of ectopic pregnancy. Obstet Gynecol 1990;77:754–757.
26. Hoppe DI, Bekkar BE, Nager CW. Single-dose systemic methotrexate for the treatment of persistent ectopic pregnancy after conservative surgery. Obstet Gyecol 1994;83:51–54.
27. Bengtsson G, Bryman I, Thorburn J, Lindblom B. Low-dose oral methotrexate as second-line therapy for persistent trophoblast after conservative treatment for ectopic pregnancy. Obstet Gynecol 1992;79:589–591.
28. Seifer DB, Barber SR, Silva PD, Grant WD, et al. Reproductive potential after treatment for persistent ectopic pregnancy. Fertil Steril 1994;62:194–195.

Avoiding Complications in Laparoscopic Management of Tubo-Ovarian Abscess

25

Scott Roberts

Laparoscopy is currently the only way to make an objective and absolute diagnosis of acute pelvic inflammatory disease (PID) (1). Its routine use for the diagnosis and management of PID remains controversial, however (2). When performed correctly, it offers an excellent and safe way to confirm diagnosis and obtain cultures (1, 3, 4).

Laparoscopy also holds promise in the treatment of pyosalpinx and pelvic abscess, with some reports of success in their laparoscopic management now emerging (5, 6). Given patient preferences for future fertility, menstrual function, and less aggressive surgical intervention, skilled gynecologists may eventually show greater willingness to use the laparoscope in initial evaluation and management of female pelvic infection.

Initial evaluation

Major considerations in PID treatment concern preoperative assessment of the need for surgical intervention. Patients refractory to initial treatment with broad-spectrum antibiotics (including anaerobe coverage) require surgical evaluation. When uncertainty persists concerning the diagnosis of pelvic infection or suspicion of rupture of pelvic abscess, immediate surgical evaluation is necessary.

Most cases of PID do not involve sequelae and respond to initial medical therapy. Routine laparoscopic evaluation of all cases of pelvic inflammatory disease is not felt to be logistically or economically feasible at this time (2). Instead, the initial pelvic examination should provide the clinician with information concerning the presence of a mass and mobility of the involved structures and can guide further evaluative efforts. Imaging studies with either ultrasound or computed tomography (CT scan) may further delineate the extent of involvement and prove helpful when patient tenderness does not permit an adequate pelvic evaluation.

Antibiotic therapy

Broad-spectrum antibiotic therapy is appropriate for all patients with PID or pelvic abscess. Initial therapy with broad-spectrum penicillins (7), penicillin/beta-lactamase inhibitor combinations (8), second-generation cephalosporins (9), carbepenams (10), clindamycin/aminoglycoside (11), and combination therapies have been found to be effective. For acute salpingitis and in the case of positive Chlamydial culture, anti-Chlamydial coverage is appropriate (12).

Unless laparoscopy is being performed for a suspect diagnosis of PID, all patients should receive therapeutic doses of appropriate antibiotics prior to surgery. Thus therapeutic levels of antibiotics should be present at the time of manipulation. For cases where PID is being ruled out, a perioperative dose of prophylactic penicillin, first-generation cephalosporin, or doxycycline may be administered after cultures from the cul-de-sac have been obtained.

Surgical intervention

Most cases that require surgical intervention may be adequately and safely evaluated with periumbilical Veress needle insertion and insufflation, followed by trocar placement with elevation of the abdominal wall. Extent of disease and further probe placement can then be performed under direct visualization.

With severe inflammatory and adhesive disease associated with pelvic abscess or an extensive history of pelvic infection, an open procedure may be the safest means of laparoscopic approach. A pneumoperitoneum may then be effected with the assurance of proper location. An open procedure may also detect those cases that do not represent good candidates for laparoscopic treatment. Careful initial dissection through a vertical subumbilical incision will detect adherent bowel and omentum. Placement of the trocar is made atraumatically to avoid injury to these structures. More probes may then be placed under direct visualization.

Microbiology

Prior to adhesiolysis, drainage, and lavage, cultures for aerobes, anaerobes, and Chlamydia should be obtained from the cul-de-sac. Normally cultures play a minor role in directing antibiotic therapy because of the delay necessary to obtain results, the polymicrobial nature of pelvic infection, and the differential sensitivity in identifying causative pathogens. Initial blood cultures may identify the patient who is bacteremic, and endocervical cultures will identify those individuals with concomitant Chlamydial and/or gonococcal infection. These results may best be used for defining prognosis, identifying a need to add Chlamydial coverage, and identifying the need to treat partners.

Adhesiolysis

A blunt probe may be used to clear away adhesions from contiguous structures involved in the inflammatory process. The surgeon should be prepared to aspirate pus, which is often concealed between contiguous structures involved with the blunt dissection. Recent infection—as evidenced by simple agglutination, pyosalpinx, and recent tubo-ovarian abscess—may be accessed with careful blunt adhesiolysis. In such cases, adhesions usually fall away quite easily. Cleavage planes within adherent bowel should be easily entered and dissected free from involved structures. For traction, atraumatic forceps can be used to grasp the round and ovarian ligaments.

Sharp dissection to achieve adhesiolysis has no place in the laparoscopic management of pelvic infection. Its apparent necessity to achieve adhesiolysis and drainage should cause the surgeon to question the safety of proceeding with laparoscopic management. Any bleeding that arises during the dissection should be managed with warm physiologic saline lavage, patience, and occasionally bipolar coagulation.

The demonstration of a heterogeneous mass in the cul-de-sac, the presence of severely adherent bowel obscuring the pelvic structures, or difficulty in achieving blunt adhesiolysis are indications of chronic pelvic abscess or infection and mandate laparotomy unless an abscess in the Pouch of Douglas has previously been identified. In the latter case, culdotomy with placement of a large-bore Malecot drain may be attempted (13).

Drainage

Direct visualization of the abscess or pyosalpinx facilitates drainage. A true pyosalpinx should be managed by making a longitudinal incision along the antimesenteric border. Expression of pus, gentle suction, and saline lavage are then undertaken. Tubal abscess may be managed with careful blunt dissection. In this instance, the surgeon grasps the ampulla with the rounded forceps, grasps and places traction on fibrinous exudate concealing pus in the tubal lumen, and then does the same for any expression of purulent exudate from the fimbriated end of the tube (14).

Recent tubo-ovarian abscess may be isolated laparoscopically with the same techniques as previously described. In such a case, rupture of the abscess will allow perioperative drainage and lavage. Chronic tubo-ovarian abscess is usually associated with severe adhesions and structural deformation of pelvic architecture. For the most part it is inaccessible by blunt dissection and not amenable to laparoscopic management. This condition should instead be managed with laparotomy.

Lavage

Irrigation and lavage of the affected areas during and after the procedure are important steps in reducing the bacterial counts left in the pelvis and peritoneal cavity. The use of warm saline can also help to achieve hemostasis. Use of antibiotic-containing solutions should not be necessary in this lavage, as the tissue concentrations needed to treat infection will already be present because of parenteral administration of broad-spectrum therapy (as previously described). The placement of active drains should be at the surgeon's discretion after optimum surgical therapy has been achieved.

Postoperative care

After laparoscopic therapy has been concluded, the patient should be carefully followed to detect any need to return to the operating room for subsequent therapy. If the treatment fails or the patient's condition worsens, laparoscopy may not be the best choice for subsequent therapy. Usually a period of 48 to 72 hours is required to evaluate the adequacy of treatment. If the patient appears to be worsening despite adhesiolysis and drainage, however, laparotomy with extirpative therapy can be life-saving.

In general, as our knowledge of pelvic infection and antibiotics improve, so should our ability to pursue conservative rather than extirpative therapy. As surgeons' laparoscopic skills and the relevant equipment improve, so should our ability to manage pelvic infections without laparotomy. It is therefore only appropriate that prospective evaluations of laparoscopic management of pelvic infection, particularly pelvic abscess, be performed and published.

REFERENCES

1. Jacobson L, Westrom L. Objectivized diagnosis of acute pelvic inflammatory disease. Am J Obstet Gynecol 1969;105:1088.
2. Sweet RL, Gibbs RS. Pelvic inflammatory disease. In: Brown CL, ed. Infectious diseases of the female genital tract, 2nd ed. Baltimore: Williams and Wilkins; 1990:254–255.
3. Chapporo MV, Ghosh S, Nashed A, et al. Laparoscopy for confirmation and prognostic evaluation of pelvic inflammatory disease. Int J Gynecol Obstet 1978;15:307–311.
4. Sweet RL, Draper DL, Schachter J, et al. Microbiology and pathogenesis of acute salpingitis as determined by laparoscopy: what is the appropriate site to sample? Am J Obstet Gynecol 1980; 138:985.
5. Adducci JE. Laparoscopy in the diagnosis and treatment of pelvic inflammatory disease abscess formation. Int Surg 1981;66:359.
6. Henry-Souchet J, Soler A-M, Laffredo V. Laparoscopic treatment of tuboovarian abscesses. J Reprod Med 1984;29:579–582.
7. Dinsmoor MJ, Gibbs RS. The role of the newer antimicrobial agents in obstetrics and gynecology. Clin Obstet Gynecol 1988;31:423–424.
8. Eschenbach D, Faro S, Postorek JH II, et al. Treatment of patients with obstetric and gynecologic infections. A scientific exhibit presented at the annual meeting of the American College of Obstetricians and Gynecologists, San Francisco, May 7–10, 1984.
9. Hemsell DL, Wendel GD, Gall SA, et al. Multicenter comparison of cefotetan and cefoxitin in the treatment of acute obstetric and gynecologic infections. Am J Obstet Gynecol 1988;158:722–727.
10. Sweet RL. Imipenem/cilistatin in the treatment of obstetric and gynecologic infections: A review of worldwide experience. Rev Infect Dis 1985;7(suppl):522–527.
11. Gall SA, Kohan AP, Ayers OM, et al. Intravenous metronidazole or clindamycin with tobramycin for therapy of pelvic infections. Obstet Gynecol 1981;57:51.
12. Centers for Disease Control. 1989 STD treatment guidelines. MMWR 1989;38(S):31–34.
13. Rivlin ME, Golan A, Darling MR. Diffuse peritoneal sepsis associated with colpotomy drainage of pelvic abscess. Obstet Gynecol 1983;61:169.
14. Bruhat M-A, Canis M, Mage G, Manhes H, Pouly J-L, Wattiez A. Pelvic inflammatory disease. In: Pennington JE, Navrozov M, eds. Duvier R, Vancaillie TG, trans. Operative laparoscopy. Paris: MEDSI/McGraw-Hill, 1992:63–64.

26 | Laparoscopic Microsurgical Tubal Anastomosis—Difficulties and Pitfalls

Charles H. Koh and Grace M. Janik

The era for gynecologic microsurgery began conceptually with Swolin (1) in 1968 and was extended to the art of microsuturing by Gomel (2) and Winston (3) when they published the first series on microsurgical anastomosis in 1977. The microsurgical principles and techniques established in these works included magnification, fine instrumentation for accuracy, and microsutures (i.e., 7-0, 8-0, 9-0, 10-0) that more closely matched the size of the tubal lumen being apposed (which could be as small as 500 microns). Concomitant with microsurgical technique came a new respect for tissue and the practice of atraumatic surgery. In April 1992 we presented the world's first laparoscopic microsurgical tubal anastomosis with 8-0 nylon (4). The technique has since evolved, with new ultramicroinstrumentation (5) for laparoscopic microsurgery being designed.

Nevertheless, many challenges remain. In this chapter we hope to highlight some of the pitfalls and how they can be overcome or anticipated.

Skills

The endoscopist embarking on laparoscopic tubal anastomosis must be both a skilled microsurgeon and an endoscopist. The former experience will provide the necessary complement to assessment of tubal normalcy and pathology, as well as anticipated results of surgery. For the initial cases, two surgeons working together is essential.

Patient selection

The ideal location for laparoscopic anastomosis is mid-tubal and ampullary. Tubal cornual anastomosis should not be attempted by any laparoscopist who has not attained considerable experience with laparoscopic anastomosis. Therefore, a preliminary hysterosalpingogram is essential to select out these cases for laparotomy. A pre-liminary microlaparoscopy is suggested for all cases of electrosurgical sterilization (especially unipolar procedures), as the tubal length available cannot be inferred from the operative report. Such preparation avoids operating room schedule disruptions.

Microinstrumentation

Micrograspers used for laparoscopic microsurgery should have a tip diameter of 250 to 500 microns and have jaw characteristics that allow the suture to be pulled without slippage or snapping. The choice of such instruments will spare hours of frustration and can make the difference between success or failure to complete surgery.

The tips of these instruments should enable the surgeon to grasp the serosa of the fallopian tube without causing petechiae. The needle holder should be able to hold the needle firmly, but at the same time not crush the microneedle. To meet these goals, specially designed microinstruments and needle holders for laparoscopic microsurgery (5) are essential. Driving the needle without causing it to bend depends on a highly developed sense of touch such that the force driving the needle is always axial and not lateral.

Needle and suture materials

For tubal anastomosis, experience at "open" microsurgery has shown that 7-0 and 8-0 sutures are adequate. For our part, the authors try to avoid going intraluminal with 7-0 sutures. The debate over using absorbable versus nonabsorbable suture seems to have evolved into two camps, with both touting data showing that their suture of choice causes less tissue reaction (2, 3). These studies apply to 8-0 and finer suture material, and thus may not have relevancy for larger sutures.

With laparoscopic microsurgery, the choice of suture

becomes more limited because of the needle characteristics. The latest generation of "tru-taper" titanium needles require less force for tissue penetration because of their design, and rigidity afforded by the titanium material prevents needle bending. We have found that the BV175-6 needle with a core diameter of 175 microns is ideal. More recently, a 135-micron 5-mm needle has been produced with the same material. As this needle is swaged to 7-0 and 8-0 prolene, this suture can be used for tubal anastomosis. From a laparoscopic standpoint, black nylon or ethilon is the most ideal for visibility. Plain Vicryl, which absorbs blood, is less discernible. All of these materials demonstrate adequate tensile strength.

For intracorporeal knot tying, the more rigid monofilament sutures have an advantage over braided sutures in forming loops. On the other hand, the monofilaments are more likely to become crinkled because of their memory. Whenever this situation arises, a new suture should be used.

Trocars and trocar sites

For secondary ports, the authors use 5-mm trocars that reduce to 3 mm for the ultramicroinstrumentation. For maximal versatility, we use three 5-mm trocars; if a fourth is needed, a 3-mm trocar can be introduced. This approach allows the substitution of suction irrigators, bipolar, and other 5-mm instruments as well as the use of the 3-mm ultramicroinstrumentation.

The trocar site is the key to successful micro—or indeed macro—suturing. Figure 26.1 illustrates placement of the lateral ports, with the lower ports being no more than 2 cm medial to the anterior superior iliac spine, and the other sites level with the umbilicus (paraumbilical) and having the same laterality as the lower ports. After abdominal wall insufflation, the lateral ports allow the surgeon to operate with the upper arm and elbows adducted so that only wrist and finger movements are needed to accomplish the microsuturing. Traditional port placement, which is more medial or even central, causes the operator to extend the upper arms away from the body. Such a position is not conducive to accurate, relaxed microsuturing, as it prohibits fine movements.

Magnification and resolution

The degree of magnification required for either open or laparoscopic microsurgery should be sufficient to allow differentiation of healthy from diseased tubal muscosa and muscularis, which at the interstitial and isthmic area may involve luminal diameters of 0.5 mm. Although the operating microscope permits magnification as high as $40\times$, $26\times$ magnification is usually adequate for examination, and $10–15\times$ normally proves adequate for suture placement and tying. Laparoscopic microsurgery requires similar magnification.

Operating from a television monitor is absolutely essential to reduce fatigue, improve fine control, and enable meaningful assistance from the assistant surgeon. The authors initially used the single-chip zoom camera system manufactured by Storz, which gave reasonable $10–15\times$ magnification. Recently, we have used a three-chip camera, which provides superior resolution at 800 lines. The Storz 0° Hopkins laparoscope offers exceptional depth of field and remains in focus at macro range, thus facilitating magnification. A digital enhancer improves contrast, thereby increasing suture visibility. The third component of the set-up consists of a Sony 20-inch monitor with 800 lines of horizontal resolution. With this combination, it is possible to make a 1-cm probe fill the whole screen horizontally, giving a magnification of $40:1$, with usable resolution (the best measure of a laparoscope's magnification) rivaling that of the operating microscope.

A good test of the adequacy of the system is to bring the laparoscope to within 1 cm of the fallopian tube for extreme magnification. In this position, the surgeon should be able to see detail of the muscularis and mucosa within individual vessel and muscle bundles. If the telescope/camera/television combination does not provide sufficiently high resolution or the auto-iris does not work well, a whiteout of the muscularis and a loss of detail will be obvious. Such a set-up is not adequate for inspection or suturing.

Although videolaparoscopy lacks stereoscopic vision, this absence should not pose a problem as the surgeon becomes accustomed to two-dimensional surgery, particularly with magnification. In fact, current three-dimensional camera systems are not recommended for microsurgery because they introduce "strobe" and other visual artifacts, which can inhibit fine movement.

Tubal preparation

For preparation of the proximal tube, dilute $1:50$ pitressin is injected to lift the serosa. This material is then incised using a 150-micron microneedle to expose the muscularis and mobilize the proximal tube from the mesosalpinx. By keeping close to the muscularis, it is possible to avoid dividing the mesosalpingeal vessel. A segment of approximately 5 to 10 mm is cut off from the proximal tube using a guillotine or sharp scissors, and the tubal muscularis and mucosa (after methylene blue instillation) are examined for normalcy and patency. Preparation of the proximal tube is easier and requires that the surgeon perform only serial cuts until satisfied that the tissue is vital. Because no true "micro" bipolar forceps are available, care is needed to avoid overcoagulation of vessels.

Preparation of the distal tube is much more difficult and critical. The laparoscopic approach is unforgiving of errors, and it is virtually impossible to repair an opening that has been made too large to achieve an equal lumen anastomosis. Therefore, time invested at this stage will ensure success. After dissecting the stump free, pitressin is injected, and the serosa of the proximal part of the distal tube is divided. With elegant microdissection, it is possible to see the blind end of the muscularis. This tissue is then picked up by the assistant's grasper, causing it to tent. With the use of a gauge that confirms whether the proximal opening is 1, 2, or 3 mm in diameter, the laparoscopist fashions the cut of the distal tube (via a guillotine) such that the lumen is no more than 1 mm larger than the proximal tube. Chromopertubation is performed through this opening and the fimbria is inspected for the emergence of dye. Unfortunately, this delicate procedure can easily cause the proximal opening to rip apart. The authors use a specially designed chromopertubator for efficiency and to prevent such accidental tearing.

Suturing difficulties and pitfalls

The most critical aspect of microsurgical anastomosis is the accurate placement of the microneedle into the tubal muscularis in a precise radial manner at 3, 6, 9, and 12 o'clock. Holding the needle with the sharp end at the concavity of the curved jaw typically provides better laparoscopic visualization of the direction of the needle and greater control over its movement. The fallopian tube can be held by the assistant grasper and positioned so that rotatory motion of the needle holder can be practiced and observation confirms that the needle is directed radially toward the tubal lumen. Following this practice motion, the actual needle insertion into tissue takes place. Because of the needle characteristics, it is not necessary to hold tissue to counterpress the needle insertion. Instead, the resistance and weight of the tissue provide the countertraction to needle entry.

For needle exit, the assistant grasper is used to counterpush the tissue against the needle. The needle holder is then released and picks up the tip of the needle, pulling it through the tissue. It is better not to attempt to grasp the tip of the needle as it emerges through the tissue with an assistant grasper before releasing the needle holder (which is often done in fear that the needle will slip back into the tissue) as this technique often leads to problems because of poor visualization, tremor, and disruption.

In midtubal anastomosis, both left and right suture placement may be undertaken with the operator standing on the right side of the patient. To avoid cornual anastomosis, it should be noted that it is very difficult to place radial sutures into the immobile tubal cornua and to visualize the cornua with the 0° umbilical laparoscope.

An attempt to use an angled laparoscope in this situation will cause further disorientation and confusion.

Figures 26.2 through 26.21 illustrate a contralateral and ipsilateral technique of suturing that is, in fact, applicable to both macro and micro suturing. As previously mentioned, the port positions are critical considerations because they can minimize surgeon fatigue and tremor. The "address" position or set-up of the "U" or "C" positions is absolutely vital to ensure easy, successful knot tying. Time invested in achieving this address will be richly rewarded.

Note that the tips of the graspers are close to one another and to the suture end to be picked up. This method ensures that after the loops have been thrown,

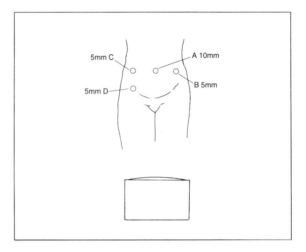

Fig. 26.1 Position of portals: 3 mm reducers are used at 5 mm ports (B, C, D) for the ultramicro instruments.

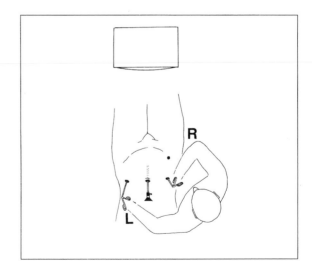

Fig. 26.2 The surgeon's left arm crosses to the opposite (contralateral) side for suturing.

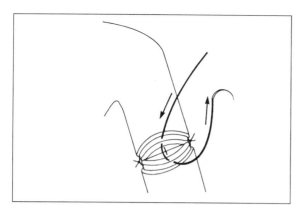

Fig. 26.3 The most important aspect is a proper initial grasper positioning similar to the address in golfing. The address for intracorporeal suturing is the "U" position as illustrated. Failure to adopt to address position as depicted will result in frustration and often failure. The 6, 3, and 9 o'clock sutures have been tied. The suturing technique is being demonstrated for the 12 o'clock suture.

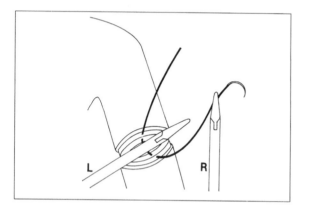

Fig. 26.4 The contralateral left grasper is positioned at the base of the "U" parallel to the long (needle) arm of the "U."

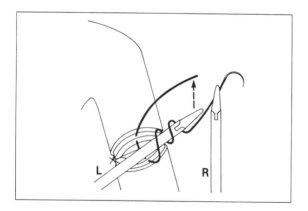

Fig. 26.5 The needle end of the suture is held with the right hand grasper, which proceeds to throw a clockwise double loop over the left grasper.

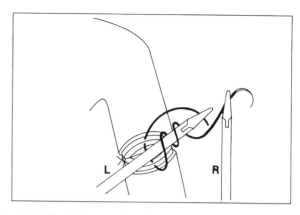

Fig. 26.6 The left (contralateral) grasper picks up the short end.

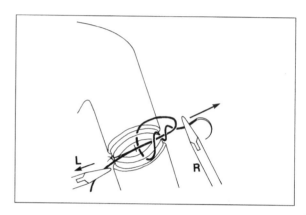

Fig. 26.7 Pull is exerted in opposite directions (note arrows) to cinch the knot squarely.

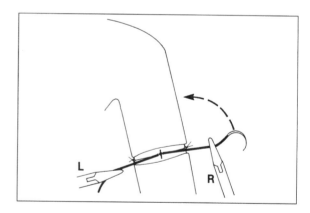

Fig. 26.8 The first knot has been tightened. Arrow shows movement of right grasper to pass the long end of the suture to the left contralateral grasper.

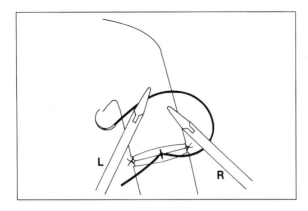

Fig. 26.9 After the left grasper picks up the long end, the address now becomes an "inverted U" or "inverted C."

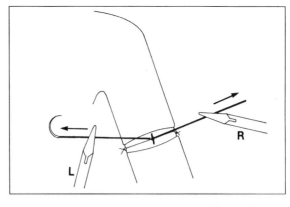

Fig. 26.12 The completed surgeon's square knot is shown.

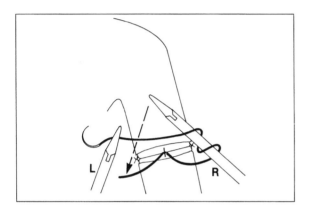

Fig. 26.10 The second knot is counterclockwise single loop over the right grasper.

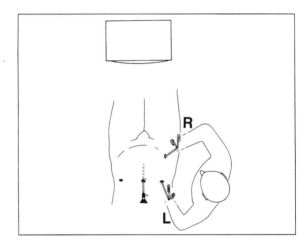

Fig. 26.13 In this method, both arms remain on the ipsilateral side of the patient. The left arm of the surgeon does not have to cross over to the contralateral side and, therefore, fatigue is decreased. This is the most advanced form of intracorporeal suturing and requires considerably more dexterity and experience than the contralateral method. When properly mastered, it is rapid and allows the assistant to assist with the contralateral grasper.

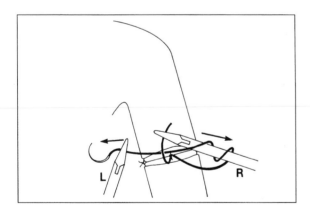

Fig. 26.11 The short end has been picked up by the right grasper and cinching begins.

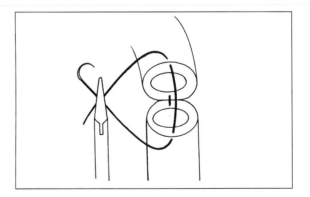

Fig. 26.14 The 6 o'clock suture has been tied. The 12 o'clock suture has been placed and is held by the contralateral grasper by the assistant.

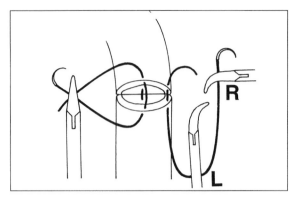

Fig. 26.15 The contralateral grasper rotates the tube counterclockwise to expose the 3 o'clock area to aid in suture placement. The suture has passed from proximal to distal tube, and pulled through. The "U" address is now prepared by the right grasper (R) holding up the needle end.

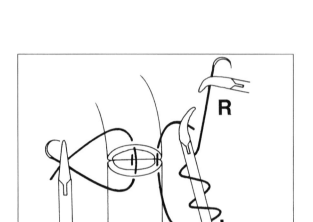

Fig. 26.16 A double clockwise loop has been thrown over the left (L) ultramicro grasper which then picks the short end of the suture.

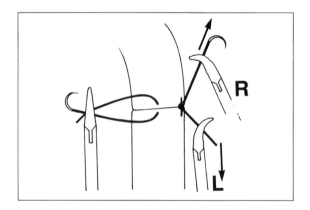

Fig. 26.17 The knot is cinched by pulling in the direction of the arrows.

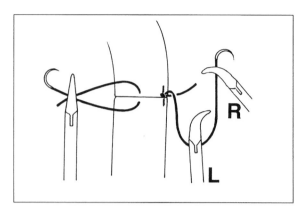

Fig. 26.18 The "U" address is again formed.

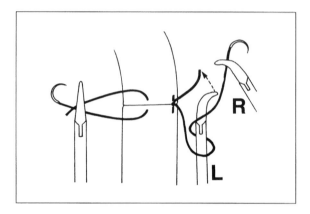

Fig. 26.19 A single counterclockwise loop is thrown over the left grasper (L) held by the left hand of the operator which then picks up the short end.

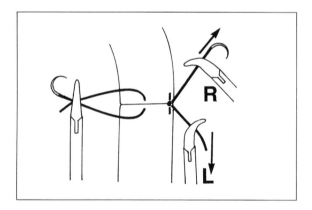

Fig. 26.20 After pulling in opposite directions the knot is completed.

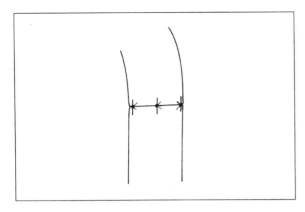

Fig. 26.21 7-0 interrupted serosa sutures complete the anastomosis.

Table 26.1. Results of laparoscopic tubal anastomosis

	Patient Data
Total patients	$n = 31$
Age (mean)	33.5 ± 3.8 years
Range	26–39 years
Total patients pregnant	$n = 22$ (71%)
Ectopic pregnancy	$n = 1$ (3.2%)
Surgery to pregnancy interval	4.3 ± 2.5 months
Range	1.5–10 months

Table 26.2. Cumulative pregnancy rates (quarterly intervals).

Interval	0–3 months	3–6 months	6–9 months	9–12 months
Pregnancy	11 (35.5%)	6 (54.8%)	4 (67.7%)	1 (71%)*

*Ectopic.

the grasper does not search for the suture end or back up on itself; such maneuvers often lead to the loop falling out of the shaft, resulting in the need to repeat the entire process.

When cinching the knot, care must be taken not to pull the suture away from the fallopian tube, as it may cause cutting out. Mesosalpingeal and serosal closure relieves tension on the completed anastomosis, which otherwise may fall apart from any accidental rough motion. It is not necessary to attempt a "perfect" serosal closure, as the breach will heal well even without suturing and the closure is needed only to maintain immediate postoperative strength.

Results

The pregnancy outcome we have achieved with this technique has been gratifying, especially the fact that pregnancies occur somewhat earlier than with other surgical approaches. Our cumulative pregnancy rates are reflected in Tables 26.1 and 26.2.

Conclusion

Laparoscopic microsurgical tubal anastomosis is a viable alternative to open laparotomy or minilaparotomy microsurgery. Its advantages over minilaparotomy include its applicability to obese patients and patients who have undergone previous surgery (6), the panoramic view of the pelvis that makes treatment of endometriosis or adhesions possible, and the relatively easy ampullary anastomosis as compared with minilaparotomy. The learning curve is long and steep, however, and specialized training and practice are essential before embarking on human anastomosis.

With judicious attention to detail and practice, we foresee laparoscopic microsurgery replacing open microsurgery in the future.

REFERENCES

1. Swolin K. Fifty fertilatiasoperationen, vols. 1–2. Microsurgical concepts for infertility surgery. Acta Obstet Gynecol Scand 1967;46(2):234–267.
2. Gomel V. Tubal reconstruction by microsurgery. Fertil Steril 1977;28:59.
3. Winston RML. Microsurgical tubocornual anastomosis for reversal of sterilization. Lancet 1977;1:284.
4. Koh CH, Janik GM. Laparoscopic microsurgical tubal reanastomosis (abstracts). The fallopian tube: advances in diagnosis and surgical treatment. Presented at the Third Conference, The Royal London Hospital, London, April 1–3, 1992.
5. Koh CH. Laparoscopic microsuturing. Culver City: Karl Storz Endoscopy-America, 1994.
6. Silva PD, Schaper AM, Meisch JK, Schauberger CW. Outpatient microsurgical reversal of tubal sterilization by a combined approach of laparoscopy and minilaparotomy. Fertil Steril 1991;55:696–699.

Endometriosis in the Cul-de-sac: Complications of Treatment

27

Gordon D. Davis

The cul-de-sac is one of the most common pelvic areas affected by endometriosis. The presence of endometriosis in the cul-de-sac may produce dyspareunia, dyschezia, or generalized pelvic pain. The diagnosis of endometriosis in this location is suggested by cul-de-sac tenderness or modularity on pelvic examination. Intervention occurs most frequently to relieve these painful symptoms, but the diagnosis of cul-de-sac endometriosis is most often made at laparoscopy for infertility (1).

Because of the proximity of the rectum, surgical treatment of endometriosis in this region takes on special considerations. Injury to the rectum in the patient without proper bowel preparation results in serious morbidity and may result in death. A through knowledge of the anatomy of this region of the pelvis is mandatory.

Characteristics of cul-de-sac endometriosis

Recognition

The posterior peritoneum covers the surface of the rectum and is reflected superiorly from the most dependent aspect of the pelvis onto the uterus as serosa. The boundaries of this peritoneum (and thus the cul-de-sac) are the rectum posteriorly, the vagina inferiorly, the cervix superiorly, and the uterosacral ligaments laterally.

Peritoneum covering the uterosacral ligaments, although visually normal, has been reported to contain endometriosis in 6% of patients. The size of the lesions varied from 88 to 720 μm. Similar findings were noted by a scanning electron microscopy study of peritoneum excised elsewhere in the pelvis (2). This result suggests that the pelvic peritoneum deserves careful scrutiny when endometriosis is suspected. The peritoneal surface may have more fibrotic and less red or other atypical lesions as a function of time (3). Infiltrating lesions may, however, be covered by a pleomorphic peritoneum.

Peritoneal lesions vary drastically in appearance, ranging from dark, cystic lesions to small, clear blebs

(4). Nodular implants may be visible or appreciated only by palpation. Lesion color changes little during the phases of the menstrual cycle but varies as a function of the patient's age (5).

Some endometriosis is palpable but not visible laparoscopically. This condition is most commonly seen with deep disease in the uterosacral ligaments, the rectum, the vagina, and the sigmoid colon. The small bowel, the appendix, and the mesentery may display puckering and no colorful changes.

Direct implantation, lymphatic spread, seeding of endometrial cells at the time of surgery, and metaplasia may all produce cul-de-sac endometriosis. Several routes of dissemination have been described and may account for the occasional finding of endometriosis in the deep pelvis, where it may be neither visible nor palpable. Endometriosis of the retroperitoneal lymph nodes is believed to be rare, but the incidence of such lesions is unknown.

Whether infiltrating (>5 mm) or superficial endometriosis of the cul-de-sac decreases fecundity is controversial. In this location, however, both forms of endometriosis may produce dyspareunia. With fibrosis and infiltration, the cul-de-sac may be completely replaced with endometriosis. The proximity of the rectum accounts for the frequent coexistence of serosal and muscularis rectal lesions.

Superficial endometriosis of the cul-de-sac most frequently arises in or penetrates the peritoneum and is confined along the fatty space below the mesothelial surface. Fibrosis, cyst formation, and penetration along the fibromuscular septae may permit cul-de-sac endometriosis to invade deeply into the rectovaginal septum and uterosacral ligaments as well as the fatty tissue of the cul-de-sac. Superficial and invasive cul-de-sac lesions behave differently, but both often require surgical intervention. Over time superficial and atypical lesions may give way to infiltrating disease (6).

Cul-de-sac obliteration

Complete anatomical distortion of the cul-de-sac was defined by Sampson (7). The severity of this surgical problem is not reflected in most staging systems. While cul-de-sac obliteration represents the most difficult challenge for the endometriosis surgeon, it also provides the greatest risk for complications to the patient.

Reich has separated partial cul-de-sac occlusion from complete cul-de-sac obliteration. This determination is made at the time of laparoscopy. Partial obliteration is separated from complete cul-de-sac obliteration by whether the vagina can be visualized by the manipulation of the vaginal fornices at laparoscopy using an intravaginal probe. The probe is placed in the posterior vaginal fornix and attempts are made to visualize the cul-de-sac. If no part of the vagina is visualized, the cul-de-sac is considered to be completely obliterated and rectal involvement is more extensive. If the lateral margin or superior aspect of the cul-de-sac permits visualization of the apex of the vagina, partial cul-de-sac obliteration is said to be present. This condition carries significant surgical implications since the bulk of the endometriotic lesion is frequently lateral to the rectum with partial cul-de-sac obliteration.

Complications

Superficial cul-de-sac lesions (1–2 mm)

Any mode of ablation is satisfactory for superficial cul-de-sac lesions (1–2 mm). Thermal energy sources and sharp excision are the most common methods of destruction of these lesions. Laser vaporization, bipolar or monopolar electrosurgery, or scissors dissection are satisfactory for such lesions as long as large surface areas are not involved. When the entire cul-de-sac is involved with superficial lesions, it is recommended that the peritoneum be excised. Excision of extensive superficial implants in the cul-de-sac is associated with a shorter healing phase than is thermal destruction. In either case, in general, the rectum is not at risk nor is any significant risk of bleeding incurred. A thorough knowledge of thermal energy sources and their depth of penetration is mandatory for safe ablation of cul-de-sac lesions.

Intermediate lesions (<5 mm)

Intermediate lesions may be managed by vaporization or coagulation if focal. More frequently, however, lesions of 5-mm diameter require excision for total ablation. If coagulation or vaporization with lasers is selected as the mode of ablation of these lesions, care should be taken to limit the amount of thermal conduction onto the surface of the rectum and surrounding tissues.

The most common complication of attempts to ablate intermediate size lesions by coagulation or vaporization is failure to completely destroy the lesion. This results in persistence of endometriosis and sometimes in excessive carbon deposition secondary to the vaporization process.

Effective ablation of intermediate size lesions is more efficiently performed by coagulation combined with excision or by excision alone. In a stepwise manner, these lesions may be elevated and excised by sharp, electrosurgical, or laser dissection.

Deeply infiltrating lesions (>5 mm)

Deeply infiltrating lesions may penetrate into the upper aspect of the vagina and involve the posterior cervix. These lesions may be excised via a combination of laparoscopic and vaginal approaches. The most common complication of dissecting a large rectovaginal nodule is bleeding from the lateral vaginal veins. When it occurs, bipolar coagulation has almost always been effective in controlling such bleeding. Occasionally the surgeon may have to resort to suturing either laparoscopically or transvaginally. Vaginal packing has not been utilized in our series of patients.

Cul-de-sac obliteration

The sigmoid colon and rectum are at risk with partial or complete cul-de-sac obliteration. The frequency of entry into the vagina depends upon the aggressiveness of the surgeon. Entry into the vagina is often required to completely excise infiltrating endometriosis or to gain access to lateral or to posterior cervical lesions. Vaginal entry is not considered to be a complication, and the vagina may be closed in a proper fashion either vaginally or laparoscopically. However, such entry exposes the pelvic tissue to contamination and the risk of pelvic abscess. This complication has been encountered in 2 per 500 cases.

Rectal entry, however, constitutes a major complication, particularly if the bowel is unprepared or if it is not anticipated and recognized by the surgeon. One may inadvertently injure the rectum by miscalculating the depth of penetration of endometriosis or the extent of cystic disease of the bowel wall. The frequency of this type of injury relates to the willingness of the surgeon to pursue deeply infiltrating rectal disease. When the rectum is adherent to the posterior aspect of the cervix or uterosacral ligaments, blunt dissection may lacerate the rectum away from the endometriosis. Therefore, we recommend sharp dissection with a mechanical (scissors) or thermal energy source (CO_2 laser).

A proper bowel preparation is mandatory in all patients with cul-de-sac occlusion and we recommend the following regimen:

1. No solid foods for at least 36 hours prior to surgery (clear liquid diet).
2. GoLytely 4 liters by mouth beginning the afternoon prior to surgery.

3. Erythromycin or neomycin base: at least six doses of erythromycin or neomycin base to be initiated just prior to beginning the mechanical bowel preparation with GoLytely.

This mechanical and chemical bowel preparation has been satisfactory in all of our patients requiring treatment for rectal nodules where entry into the bowel is a risk. We also utilize this regimen when bowel resection and end-to-end anastomosis are planned. This preparation will diminish but not eliminate cellulitis and abscess formation.

If the patient cannot tolerate a bowel preparation in the outpatient setting, it is unwise to proceed with surgery. The patient should instead be admitted to the hospital for supervised bowel preparation.

Avoidance of entry into the bowel is facilitated by beginning the cul-de-sac dissection at the rectal border of the lesion. Often a curvilinear incision is made at the level of the arch of the uterosacral ligaments at the posterior aspect of the cervix in normal tissue. Nodules are dissected free from the ligaments and the uterus. The operator may be surprised to find that it is then difficult to identify completely the rectal component of the lesion. It is more common for endometriosis to infiltrate along the uterosacral ligaments and into the posterior aspect of the cervix or superior aspect of the vagina than to be full thickness through the bowel. If the rectal lesion is superficial, the risk of entry into the rectum is dramatically decreased. If deep rectal involvement is present, it should be visible or palpable early in the dissection and carries a high risk of rectal entry.

A rectal probe and a vaginal probe are mandatory for the identification of structures at the time of dissection. The vagina is reflected anteriorly and cephalad, and the rectum is displaced posteriorly. Although almost any instrument that does not cause significant trauma to the mucosa of the rectum may be used as a rectal probe, the more oval, smooth instruments are recommended. For the vaginal probe, a ring forceps or other instrument with a blunt end may serve as a probe. It is often helpful to place a folded sponge in the jaws of the ring forceps.

Rectal and vaginal examination is an indispensable component of cul-de-sac surgery. A qualified assistant may be able to palpitate nodules or extensions of fibrotic disease not visible at laparoscopy. A thorough recto-vaginal examination prior to and following completion of cul-de-sac dissection is mandatory.

Avoidance of entry into the rectum during resection of cul-de-sac endometriosis is dependent upon careful visualization of the tissue planes with the magnification afforded by the laparoscope and good lighting. Should inadvertent entry into the rectum occur in the patient who has undergone the proper bowel preparation, primary closure with proper surgical consultation may be performed laparoscopically.

Pockets

In the cul-de-sac near the uterosacral ligaments, invaginations of peritoneum (peritoneal defects) are found in a significant number of patients with endometriosis (8). In our series of patients the incidence of such pockets approximates 10%. When excised, the peritoneum lining these pockets is usually positive for endometriosis if endometriosis is noted elsewhere. Peritoneal pockets may extend into the avascular spaces in the lateral and dependent pelvis. Pockets have been described lateral to the ureter, although this finding is rare. Peritoneal pockets may be considered to be hernias with a very low incidence of bowel entrapment. They are most commonly found just under the medial aspect of the uterosacral ligaments.

"Secondary" peritoneal pockets refers to pockets formed by fibrosis from endometriosis. True peritoneal pockets, however, are probably developmental anomalies. They may be quite subtle; their peritoneal ostia may be mere pinpoints. The application of pressure following the instillation of fluid into the cul-de-sac and its subsequent aspiration may be helpful in identifying subtle peritoneal pockets. Such fluid may be seen to escape from the ostia of pockets.

Complications of the management of cul-de-sac endometriosis in peritoneal pockets are uncommon. The peritoneal pocket should be grasped at or near its base, gently everted, and explored. Laser dissection or sharp dissection may be used to open the pocket. Subtle pockets with small ostia may require an incision or other dissection to increase the size of the pocket opening. After grasping forceps are used to evert the pocket, the peritoneum may be dissected free. If the ostium of the pocket is small, the pocket will usually close with the fibrosis of healing after removal of its peritoneal lining. Large pockets may become reperitonealized and serve as a site of recurrent endometriosis. For this reason, it is prudent to close large pockets after resection of their peritoneal component and any associated infiltrating endometriosis.

Complications related to excision of peritoneal pockets generally involve bleeding. Veins or small arteries are sometimes encountered and require desiccation. This finding occurs in approximately one per ten peritoneal pockets, but is related to the depth of the pocket, since deeper peritoneal pockets have been noted to be associated with more peritoneal surface area and, therefore, more subperitoneal supportive tissue that is likely to contain blood vessels. Most often after eversion of the pocket and while dissecting the peritoneum from the pocket or excising a nodule from the base of the pocket, a vein is entered and bipolar coagulation is utilized to desiccate the vein or small artery. Alternatively, sutures or loop ligatures may be used prophylactically, particularly if a nodule of significant size is present and bleeding is anticipated. Avoidance of such complications requires the surgeon to confine the dissection to the peritoneum or nodule only, restricting entry into the pelvic supportive tissue through which the pocket penetrates. The lateral sulcus veins of the paravaginal tissue and the blood supply to the rectal wall are generally not at risk when dissecting peritoneal pockets.

Injury to the rectum

Injury to the rectum is extremely rare as related to removal of peritoneal pockets. We have not encountered this complication, but the rectum is theoretically at risk with some broad-based pockets. Pockets, in general, descend in a lateral position to the rectum. Care must be taken, however, to maintain good visualization when dissecting peritoneum from pockets in the perirectal tissue.

Ureteral injury

In our experience, the ureter is not at significant risk when dissecting the more dependent primary peritoneal pockets. When a secondary pocket of the pelvic side wall superior to the uterosacral ligaments is encountered, the ureter is theoretically at risk and should be isolated by dissection. The ureter has been superior to every pocket thus far encountered in our series. Sampson described a peritoneal pocket that communicated with the sciatic nerve, indicating that variation may be extreme. Avoidance of complications when dissecting peritoneal pockets is dependent upon careful delicate dissection of the involved peritoneum.

Cul-de-sac healing

Complications such as scarring or adhesions of the cul-de-sac occur in as many as 10% to 20% of patients with cul-de-sac obliteration. With extensive electrosurgical applications to endometriosis lesions of the cul-de-sac, granulation tissue forms that may persist. Similarly, with vaporization with lasers or desiccation with electrosurgery, granulation tissue may develop from the carbon deposited. With sharp excision, cul-de-sac adhesions may form. When excision of the cul-de-sac peritoneum is performed by any method, healing usually occurs without significant granulation tissue. Occasionally, anteroposterior adhesions may form between the uterus and the regenerated peritoneum. These adhesions are usually of minimal clinical consequence. They may, however, obscure visualization of residual or recurrent endometriosis.

After excision of the cul-de-sac peritoneum, we have found it beneficial to plicate the uterosacral ligaments with sutures. This strategy reduces the amount of healing time and preserves a more normal anatomical relationship between the apex of the vagina, the rectum, and the uterus. One or two sutures placed laparoscopically have sufficed in such plications. We do not advocate producing a shelf that might be palpable vaginally.

REFERENCES

1. Wild RA, Wilson EA. Clinical presentation and diagnosis. In: Wilson EA, ed. Endometriosis. New York: Liss, 1987:53.
2. Murphy AA, Green WR, Bobbie D, *et al*. Unsuspected endometriosis documented by scanning electron microscopy in visually normal peritoneum. Fertil Steril 1986;46:522–524.
3. Koninckx PR, Meuleman C, Demeyers S, *et al*. Suggestive evidence that pelvic endometriosis is a progressive disease, whereas deeply infiltrating endometriosis is associated with pelvic pain. Fertil Steril 1991;55:759–766.
4. Jansen PS, Russel P. Nonpigmented endometriosis: clinical laparoscopy and pathological definition. Am J Obstet Gynecol 1986;155:1154–1159.
5. Redwine DB. Age-related evolution and color appearance of endometriosis. Fertil Steril 1987;48:1062–1063.
6. Koninckx PR. Cornillie FJ. Deeply infiltrating endometriosis: a new entity. In: Shaw RW, ed. Advances in endocrinology I: endometriosis. Lancaster: Parthenon Publishing Group, 1990:31.
7. Sampson JA. Heterotrophic or misplaced endometrial tissue. Am J Obstet Gynecol 1925;10:649–651.
8. Chatman DL, Lbella EA. Pelvic endometrial defects and endoscopy: further observations. Fertil Steril 1986;46:711–714.

Intestinal Endometriosis: Diagnosis and Endoscopic Treatment with Attention to the Prevention, Recognition, and Management of Complications

28

George M. Grunert and Robert R. Franklin

Introduction

With the rapid evolution of operative and laser laparoscopic technology, an increasing emphasis has been placed on use of this approach for surgical treatment of endometriosis. In this chapter, we will discuss the presentation, diagnosis, preoperative evaluation, and laparoscopic treatment of endometriosis involving the bowel. In addition, we will review the prevention, recognition, and management of bowel injuries at operative laparoscopy for endometriosis.

Diagnosis of intestinal endometriosis

Between 5% and 37% of patients with pelvic endometriosis have been found to have involvement of the bowel (1, 2). In patients with severe-stage endometriosis, this figure approaches 50% (3, 4). In a study of 1519 patients with all stages of endometriosis, Redwine and Sharpe found biopsy-proven endometriosis of the sigmoid in 17.8%, rectum in 13.2%, ileum in 4.1%, appendix in 2.5%, and cecum in 1.4% (5). The authors felt that the frequency of appendix involvement was artificially lowered by previous appendectomy in a significant number of patients.

Given these statistics, it is important to maintain a high degree of suspicion of bowel involvement for any patient with confirmed or suspected endometriosis. This approach allows appropriate preoperative patient evaluation and preparation. The most common presenting symptoms are abdominal pain, nausea, vomiting, diarrhea, constipation, tenesmus, small caliber stools, abdominal distention, passage of blood per rectum, or nonspecific change in bowel habit (6). A history of chronic laxative use with futile attempts at management via dietary change is often seen. Occasionally patients will present with end-stage symptoms of complete obstruction of the small or large bowel (7) or with peritonitis secondary to perforation (8). In a significant minority of patients, no gastrointestinal symptoms are elicited, and the complaints are related to gynecological pain, vaginal bleeding, infertility, or the presence of a pelvic or rectal mass. Although classically endometriosis is thought to produce cyclic symptoms, menstrual-related gastrointestinal symptoms appear in only a minority of patients (9). To obtain an accurate history, patients should be queried specifically about these symptoms.

Active intestinal endometriosis causes symptoms by producing irritation and inflammation of the bowel wall. Intraluminal bleeding can occur as a result of direct mucosal penetration of endometriosis or from mucosal ulceration overlying an area of fibromuscular inflammation. Because mucosal involvement is not a prerequisite for rectal bleeding, sigmoidoscopy or colonoscopy may miss significant colonic disease (10). Intramural infiltration elicits an inflammatory response by the bowel wall that causes progressive fibrosis and eventually narrowing of the lumen obstruction. Symptoms from scarring may persist in post-oophorectomized or postmenopausal patients even though no active endometriosis is present.

A careful bimanual and rectovaginal examination should be performed to detect uterosacral nodularity, cul-de-sac fixation or nodularity, or a pelvic mass. All patients with historical or physical findings suggestive of bowel endometriosis and all patients with severe endometriosis should undergo a preoperative colonoscopy, barium enema, and IVP. Unfortunately, as noted earlier, colonoscopy is frequently unrewarding in the absence of mucosal endometriosis, except for the frequent finding of stenosis or fixation of the sigmoid. In addition, it may prove difficult to obtain histologically satisfying biopsy specimens at colonoscopy. Although barium enema frequently reveals a mass, endometriosis is not associated with any pathognomonic X-ray change, making it impossible to exclude a malignancy (11). IVP may be employed to detect ureteral deviation, duplication, or obstruction so that care can be taken in identifying and safeguarding the ureter at surgery. The authors have not found MRI or CT scanning helpful in such cases. Indeed, the correct diagnosis is made preoperatively in only a minority of patients (12).

In confirmed cases, it may prove helpful to treat the patient preoperatively with a GnRH agonist for two to three months. If severe endometriosis with significant intestinal involvement is noted at initial laparoscopy in a patient without a proper bowel preparation, definitive surgery should be delayed until after a period of medical suppression. Down-regulation via a GnRH agonist decreases the volume and vascularity of endometriotic lesions and may enable laparoscopic treatment of patients who were not good candidates prior to suppression. Patients should have a preoperative mechanical and antibiotic bowel preparative assessment and should be apprised of the possibility of laparotomy and bowel resection if necessary for treatment of their disease. Although it should be discussed with all patients, colostomy is a rare necessity. If the gynecologist is not trained in and comfortable with bowel surgery, a colonrectal surgeon should be available to direct or perform the definitive surgery should involvement of the bowel be identified. In the latter case, the patient should see the surgeon prior to surgery.

The accurate diagnosis of intestinal endometriosis can prove challenging even under direct vision at laparoscopy. Ovarian endometriomas adherent to the rectosigmoid often signal local infiltration of the colon, which can be difficult to appreciate. Palpation of the bowel with a probe aids in diagnosing and demarcating the extent of involvement. In many cases, lower colon lesions can be palpated by rectal examination while observing the cul-de-sac and colon through the laparoscope. Areas of localized thickening, kinking, and stenosis should be considered to contain endometriosis. Not infrequently, microscopic examination will reveal that areas of induration or fibrosis in the bowel wall harbor endometriosis. Because endometriosis can resemble other pathologic entities, and differentiation from primary colon malignancy may be difficult, a histologic diagnosis should always be made before definitive treatment (13).

Laparoscopic management of intestinal endometriosis

The primary aim of surgery for endometriosis is the complete removal of all diseased tissue, and the restoration of normal anatomy and function. No laparoscopic procedure taxes the surgeon more than the treatment of bowel endometriosis. Intestinal endometriosis can be classified into three categories based on the degree of involvement of the bowel wall:

- Serosal lesions are attached to the peritoneal surface, but do not involve the muscularis.
- Intramural lesions involve the muscularis, but do not penetrate to the mucosa.
- Transmural endometriosis infiltrates the full thickness of the wall, producing mucosal endometriosis, ulceration, or luminal constriction (Fig. 28.1).

Superficial serosal involvement can be managed laparoscopically by sharp local excision, bipolar electrocautery, or laser excision or vaporization. Care must be taken—especially in small bowel lesions—not to penetrate beneath the serosal surface. Repair of small, hemostatic serosal defects is not necessary, but large defects or those adjacent to the tubes or ovaries should be closed. To reduce the chance of postoperative adhesion formation, a meticulous approach to hemostasis is necessary. The peritoneum should be reapproximated only where it can be accomplished without tension on suture lines. In our practice, we make liberal use of oxidized regenerated cellulose (Interceed, Johnson & Johnson) over suture lines and areas of incomplete reperitonealization.

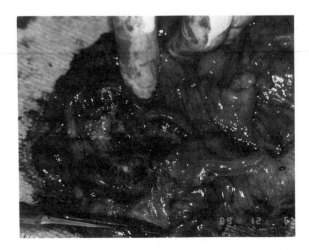

Fig. 28.1 This specimen from a low anterior rectosigmoid resection and primary anastomosis demonstrates transmural endometriosis with involvement of the intestinal mucosa.

Endoscopic treatment of intra- or transmural endometriosis remains controversial. Its applicability depends on the location and size of implants as well as the skill, training, and experience of the endoscopist. The same approach to excision described for serosal lesions can be employed if care is taken to stop the dissection short of the lumen and to carefully repair defects in the bowel wall. Palpation with laparoscopic instruments or with a rectal finger or probe may help ensure the removal of all endometriosis and avoid inadvertent enterotomy. If questions arise about a colorectal enterotomy, a Betadine enema may be used to detect leakage. Lesions that extend through the muscularis or that leave large serosal defects should be sutured.

Traditional management of transmural endometriotic lesions involves one of two options: (1) laparotomy and either disk excision with closure of the enterotomy, or (2) segmental resection and primary anastomosis. In a properly prepared patient, colostomy should not be necessary. With the evolution of endoscopic surgical techniques, these procedures are now being performed laparoscopically. Nezhat et al. described a novel approach to lesions of the anterior rectal wall. In this procedure, the rectum was mobilized laparoscopically, the anterior rectal wall everted through the anus, the lesion excised and the rectum repaired under direct vision, and the rectal wall inverted back through the anus (14). A similar technique for transrectal segmental resection has been reported by Redwine and associates (15). For more proximal lesions, Nezhat et al. have reported disk excision with primary endoscopic repair in eight patients with no complications or subsequent stricture (16).

Patients requiring large bowel resection and anastomosis have also been managed laparoscopically. In these cases, the segment to be resected is isolated laparoscopically, the vascular supply to the segment isolated and either ligated or cauterized, the segment excised and removed through the rectal stump or a separate abdominal incision, and anastomosis performed using a staple device inserted through the anus (17). Results, complications, and healing compare favorably with those seen with resection and anastomosis at laparotomy (18). Redwine and Sharpe used this approach to excise a 5-cm endometriotic lesion of the mid-sigmoid (19). In addition to its application in patients with benign diseases such as endometriosis, this technique has also proved useful for patients with premalignant lesions of the colon (20) as well as colon carcinoma. Surgical specimens, lymph node samples, morbidity, mortality, hospital stay, and recurrence were all comparable to laparotomy (21).

Endometriotic involvement of the small bowel is less common that that of the colon. Because of the thin wall and relatively small lumen of the small bowel, this condition frequently presents as obstruction. Superficial lesions are managed as outlined earlier, keeping in mind that entry into the lumen is always a possibility. The principles of resection and repair of transmural or obstructive lesions are the same as for colon lesions. Using endoscopic suturing techniques, laparoscopic resection and anastomosis are possible. Even acute small bowel obstruction—once considered an absolute contraindication for laparoscopy—has been successfully managed laparoscopically in 20 of 23 patients by Franklin et al. (22).

Endometriosis involves the appendix in 15% of all patients with severe-stage disease. Laparoscopic appendectomy is now a standard procedure in endoscopic surgery, with low complication rates if the appendix base and cecum are normal (23). If the patient has necrosis or gangrene of the base or cecum, or invasive disease of the terminal ileum, then laparotomy for resection is advised.

Prevention, recognition, and management of intestinal injuries

Three potential sources of bowel injury at the time of laparoscopic treatment of endometriosis exist: (1) injury due to the skin incision, insufflation, or trocar insertion; (2) injury resulting from endoscopic surgery; and (3) postoperative herniation through one of the laparoscopic incision sites. Krebs, in a study of intestinal injuries in gynecological surgery, found that patients with endometriosis had a significantly higher incidence of bowel injury than patients with other benign conditions. The majority of injuries were suffered at entrance into the peritoneal cavity or at lysis of adhesions (24).

Prevention of bowel injury is best accomplished by the anticipation of bowel adhesions to the anterior abdominal wall and of bowel endometriosis and/or adhesions. As discussed earlier, proper preoperative evaluation and preparation are essential to decrease the incidence of injury as well as facilitate appropriate treatment. Open laparoscopy, while not guaranteeing safety, may potentially reduce the chance of inadvertent injury at initial peritoneal entry. At endoscopic surgery, meticulous technique, careful tissue handling without excessive tension, positive identification of pelvic structures, blood vessels, and ureters prior to making incisions or cauterizing or vaporizing lesions, and an appreciation for the fact that endometriosis may obscure normal tissue planes are all critical factors in minimizing injuries. Finally, the surgeon must assess his or her own technical skill and experience as well as the extent of the disease encountered before embarking on an overly ambitious laparoscopic resection. One must never exceed the limits of common-sense safety to avoid a laparotomy. In particular, the surgical team should never begin treatment of intestinal endometriosis unless the surgeon or an immediately available consultant can manage untoward events.

Because injuries to the abdominal wall, blood vessels, and urinary tract are covered elsewhere in this book, we will limit our discussion to complications related to enterotomy and hernia formation. If an enterotomy occurs, immediate recognition of the injury is essential to prevent long-term sequelae. We make it a practice to carefully examine the abdominal wall circumferentially around the laparoscopy site as well as structures immediately beneath the insertion incision. All secondary ports should be introduced under direct laparoscopic control to minimize the chance of trocar injury. While the use of disposable, auto-retracting trocar points may reduce the incidence of injury, instrumentation cannot eliminate all potential problems. In using intraabdominal cautery, use bipolar cautery if at all possible. A 40-year survey of laparoscopic complications in Germany revealed that monopolar electrocautery burns were second only to mechanical trauma in producing complications (25). Even though bipolar forceps are associated with a lesser chance of adjacent injury, the complete electron path must be appreciated to avoid transmural desiccation of the bowel wall. In laparoscopic laser cases, the complete path of the laser beam must be clearly seen and the beam backstopped to prevent injury distal to the target site. All bowel at or adjacent to the site of excision should be explored to ensure that it has not been entered or devitalized.

Small serosal injuries without enterotomy may be managed by expectant observation. The same course can be used for small needle puncture injuries without spillage of intestinal contents (26), but care must be taken to ensure that no deeper, more extensive penetration occurs. Vascular lesions may be cauterized or sutured, taking care not to devitalize any segment of bowel. Small hematomas should be observed after partially deflating the abdomen to lessen the compression effect of the pneumoperitoneum. If stable and without impairment of bowel perfusion, then this condition may be managed by observation.

If the extent of damage cannot be determined, if evidence of bowel devitalization (especially with unipolar cautery) appears, or if the bowel lumen has been entered with or without spillage of contents, the "gold standard" of management is immediate laparotomy. If the possibility of a through and through injury or damage to multiple loops of bowel exists, all trocars should be left in place to assist in locating defects at laparotomy. Once an injury has been recognized, treatment must be prompt to avoid peritonitis. Intravenous broad-spectrum antibiotics to cover both *E. coli* and bacteroides species should be administered. We use a second- or third-generation cephalosporin or the combination ampicillin/sulbactam for this purpose.

The principles of bowel repair in the acute setting include meticulous hemostasis, debridement of devitalized tissue, generous irrigation, and prompt closure of healthy wound edges. To prevent additional abdominal contamination at laparotomy, the injury site should be isolated with lap pads and massive irrigation used to reduce fecal contamination. Both small bowel and colon injuries can be closed with a primary repair. The bowel should be approximated in a transverse fashion with either a single- or double-layer closure. The authors prefer a two-layer closure, with the first line of sutures passing through all layers, followed by a layer of interrupted inverting seromuscular sutures, using either a 3–0 polyglycolic acid or absorbable monofilament suture. If a significant segment of bowel has been injured or rendered ischemic, a segmental bowel resection and anastomosis is indicated. A colostomy is rarely necessary (27). On closing, the abdomen is flooded with 1 liter of irrigation containing 1 g of kanamycin and 50,000 units of bacitracin.

Increasingly, laparoscopic repair of enterotomies has been attempted. Nezhat *et al.* reported primary laparoscopic closure of enterotomies in 26 women without complication. All of these patients had undergone preoperative mechanical and antibiotic bowel preparation, however. Elkus reported repair of a small bowel enterotomy at laparoscopic cholecystectomy by bringing the loop of bowel through the umbilical incision, repairing it under direct vision, and replacing it in the abdomen.

The patient with an unrecognized traumatic perforation will usually present with symptoms of localized or generalized peritonitis within 12 to 36 hours after surgery. Fever and leukocytosis are variable signs, and the presence of free gas in the peritoneum on X ray is not a useful indicator because of the recent pneumoperitoneum. If symptoms do not regress promptly, exploration is mandatory. Patients with intestinal devitalization without direct enterotomy (such as that following laparoscopic unipolar cautery injuries or vascular injury with delayed bowel necrosis) may present as late as 4 to 10 days postoperatively. The principles of management are the same as outlined above. Primary resection and repair are usually possible as long as healthy bowel can be approximated.

Postoperatively, antibiotics are continued until the patient has begun eating and has been afebrile for more than 24 hours. Constant decompression by continuous gastric suction through a nasogastric (NG) tube is maintained until the patient passes flatus. In patients with peritonitis and severe inflammation where a prolonged recovery period is anticipated, it may be desirable to use a gastrostomy tube in place of the NG tube. Careful attention must be paid to appropriate fluid and electrolyte replacement. In cases requiring prolonged recovery, total parenteral nutrition may be indicated.

Although seen on only rare occasions with single puncture laparoscopy (28), the incidence of postoperative small bowel herniation through 10-mm and larger laparoscopic port sites has been increasing. Boike *et al.* reported 19 such cases, presenting with small bowel obstruction or strangulation an average of 8.5 days postoperatively (29). To prevent this complication, the defects created by large secondary trocars and 12-mm umbilical trocars should be closed (30, 31). Because many of these defects have been reported in patients over age 50, special consideration should be given to closing the umbilical site in such women. A relatively simple procedure is to pass a suture end into the peritoneum lateral to the fascial incision by placing the suture in a Veress needle, inserting the needle so that the blunt end does not retract and cut the suture. The end can then be grasped and brought out through the operative sleeve. The other end of the suture is placed on the opposite side of the incision in a similar fashion. The suture is tied after removal of the trocar sleeve. A variety of specialized surgical suture placement devices are also marketed for this purpose.

Conclusion

With appropriate forethought and preparation, the skilled laparoscopist can diagnose and manage many women with intestinal endometriosis. If the surgeon recognizes the risks of laparoscopic surgery for endometriosis, is cognizant of his or her own skills and abilities, and carefully considers the degree of intestinal involvement, a decision can be made about the appropriateness of endoscopic management of an individual patient. It must be remembered that the main aim is to treat the patient and remove her disease, not to perform surgical heroics thorough a small incision. It is far better to stop, properly prepare the patient (and the operating room team), and delay definitive surgery than risk bowel injury in the unprepped patient. Similarly, one should not apologize for a laparotomy if it is in the best interests of the patient.

The keys to the management of bowel injuries are recognition and anticipation. Injuries can and will happen, despite the most careful technique. There is no excuse for being unprepared to immediately and appropriately treat such complications.

We express our appreciation to Gary Skakun, M.D., for his assistance in the compilation and preparation of this chapter.

REFERENCES

1. Prystowsky JB, Stryker SJ, Ujiki GT, Poticha SM. Gastrointestinal endometriosis: incidence and indications for resection. Arch Surg 1988;123:855–858.
2. Macafee CH, Greer HL. Intestinal endometriosis: a report of 29 cases and a survey of the literature. J Obstet Gynaecol Br Emp 1960;67:539–543.
3. Buttram VC Jr, Reiter RC. Endometriosis. In: Buttram VC Jr, Reiter RC, eds. Surgical treatment of the infertile female. Baltimore: Williams & Wilkins, 1985:89.
4. Kistner RW. Endometriosis. In: McElin TW, Sciarra JJ, eds. Gynecology and obstetrics. Hagerstown, Md.: Harper and Row, 1981:1–44.
5. Redwine DB, Sharpe DR. Laparoscopic surgery for intestinal and urinary endometriosis. In: Sutton CJG, ed. Advanced laparoscopic surgery, vol. 19, no. 4. London: Balliere Tindall, 1995:775–794.
6. Cameron JC, Rogers S, Collins MC, Reed MW. Intestinal endometriosis: presentation, investigation, and surgical management. Int J Colorectal Dis 1995;10:83–86.
7. Eyers T, Morgan B, Bignold L. Endometriosis of the sigmoid colon and rectum. Aust N Z J Surg 1978;48:639–643.
8. Goodman P, Raval B, Zimmerman G. Perforation of the colon due to endometriosis. Gastrointest Radiol 1990;15:346–348.
9. Collin GR, Russell JC. Endometriosis of the colon. Its diagnosis and management. Am Surg 1990;56:275–279.
10. Levitt MD, Hodby KJ, van Merwyck AJ, Glancy RJ. Cyclic rectal bleeding in colorectal endometriosis. Aust N Z J Surg 1989; 59:941–943.
11. Athmanathan N, Sehdev VK, Walsh TH. Endometriosis of the sigmoid colon: a diagnostic problem. Br J Clin Pract 1990; 44:658–660.
12. Rowland R, Langman JM. Endometriosis of the large bowel: a report of 11 cases. Pathology 1989;21:259–265.
13. Parr NJ, Murphy C, Holt S, Zakhour H, Crosbie RB. Endometriosis and the gut. Gut 1988;29:1112–1115.
14. Nezhat F, Nezhat C, Pennington E. Laparoscopic proctectomy for infiltrating endometriosis of the rectum. Fertil Steril 1992;57: 1129–1132.
15. Redwine DB, Koning M, Sharpe DR. Laparoscopically assisted transvaginal segmental resection of the rectosigmoid colon for endometriosis. Fertil Steril 1996;65:193–197.
16. Nezhat C, Nezhat F, Pennington E, Nezhat CH, Ambroze W. Laparoscopic disk excision and primary repair of the anterior rectal wall for the treatment of full-thickness bowel endometriosis. Surg Endosc 1994;8:682–685.
17. Franklin ME Jr, Ramos R, Rosenthal D, Schuessler W. World J Surg 1993;17:51–56.
18. Van Ye TM, Cattey RP, Henry LG. Laparoscopically assisted colon resections compare favorably with open technique. Surg Laparosc Endosc 1994;4:25–31.
19. Redwine DB, Sharpe DR. Laparoscopic segmental resection of the sigmoid colon for endometriosis. J Laparoendosc Surg 1991; 1:217–220.
20. Chen WS, Tzeng KH, Leu SY, Hsu H. The application of laparoscopy in colorectal surgery: a preliminary report of twelve cases. Chung Hua I Hsueh Tsa Chin 1994;53:357–362.
21. Vara-Thorbeck C, Garcia-Caballero M, Salvi M, Gutstein D, Toscano R, Gomez A, Vara-Thorbeck R. Indications and advantages of laparoscopy-assisted colon resection for carcinoma in elderly patients. Surg Laparosc Endosc 1994;4: 110–118.
22. Franklin ME Jr, Dorman JP, Pharand D. Laparoscopic surgery in acute small bowel obstruction. Surg Laparosc Endosc 1994; 4:289–296.
23. Ludwig KA, Cattey RP, Henry LG. Initial experience with laparoscopic appendectomy. Dis Colon Rectum 1993;36:463–467.
24. Krebs HB. Intestinal injury in gynecologic surgery: a ten-year experience. Am J Obstet Gynecol 1986;155:509–514.
25. Lehmann-Willenbrock E, Riedel HH, Mecke H, Semm K. Pelviscopy/laparoscopy and its complications in Germany, 1949–1988. J Reprod Med 1992;37:671–677.
26. Reich H. Laparoscopic bowel injury. Surg Laparosc Endosc 1992;2:74–78.
27. Burch JM, Brock JC, Gevirtzman L, Feliciano DV, Mattox KL, Jordan GL Jr, DeBakey ME. The injured colon. Ann Surg 1986;203:701–711.

28. Thomas AG, McLymont F, Moshipur J. Incarcerated hernia after laparoscopic sterilization. A case report. J Reprod Med 1990;35:639–640.

29. Boike GM, Miller CE, Spiritos NM, Mercer LJ, Fowler JM, Summitt R, Orr JW Jr. Incisional bowel herniations after operative laparoscopy: a series of nineteen cases and review of the literature. Am J Obstet Gynecol 1995;172:1726–1731.

30. Patterson M, Walters D, Browder W. Postoperative bowel obstruction following laparoscopic surgery. Am Surg 1993;59: 656–657.

31. Storms P, Stuyven G, Vanhemelen G, Sebrechts R. Incarcerated trocar-wound hernia after laparoscopic hysterectomy. Is closure of large trocar fascia defects after laparoscopy necessary? Surg Endosc 1994;8:901–902.

Endometriosis: Ureteral Injuries

Linda M. Chaffkin and Anthony A. Luciano

Introduction

Endometriosis is a common pathological disorder that is found in 18.7% of laparotomies performed for gynecological indications (1). Ectopic endometrium has been described in a wide variety of locations but most commonly affects the ovaries, uterine ligaments, cul-de-sac, recto- and vesicovaginal septum, and pelvic peritoneum.

Many theories have been proposed for the etiology of endometriosis including the transport theory first proposed by Sampson (2) in 1921 and the coelomic metaplasia theory (3). The transport theory incorporates both retrograde regurgitation of endometrium through the oviducts and the transport of endometrium via blood vessels or the lymphatic system. The former mechanism accounts for pelvic endometriosis, while the vascular transport explains the occurrence of endometriosis outside of the abdominal cavity (4). Coelomic metaplasia is an alternative theory describing metaplasia of peritoneum of the abdomen or pelvis into a Mullerian element such as endometrium. Experimental proof of these theories has been difficult to establish. Neither theory can fully account for the vastly divergent sites of endometriosis, suggesting that a combination of these etiologies may be appropriate (4).

Endometriosis of the pelvic retroperitoneal space is rare, with the incidence of urinary tract endometriosis reported at approximately 1% of endometriosis in general (5–7). The urinary bladder is by far the most common site of urinary tract involvement by endometriosis; it is affected in approximately 84% of cases (8). Endometriosis of the urethra, kidneys, and ureters has also been reported (9). In their evaluation of 1000 consecutive celiotomies, Williams and Pratt (10) noted the involvement of small or large bowel in 33% of women with pelvic endometriosis. In this group only 16% of patients had urinary involvement, with 1.5% exhibiting endometriosis of the ureter. Endometriosis of the ureter has recently been reported with increasing frequency (11), perhaps reflecting heightened awareness of this particular manifestation of the disease (12).

The intrapelvic segment is in close proximity to the broad ligament, ovaries, and uterosacral ligaments, the most commonly affected sites for endometriosis. Consequently, the ureter is at risk for invasion or extrinsic compression (7). Kerr (13) reported a series of 47 cases of endometriosis involving the ureter in which severe and irreversible renal damage was noted in 28% of patients at the time of diagnosis. Bilateral ureteral involvement was found in 11% of cases in this series. Moore and colleagues (7) described eight cases of ureteral obstruction secondary to endometriosis. In their study, they found a 25% rate of severe renal damage when ureteral obstruction was present.

In their excellent review, Bradford and associates (12) noted that the relatively poor salvage rate may reflect diagnoses made late in the course of the disease. They proposed three general reasons for delayed diagnosis. First, ureteral obstruction often occurs by a gradual, and often asymptomatic, process of extrinsic compression (7, 15). Thus, discovery may be made either as an incidental finding or when symptoms have progressed to a degree where hydronephrosis, hypertension, or other evidence of renal failure is present. Second, delayed diagnosis may result from a low index of suspicion in the minds of the treating physician. Consequently, some authors (7, 14–16) advocate an intravenous pyelogram in women with severe endometriosis prior to surgery. In a prospective study, Maxson and colleagues (17) evaluated the occurrence of ureteral abnormalities by intravenous pyelography in 63 women with documented endometriosis before surgery. They reported an incidence of subtle ureteral abnormalities, including extrinsic compression and kinking and narrowing of the ureteral lumen, in 15.9% of these women, none of whom had urologic symptoms. Third, failure to recognize ureteric compression leading to obstruction may occur when only minimal pelvic disease is present. Kane (16) and associates reported that 50% of their patients with obstructive uropathy secondary to endometriotic involvement of the ureter were diagnosed as not having endometriosis prior to surgery. Other authors (11, 12) have also described ureteric obstruction in the presence of mild endometriosis when few clinical symptoms were manifest.

Although most cases of endometriosis with ureteral involvement are asymptomatic, the clinician must be alert to symptoms that may suggest involvement of the genitourinary tract (Table 29.1). Ureteral obstruction may lead to flank or abdominal pain; dysuria, hematuria, pyelonephritis, or hydronephrosis. These symptoms, which typically occur in a cyclic fashion, are exacerbated by the onset of menses. A pelvic mass or signs of peritonitis may be present. Endometriosis involving the urinary bladder most commonly presents as vesical discomfort (i.e., sense of heaviness, pain, or pressure in the bladder region), occurring in 78% of cases (8). Other symptoms include cyclic dysuria, hematuria, frequency, and urgency. Although endometriosis of the kidney is extremely rare, it should be considered in the differential diagnosis of the patient who presents with cyclic lumbar pain and hematuria (4).

Diagnosis

Differential diagnosis of endometriosis involving the genitourinary system includes both benign and malignant disease (9). One must rule out inflammatory disorders, papilloma, varices, and primary or metastatic carcinoma as an etiology for the patient's symptoms. The correct diagnosis will most often be made by the clinician who elicits careful history of urinary symptoms and who performs a thorough and complete pelvic examination with the routine use of biopsies as indicated.

Although endometriosis can occur anywhere along the course of the ureter, it is most often observed on the pelvic side wall lateral to the ureterosacral ligaments. Endometrial implants involving the uterosacral ligament may affect the paracervical tissue, inducing a thick

Table 29.1. Genitourinary endometriosis: symptoms.

Flank pain
Abdominal pain
Peritonitis
Pyelonephritis
Vesical discomfort
Hematuria
Cyclic dysuria
Urinary frequency or urgency

fibrous reaction involving the ureter, cervix, and vaginal fornix. Such growths may also occur lateral to the ureter, extending into the obturator fossa below the bifurcation of the common iliac artery with involvement of the distal ureter (18).

Appearance of endometriotic implants varies, ranging from the characteristic "powder burn" lesions and scarring of deep endometriosis to purple, red or clear superficial implants. Martin *et al.* (19) have described 20 variations in the morphological appearance of endometriosis. It is becoming increasingly apparent that the atypical or nonpigmented lesions contain active endometriotic glands and stroma and that the bluish "powder burn" lesions contain inactive glands and stroma in which hemosiderin is embedded (20, 21). Histologic examination of long-standing endometriotic implants causing periureteral fibrosis typically reveals minimal stroma and glandular tissue with large amounts of collagen and scarring (22).

Treatment

The management of endometriosis involving the urinary tract is a subject of ongoing debate. The decision to perform extirpative surgery is a difficult one, especially in women who desire continued reproductive potential. Some attempts have been made to alleviate ureteral obstruction using medical therapy alone. Isolated reports of reversal of ureteral obstruction documented by roentgenography using hormonal suppressive therapy have been described (23, 24). Gantt (23) described complete resolution of unilateral ureteric obstruction in a patient treated with depo-medroxyprogesterone acetate (400 mg/2 week). Lavelle *et al.* (24) reported success in relieving ureteral obstruction in a patient treated with four to six tablets daily of 0.5 mg norgestrel and 0.5 mg ethinyl estradiol (Wyeth Laboratories) orally for seven weeks. This patient subsequently developed hydronephrosis on the opposite side, however, and underwent definitive surgery. Others (25–29) have evaluated the role of danazol, an isoxazol derivative of the synthetic steroid 17α-ethinyl testosterone (30) in the management of endometriosis with ureteral involvement.

Two authors (27, 28) report successful resolution in three cases of endometriosis associated with ureteral obstruction following therapy with danazol alone. Solid documentation of the efficacy of danazol against ureteral endometriosis is lacking (29), however, and reports indicate that ureteral obstruction may recur upon discontinuation of danazol (26, 31) or that no response may occur if associated fibrosis is present (25).

In a recent report, Rivlin and associates (32) describe their experience with three patients with endometriotic ureteral obstruction who were treated preoperatively for six to nine months with leuprolide acetate, a GnRH agonist. Two patients had unilateral obstruction, and one patient had bilateral obstruction. Obstruction was relieved in one patient with bilateral disease and one patient with unilateral changes. Therapy failed in a patient with intrinsic ureteric endometriosis. The authors suggest that GnRH agonist therapy may play a role in patients with ureteric obstruction due to endometriosis "probably but not necessarily in conjunction with a planned surgical procedure." They caution that if medical therapy is attempted "close surveillance of renal function is mandatory."

Davis and Shiff (33) reported a case of endometriosis and unilateral ureteral obstruction in which a patient was treated with 0.1 mg leuprolide subcutaneously daily for three to four months before definitive surgical therapy. Operative findings included a left adnexa that was firmly fibrotically adherent to the distal left ureter. Because duration of medical therapy prior to surgery was short, it is difficult to adequately evaluate therapeutic response.

Treatment decisions for the medical management of ureteric endometriosis must take into account the patient's age, parity, symptoms, and extent and location of disease. While isolated reports of success have been described with medical therapy, nonsurgical management may not be efficacious in the presence of fibrosis. Hormonal therapy may also delay treatment, potentially leading to progression of hydronephrosis and renal damage. Consequently, renal function must be closely monitored in these patients. Nonoperative management may have a role in a carefully selected patient population, however, but further studies are needed to assess this treatment option. Preservation of renal function must be the highest priority when making any management decision.

Several basic procedures have been employed in the surgical management of endometriosis involving the genitourinary system. Implants of endometriosis may be sharply resected with scissors or coagulated or vaporized using electricity or laser. Superficial endometriotic implants on the peritoneum covering the ureter may be managed by hydrodissection and resection (34). After a small entry port is made into the retroperitoneum using laser or laparoscopic scissors, 50–100 cc of Ringer's lactate is injected along the course of the ureter. This procedure results in lateral displacement of the ureter, providing a plane for safe ablation of endometriotic implants or resection of the involved peritoneum. Additionally, the fluid absorbs the laser energy, thereby serving as a buffer to lessen the risk of thermal damage to underlying tissue (20). This procedure is applicable only when the peritoneum is not densely adherent to the underlying ureter. Indeed, critics have pointed out that this technique may not be successful when the endometriosis is subperitoneal (35). Bakri and colleagues caution that the beneficial effects of hydrodissection may be mitigated in the presence of severe endometriotic adhesions and fibrosis, as an adequate "water bed" may not be created beneath the endometriotic implants (36).

With ureteral obstruction, many authors (13, 14, 34) advocate a surgical approach, which may involve ureteral lysis, primary urinary diversion, resection of endometriosis, and total abdominal hysterectomy with bilateral salpingo-oophorectomy. Because of the dense fibrosis that accompanies ureteric endometriosis, early surgical excision of the ureteric stricture may permit effective resolution of upper tract dilatation and improve renal salvage (37).

Recently, Nezhat and colleagues (38) described a case of long-term ureteral obstruction due to endometriosis that was managed laparoscopically using the laser. A 2-cm fibrotic nodule was noted on the left ureter, approximately 4 cm above the bladder, that distorted the course of the ureter corresponding to the level of obstruction. Under laparoscopic visualization, a cystoscopic attempt at retrograde ureteral catheterization was unsuccessful. The technique of video laseroscopy and hydrodissection was used to enter the left retroperitoneal space at the pelvic brim. The ureter was then dissected free with the CO_2 laser. Because the nodule involved the entire thickness of the ureter, partial resection was elected. Under cystoscopic guidance, a 7 French ureteral catheter was passed through the ureterovesical junction and the CO_2 laser was used to enter the bladder at this level. The catheter was advanced up through the proximal portion of the ureter to the left renal pelvis. Using three interrupted 4-0 PDS sutures, the edges of the ureter were reapproximated to the neocystostomy. The postoperative course was uncomplicated, with intravenous pyelogram confirming ureteral patency.

Few endoscopists possess the surgical skill to duplicate Dr. Nezhat's feat. Most gynecologists should, however, feel comfortable ablating endometriosis and scars compressing the ureter to destroy the lesion and relieve the pressure.

Complications of surgical management of ureteral endometriosis

Laparoscopic management of endometriosis may eliminate the need for laparotomy in some cases, thereby reducing operative time, shortening hospital stay, and minimizing blood loss. The risk of inadvertent injury to blood vessels, bowel, bladder, or other intra-abdominal organs is present with laparoscopy just as it is with laparotomy. Additional risks include general anesthesia, burns to pelvic viscera and abdominal wall (39, 40), and electrical burn injury of the ureter (35, 40–43).

The embryologic development of the ureter is intimately associated with the development of the female genital tract (44). Consequently, surgical procedures of the female reproductive system predispose this area to injury. Ureteral injury—a serious complication of surgical intervention—has been estimated to occur in 0.5% to 1.5% of pelvic operations (40, 45, 46). Identification of the ureter as it courses along the pelvis is crucial for safe laparoscopic management of endometriosis and avoidance of ureteral damage (Figs. 29.1 and 29.2).

Kadar has described a laparoscopic technique for dissecting the pelvic retroperitoneum and identifying the ureters. His technique involves tracing the obliterated hypogastric artery proximally to its junction with the uterine artery to form the internal iliac artery. Blunt dissection proximal and medial to the uterine artery opens the pararectal space, the medial portion of which is bound to the ureter (47).

Diseases such as endometriosis may potentially thicken the peritoneum, obscuring the location of the ureter (especially in the area of the uterosacral ligaments). The surgeon should stay alert for potential anatomical distortions when nodularity and thickening

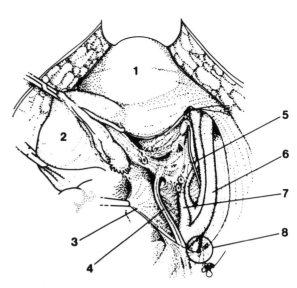

Fig. 29.2 Retroperitoneal identification of the ureter: 1. bladder; 2. uterus; 3. medial leaf of the broad ligament; 4. ureter; 5. obturator nerve; 6. external iliac artery; 7. hypogastric artery; 8. ligated and cut infundibulopelvic ligament. (Reprinted with permission from Daly JW, Higgens KA. Injury to the ureter during gynecologic surgical procedures. Surg Gynecol Obstet 1988;167:20.)

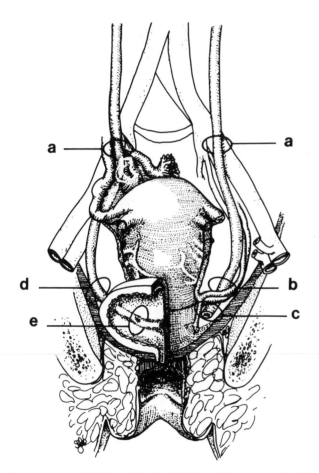

Fig. 29.1 Reported sites of ureteral injury during gynecologic procedures: (a) injury at the pelvic brim; (b) injury where ureter crosses under the uterine artery; (c) injury near the anterior fornix of the vagina; (d) injury at the lateral pelvic sidewall; and (e) injury in the intramural portion of the bladder. (Reprinted with permission from Daly JW, Higgens KA. Injury to the ureter during gynecologic surgical procedures. Surg Gynecol Obstet 1988;167:20.)

are present in the area of the uterosacral ligaments (37). The average length of the ureter ranges from 25 to 30 cm. As the ureter enters the pelvis, it passes over the iliac artery at the bifurcation point of the common iliac vessel into the internal and external iliac vessels. It then courses along the lateral pelvic wall anterior to the internal iliac artery and is attached to the medial leaf of the broad ligament. The ureter, which passes beneath the uterine artery at this point, is located approximately 1.5 cm lateral to the cervix. It then courses medially over the anterior fornix of the vagina before entering the bladder.

Although Seiler and colleagues (48) reported no complications in 45 patients undergoing laparoscopic electrocoagulation of endometriosis, most reported cases of ureteral injury during laparoscopic procedures involve the use of electrocoagulation. This type of damage is more likely to reflect excessive or improper cauterization than inherent danger of the electrocautery technique per se. As electrocoagulation is the most reliable technique to arrest bleeding by laparoscopy, it is not surprising that electricity is most frequently involved in these complications. Given the increasing popularity of laser coagulation, additional reports of ureteral injury may be expected to surface in the future.

Injury to the ureter during laparoscopic surgery may occur as a direct result of removing endometriotic implants or fibrosis from the ureter (43). Alternatively, injury may result indirectly (e.g., while transecting uterosacral ligaments). Gomel and associates (42) reported a case of ureteral injury that arose during operative laparoscopy for pelvic endometriosis. Electrosurgical ablation of the left uterosacral ligament produced a ureteral laceration. The ureter was located medial to the uterosacral ligament, a variant from its normal lateral position. Anomalies in location of the ureter, if unrecognized at the time of surgical procedure, may carry a higher risk for operative injury. To avoid such injuries, the surgeon must clearly identify the tissue being destroyed or removed. Such meticulous dissection will pinpoint anomalous locations or displace structures such as the ureter or large blood vessels, enabling these complications to be avoided.

The incidence and diagnosis of serious urinary complications after major operative laparoscopy was recently reported by Saidi and colleagues, who found that these injuries occur most frequently in patients with endometriosis. These researchers also reported that ureteral injuries occurred more frequently after adnexectomy for endometriosis (6.25%) than laparoscopic-assisted vaginal hysterectomy for endometriosis (3%). Ureteral injuries were encountered with the use of an endoscopic linear stapler, sharp dissection, endoloop, or electrosurgery (46).

Diagnosis of complications

Early recognition of ureteral injury is critical to a successful management. Ideally ureteral injuries should be identified intraoperatively by dissection of the ureter, leakage of urine, or intravenous instillation of indigo carmine with intraperitoneal spillage. Once identified, such complications can then easily be corrected with minimal adverse consequences to the patient and subsequent compromise.

Unfortunately, a diagnosis is usually made postoperatively by intravenous pyelography. Symptoms of fever, abdominal or flank pain, and abdominal distention, occurring within 48 to 72 hours after surgery, should alert the clinician to the presence of ureteral damage (see Table 29.1). Leukocytosis and hematuria may also be present. The use of high-molecular-weight dextran or other adjuvants that induce osmotic ascites may mask symptoms of ureteral injury (35). While injury may present with abdominal pain, fever, and peritonitis and may symptomatically mimic ureteral injury, performing an intravenous pyelogram will help to make the differential diagnosis (35) (Table 29.2).

Although manifestations of ureteral injury are usually evident within the first postoperative week, delayed symptomology occurring four to six weeks postoperatively has been reported in two patients. Both patients, who presented at four and six weeks postoperatively with abdominal distention and pain, were found to have peritoneal ascites, urinoma, and ureteral-peritoneal fistula located 2 cm from the bladder. The ureteral injuries were most likely caused by the thermal effects of bipolar electrodes during coagulation of uterine vessels. Such thermal injury may cause vascular compromise or ureteral wall necrosis, resulting in ureteral fistula with delayed urine spillage into the peritoneal cavity and delayed symptomology (49).

In cases of recognized ureteral complications, several therapeutic options are available, including ureteroureterostomy and ureteroneocystotomy. These procedures require stenting and draining with the ureteral catheter to facilitate healing at the site of injury. Winslow and associates (41) reported a case of conservative management of a patient who sustained an electrical burn injury to the left ureter secondary to laparoscopy performed for an infertility evaluation. Postoperative retrograde ureteral stenting was performed for 18 days. Following removal of the catheter, an intravenous pyelogram demonstrated a grade III left hydronephrosis secondary to a ureteral stricture that had developed at the pelvic brim. The patient eventually underwent cystoscopy and left retrograde catheterization with placement of a J-stent. Marked improvement of renal function was noted after this procedure. Percutaneous or cystoscopic techniques can also be used to manage certain types of ureteral injuries, avoiding the need for an open surgical procedure.

Meticulous identification of the course of the ureter during surgery for endometriosis, a high index of suspicion for ureteral injury, and prompt relief of ureteral obstruction are essential to minimize the occurrence of renal damage resulting from injuries inflicted during laparoscopic surgery. Prior disease processes, which may distort the anatomy of the ureter, increase the potential for ureteral injury and must be considered when performing laparoscopic procedures.

Table 29.2. Genitourinary endometriosis: findings.

Cystic pelvic mass
Fibrous reaction involving ureter

IVP
Ureteral stenosis
Hydroureter
Hydronephrosis

Laparoscopy
Powder burn or atypical appearing implants over ureter, lateral to the uterosacral ligaments or along pelvic sidewall
Stellate scarring

IVP, intravenous pyelogram.

REFERENCES

1. Schneider GT. Endometriosis: an update. In: Studd J, ed. Progress in obstetrics and gynecology, vol III. Edinburgh: Churchill Livingston, 1983:246.
2. Sampson JA. Perforating hemorrhagic (chocolate) cysts of the ovary. Arch Surg 1921;3:245.
3. Duson CK, Zelenik JS. Vulvar endometriosis. Obstet Gynecol 1954;3:76.
4. Rock JA, Markham SM. Extrapelvic endometriosis. In: Wilson EA, ed. Endometriosis. New York: Liss, 1987:185.
5. Dockerty MB. Pathological aspects of endometriosis. Minnesota M 1949;32:806.
6. Ball TL, Platt MA. Urological complications of endometriosis. Am J Obstet Gynecol 1962;84:1516.
7. Moore JG, Hibbard LT, Growdon WA, et al. Urinary tract endometriosis: enigmas in diagnosis and management. Am J Obstet Gynecol 1979;134:162.
8. Neto WA, et al. Vesical endometriosis. Urology 1984;24:271.
9. Abeshouse BS, Abeshouse G. Endometriosis in the urinary tract. J Int Coll Surg 1960;34:43.
10. Williams TJ, Pratt JH. Endometriosis in 1000 consecutive celiotomies: incidence and management. Am J Obstet Gynecol 1977;129:245.
11. Yates-Bell AJ, Molland EA, Prior JP. Endometriosis of the ureter. Br J Urol 1972;44:58.
12. Bradford JA, Ireland EW, Warwick BG. Ureteric endometriosis: 3 case reports and a review of the literature. Aust NZ J Gynaecol 1989;29:421.
13. Kerr WS. Endometriosis involving the urinary tract. Clin Obstet Gynaecol 1966;9:331.
14. Langmade CF. Pelvic endometriosis and ureteral obstruction. Am J Obstet Gynecol 1975;122:463.
15. Stanley KE, Utz DC, Dockerty MB. Clinically significant endometriosis of urinary tract. Surg Gynecol Obstet 1965;120:491.
16. Kane C, Drouin P. Obstructive uropathy associated with endometriosis. Am J Obstet Gynecol 1985;151:207.
17. Maxson WS, Hill GA, Herbert CM, et al. Ureteral abnormalities in women with endometriosis. Fertil Steril 1986;46:1159.
18. Bates JS, Beecham CT. Retroperitoneal endometriosis with ureteral obstruction. Obstet Gynecol 1969;34:242.
19. Martin DC, Hubert GD, Vander Vaag R, et al. Laparoscopic appearance of peritoneal endometriosis. Fertil Steril 1989;51:63.
20. Cook AS, Rock JA. The role of laparoscopy in the treatment of endometriosis. Fertil Steril 1991;55:663.
21. Jansen RP, Russell P. Nonpigmented endometriosis: clinical laparoscopic and pathologic definition. Am J Obstet Gynecol 1986;155:1154.
22. Laube DW, Calderwood GW, Benda JA. Endometriosis causing ureteral obstruction. Obstet Gynecol 1985;65(suppl):69.
23. Gantt PA, Hunt JB, McDonough PG. Progestin reversal of ureteral endometriosis. Obstet Gynecol 1981;57:665.
24. Lavelle KJ, Melman AW, Cleary RE. Ureteral obstruction owing to endometriosis: reversal with synthetic progestin. J Urol 1976;116:665.
25. Rivlin ME, Krueger RP, Wiser WL. Danazol in the management of ureteral obstruction secondary to endometriosis. Fertil Steril 1985;44:274.
26. Pittaway DE, Daniell JF, Winfield AC, et al. Recurrence of ureteral obstruction caused by endometriosis after danazol therapy. Am J Obstet Gynecol 1982;143:720.
27. Matsuura K, Kawasaki N, Oka M, et al. Treatment with danazol of ureteral obstruction caused by endometriosis. Acta Obstet Gynecol Scand 1985;64:339.
28. Gardner B, Whitaker RH. The use of danazol for ureteral obstruction caused by endometriosis. J Urol 1981;125:117.
29. Jepsen JM, Hansen KB. Danazol in the treatment of ureteral endometriosis. J Urol 1988;139:1045.
30. Dmowski WP. Endocrine properties and clinical applications of danazol. Fertil Steril 1979;31:237.
31. Wood GP, Wu CH, Flickinger GL, et al. Changes associated with danazol therapy. Obstet Gynecol 1975;45:302.
32. Rivlin ME, Miller JD, Krueger RP, et al. Leuprolide acetate in the management of ureteral obstruction caused by endometriosis. Obstet Gynecol 1990;75:532.
33. Davis OK, Schiff I. Endometriosis with unilateral ureteral obstruction and hypertension—a case report. J Reprod Med 1988;33:470.
34. Nezhat C, Nezhat, FR. Safe laser endoscopic excision or vaporization of peritoneal endometriosis. Fertil Steril 1989;52:149.
35. Granger DA, Soderstrom RM, Schiff SF, et al. Ureteral injuries at laparoscopy: insights into diagnosis, management, and prevention. Obstet Gynecol 1990;75:839.
36. Bakri YN, Sundin T, Mansi M. Ureteral injuries secondary to laparoscopic CO_2 laser. Acta Obst Gynecol Scand 1994;73:655–667.
37. Patel A, Thorpe P, Ramsay J, et al. Endometriosis of the ureter. Brit J Urol 1992;69:495–498.
38. Nezhat C, Nezhat F, Green B. Laparoscopic treatment of obstructed ureter due to endometriosis by resection and ureterureteostomy: a case report. J Urol 1992;148:865–868.
39. Schwimmer WB. Electrosurgical burn injuries during laparoscopy sterilization: treatment and prevention. Obstet Gynecol 1974;44:526.
40. Soderstrom RM. Hazard of laparoscopic sterilization. In: Sciarra JW, ed. Gynecology and obstetrics. Philadelphia: Harper & Row, 1982:1–6.
41. Winslow PH, Kreger R, Ebbesson B, et al. Conservative management of electrical burn injury of ureter secondary to laparoscopy. Urology 1986;27:60.
42. Gomel V, James C. Intraoperative management of ureteral injury during operative laparoscopy. Fertil Steril 1991;55:416.
43. Cheng YS. Ureteral injury resulting from laparoscopic fulguration of endometriotic implant—letter. Am J Obstet Gynecol 1976;126:1045.
44. Moore KC. The developing human, 2nd ed. Philadelphia: WB Saunders, 1977:220–257.
45. Daly JW, Higgins KA. Injury to the ureter during gynecologic surgical procedures. Surg Gynecol Obstet 1988;167:29–22.
46. Saidi MH, Sadler RK, Vancaillie TG, Akright BD, Farhart SA, White JA. Diagnosis and management of serious urinary complications after major operative laparoscopy. Obstet Gynecol 1996;87:272–276.
47. Kadar N. Dissecting the pelvic retroperitoneum and identifying the ureters: a laparoscopic technique. J Reprod Med 1995;40:116–122.
48. Seiler JC, Gidwani G, Ballard L. Laparoscopic cauterization of endometriosis for fertility: a controlled study. Fertil Steril 1986;46:1098.
49. Albini SM, Karolicki B, Chere M, Polke DR, Feldman RA, Luciano AA. Delayed ureteral injury after laparoscopic surgery. J Am Assoc Gynecol Laparosc 1995;2(suppl):S1–S2.

Endometriosis: Ovarian Involvement | 30

Joseph R. Feste

The complications plaguing any surgeon at the time of an operative laparoscopy are hemorrhage, postoperative infections, adhesion formation, and damage to normal adjacent organs, such as the uterus, fallopian tubes, bowel, ureter, bladder, or major vessels. The actual incidence of injuries occurring as a result of treating endometriomas has not been reported. However, articles by Jenkins *et al.* (1) and by Hori *et al.* (2) reported that the most common site of endometriosis is the ovary (Table 30.1). In the case of ovarian endometriosis, one would need to consider the incidence of complications based upon the size of the endometrioma and whether it is associated with adhesions to any organ in the pelvis or on the pelvic walls.

The issue of infection can be resolved easily by the use of prophylactic antibiotics and careful adherence to sterile technique while performing surgery on the ovary. This approach would obviously mean draping laparoscopes, laser arms, and cameras. In those cases requiring several hours for completion, prophylactic antibiotics are certainly recommended. Needless to say, frequently used instruments must be properly cleaned before sterilization by soaking in various solutions, and rinsed before use. More frequent use of disposable instruments, including trocars, probes, and irrigating systems, would reduce the risk of infection.

Another complication that can be addressed fairly easily is the formation of adhesions following laparoscopic removal of ovarian endometriomas. Even though not classified as a "severe injury," adhesions can cause both pain and infertility. Therefore, the need for prevention becomes very important. Several generally accepted methods for preventing adhesion formation are listed in Table 30.2. Of all the methods used, several are used more frequently than others. These include heparinized Ringer's lactate for irrigation solutions, dexamethasone given intravenously immediately preoperatively and up to 72 hours postoperatively (a modified Horne regimen) (3), barrier grafts including Interceed (4) and Gore Tex,

and the more liberal use of second-look laparoscopies (5). Complete discussion of the efficacy of any one of these adjunctive therapies would require more detail than can be provided in the scope of this chapter. The author's choice is to irrigate with heparinized Ringer's lactate (5000 units/liter), to use Interceed as a barrier method, and to recommend a second-look laparoscopy in those patients with a high risk of developing adhesions. Interceed, being a biodegradable cellulose product, does not have to be surgically removed as does Gore Tex. However, studies of the use of Gore Tex in gynecology have not yet been published and, therefore, valid conclusions cannot be reached concerning this product. Those patients most at risk for adhesions are those with Stage III or IV endometriosis or adhesive disease.

Another factor in the development of adhesions in patients with endometriomas is the way these masses are treated at the time of the initial laparoscopy. Several methods have been advocated that might limit the formation of adhesions in patients with more advanced endometriosis. The first was described by Brosens (6). At the time of diagnostic laparoscopy, he entered the capsule of the endometrioma with a specially adapted laparoscope system called an ovarioscope. The chocolate material was drained from the endometrioma, and the entire interior of the cyst was irrigated. He theorized that the endometriosis begins on the surface of the ovary, pushing the cortex down into the ovarian stroma in front of the developing cyst. A pseudomembrane forms over the small cyst that eventually fills up with old oxidized blood (Fig. 30.1). Looking for the active area of endometriosis in the endometrioma, he would destroy this area with the energy of a fiberoptic laser, speculating that this active implant was responsible for the development of the endometrioma. The remainder of endometriosis and the adhesions were vaporized and the patient was followed up for three to six months. In most instances, second-look laparoscopy should show no evidence of residual disease in the ovary. Adhesion formation was minimal because the capsule of the endometrioma was opened less than a centimeter. Even though the numbers of cases reported are small, the treatment certainly should be considered as an alternative method for treating ovarian endometriosis.

Table 30.1. Common sites of endometrial implants.

Author and site	%
Jenkins et al. (1)	
Ovary	54.9
Posterior broad ligament	35.2
Anterior cul-de-sac	34.6
Posterior cul-de-sac	34.0
Uterosacral ligament	28.0
Hori et al. (2)	
Ovary	77.9
Peritoneum	42.1
Uterosacral ligament	42.1

Table 30.2. Most popular methods for prevention of adhesion formation.

Glucocorticoid/antihistamine regimens
Nonsteroidal antiinflammatory agents
Progesterone injections
Colchicine
Dextran
Oxidized regenerated cellulose (Interceed)
Gore Tex mesh

Another alternative treatment would be to perform the same ovarioscopy, drain out the chocolate material, vaporize the vascular bed, but give the patient a gonadotropin-releasing hormone (GnRH) agonist for three to six months. At the time of the second-look laparoscopy, the remainder of the suppressed endometrioma could be vaporized with ease. This method of treatment is more logical than expecting the thick chocolate material to be absorbed through a universally sclerotic endometriotic capsule. No significant evidence has been found to suggest that either analogs or danocrine can actually decrease the size of an endometrioma over 3–4 cm. Rather they may reduce the number of active follicles or corpora lutea and thus give the impression that the endometrioma is being reduced in size.

A final alternative is that of stripping the capsule of the endometrioma from within the ovary, achieving the best hemostasis possible, and then leaving the ovarian capsule open. The unfortunate sequelae of the technique without excellent hemostasis is that postoperative adhesions are seen in an overwhelming number at second-look laparoscopy. This procedure least adheres to the principles of microsurgery and results in large gaping holes in the ovary and sometimes inadequate hemostasis. Evaluation of the efficacy of all of these procedures will require a significant period of time, and prospective studies will be needed before the correct approach can be identified. With impeccable hemostasis, closure of the ovarian stroma with 0–3 PDS suture (no suture on the cortex) and the use of adhesion barriers, such as Interceed, adhesion formation can be decreased.

The third and probably most difficult complication to deal with—but one easy to diagnose—is hemorrhage. Hemorrhage may arise from the ovary or an adjacent structure. Even with the largest endometriomas, there are not any large vessels that can be damaged as long as one "hugs" the surface of the ovary while lysing adhe-

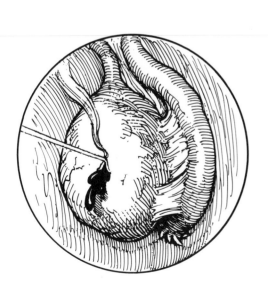
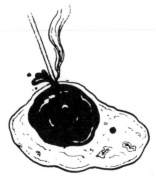

Fig. 30.1 Ovarioscopy: removing the contents of the endometrioma and vaporizing the base of the endometrioma.

sions to bring the ovary into an anterior position. Should the lateral pelvic wall be intimately involved with the wall of the endometrioma, damage to retroperitoneal vessels can be prevented by using "aquadissection" or hydrodissection (7, 8). This procedure simply employs the injection of fluid, specifically Ringer's lactate or any other irrigating solution, into the retroperitoneal space using either a blunt irrigation tube placed in a small hole in the peritoneum (Fig. 30.2) or a long 22-gauge spinal needle to inject the solution into the retroperitoneal space. This procedure essentially raises the peritoneum off the underlining vessels or ureter, acting as a backstop, for instance, when the CO_2 laser is used to dissect. One may also simply use a pair of microscissors through the laparoscope.

As the endometrioma is stripped from its attachment to the ovary, there will be unavoidable bleeding where it is attached to the stroma of the ovary. This bleeding can be minimized, however, in two ways. It has become obvious that the ovary would be less vascular if it were inactive, void of all follicular and corpus luteal activity. This inactivity can be achieved by using either a GnRH analog or danazol preoperatively, usually for no more than six to eight weeks. It has been the author's experience that one cannot completely eliminate an endometrioma with medical therapy. The reason is the extreme thickness of the endometrioma's capsule and the thick chocolate material with which it is filled. The only effect is that of decreasing both the follicular and corpus luteal activity of the ovary during the time the patient is taking the medication.

Another issue is not preventive but therapeutic. When bleeding or oozing occurs, a bipolar cautery may be used to provide hemostasis. However, on occasion, it is difficult to find the vessels to coagulate. In these cases, one would profit by the use of a new coagulator, the argon beam coagulator. This new method of coagulation produces a uniform thickness of coagulation on the surface to which it is directed. The argon gas is ionized by the monopolar current through which the gas is directed. This action essentially breaks up the current into millions of smaller, less invasive currents to give symmetrical superficial area of coagulation (Fig. 30.3). It has been shown to have an average depth of penetration of only 1–3 mm depending upon the amount of current and the time of exposure to the tissue (9). With this coagulator, one can easily provide hemostasis without any significant injury to any other tissue. This is possible because the ovary, as thick as it is, acts as its own backstop. When hemostasis is once achieved, adjunctive therapy, Interceed (as suggested previously), can be placed around the ovary to discourage formation of adhesions.

The most severe complications associated with ovarian laparoscopy are injuries to adjacent structures. The ovaries are bounded laterally by the pelvic wall that

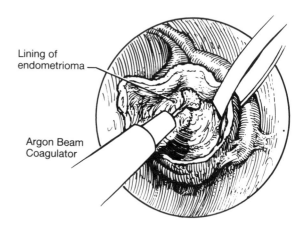

Fig. 30.3 Vaporization of the interior lining of an endometrioma for hemostasis and destruction of active endometriosis.

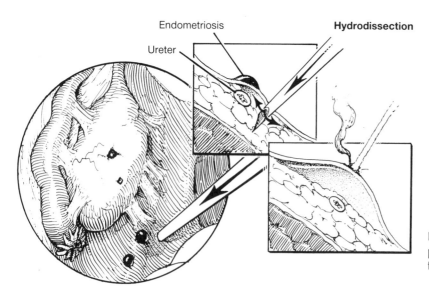

Fig. 30.2 Hydrodissection: method of raising the peritoneal lesion off the ureter to prevent injury with the CO_2 laser.

contains the uterus, common iliac, internal iliac vessels, and the obturator nerve. Medially there is the rectosigmoid colon; caudally there are the uterine vessels, ureter, and vagina, and cephalad there are the cecum, or sigmoid colon, the ureter, and iliac vessels. There is little likelihood of an injury to the anterior abdominal wall, but posteriorly there are many venous and nerve plexuses that could be damaged. The safest way to prevent damage to any of these structures is not to operate around them if their location is not clearly apparent. In such a situation, performing a laparotomy would be preferable to taking a chance on any injury. Certainly, the experience of the operator frequently will dictate the avenue to be taken when the anatomy presents a problem. Proper selection of patients is clearly the most important decision to make in endoscopic surgery.

Injury to adjacent structures can be minimized by shrinking the ovary to its smallest size by using either a GnRH agonist or similar medication. This will increase the pelvic space in which to work and reduce the vascularity of the ovary so that dissection will be easier. However, there are several precautions to be taken to minimize complications resulting from injury to a particular organ. A bowel preparation is mandatory when bowel involvement is suspected or known. In this way, if bowel is inadvertently entered, there will be no contamination or infection. The bowel can be dealt with immediately without the need for a diverting colostomy. This complication can be prevented by dissecting on top of the ovarian capsule rather than incising the bowel side of the adhesion. "Hugging" the surface of the ovary makes perforation highly unlikely.

Injury to the ureters can be prevented by making careful dissections over the peritoneum just above the ureters and carefully identifying the full extent of the ureter. If the lesion is over the top of the ureter, the retroperitoneal space can be injected with a solution of Ringer's lactate with a 22-gauge spinal needle to protect the ureter from the CO_2 laser only. This process has been termed "aquadissection." If a cautery or one of the fiberoptic lasers is used, then the ureter will not be protected. Injury to ureters is not very common. An article written by Grainger *et al.* (10) reported that the most common site of injury is at the ureterovesicle junction (Table 30.3). Lateral pelvic wall ureteral injury fortunately is less common. Should an injury occur, immediate urologic consultation must be obtained. Should there be a delay in diagnosis, most patients will manifest symptoms of lower quadrant pain within two to three days following surgery. This pain is usually associated with fever, most often mild but occasionally high, and a cystic structure giving the impression of a pelvic abscess. Should these symptoms occur, an intravenous pyelogram (IVP) is the diagnostic tool of choice. Extravasation of urine outside the boundaries of the bladder or course of the ureter will

Table 30.3. Ureteral injury at laparoscopy.

Indications for initial procedures (number)	
Endometriosis	5
Adhesions	2
Uterosacral transection	1
Sterilization	4
Diagnostic laparoscopy	1
Treatment modality (number)	
Unipolar cautery	7
Bipolar cautery	4
Laser	1
Trocar	1
Method of diagnosis (number)	
IVP	10
Laparoscopy	2
Laparotomy	1
Site of urethral injury (number)	
2 cm UVJ	5
3 cm UVJ	1
5 cm UVJ	1
Pelvic brim	6
Treatment (number)	
End-to-end anastomosis	3
Transverse ureteroureterostomy	4
Percutaneous stent	2
Boari flap	1
Ileal interposition	1
Stent at laparotomy	1
Retrograde stent	1

IVP, intravenous pyelogram.
UVJ, urethral–vesicle junction.

establish the diagnosis. The urologist should obviously be consulted at this time.

Injury to the iliac vessels is highly unlikely unless the ovarian adhesions attached to the pelvic brim are treated carelessly. This injury certainly can be prevented, either by using hydrodissection to raise the attached ovary off the vessel, or by incising the peritoneum over the vessel and tracing it out to its full extent. Retroperitoneal dissection will always allow the surgeon to visualize any vital structure, preventing inadvertent injury. It also is very rare for the common iliac or aorta to be injured during an operation on the ovary because of the usual position of the ovary in the pelvis. These injuries would more likely be associated with the insertion of the Veress needle or abdominal trocar.

Even though the literature does not contain articles concerning injury to the obturator nerve or other nerves in the pelvis, theoretically any nerve injury could be prevented by careful dissection in the cul-de-sac with the ovary used as the backstop when a laser is used. Liberal use of irrigating fluid in the lateral pelvic wall would invariably prevent such an injury.

Summary

Since the ovary is the most common place for endometriosis to occur, reasons for and frequency of occurrence, methods of recognition, and treatment methodology are obviously important. To prevent complications following treatment, it is imperative that the ovary be devoid of activity prior to surgical intervention. The ovaries must be freed from their attachments with the utmost care. The liberal use of retroperitoneal fluid to protect vital structures and complete visualization of the vital structures are mandatory to prevent unnecessary injury. Protecting the ovary from inevitable formation of adhesions is essential to protect fertility and decrease the potential of pain. Adjunctive therapy at the time of an operative laparoscopy will help in preventing formation of adhesions postoperatively. However, there is no substitute for meticulous dissection, impeccable hemostasis, and good judgment. Proper selection of patients and realistic appraisal of one's skills will ultimately result in successful treatment of endometriosis of the ovary.

REFERENCES

1. Jenkins S, Olive DL, Haney AF. Endometriosis: pathogenetic implications of the anatomic distribution. Obstet Gynecol 1986; 67:335–338.
2. Hori M, Kikkawa F, Suganuma N, et al. Conservative surgery of infertile patients with pelvic endometriosis—factors affecting the pregnancy rate and expectancy. Nippon Sanka Fujinka Gakkai Zasshi 1986;38:1763–1769.
3. Horne HW, Clyman M, Debrovren C, et al. The prevention of postoperative pelvic adhesions following conservative operative treatment for human infertility. Int J Fertil 1973;18: 109.
4. Interceed (TC7) Adhesion Barrier Study Group. Prevention of postsurgical adhesions by Interceed (TC7), an absorbable adhesion barrier: a prospective randomized multicenter clinical study. Fertil Steril 1989;51:933.
5. Evers JL. The second-look laparoscopy for evaluation of the result of medical treatment of endometriosis should not be performed during ovarian suppression. Fertil Steril 1987;47:502–504.
6. Brosens IA. New concepts in the pathophysiology and treatment of pelvic endometriosis. Contrib Gynecol Obstet 1989;17:36–43.
7. Nezhat C, Crowgey S, Nezhat F. Videolaseroscopy for the treatment of endometriosis associated with infertility. Fertil Steril 1989;51:237–239.
8. Reich H, McGlynn F. Treatment of ovarian endometriosis using laparoscopic surgical technique. J Reprod Med 1986;31: 557.
9. Rusch VW, Schmidt R, Shojl Y, Fujimura Y. Use of the argon beam electrocoagulator for performing pulmonary wedge resections. Ann Thorac Surg 1990;49:287–291.
10. Grainger DA, Soderstrom RM, Schiff SF, et al. Ureteral injuries at laparoscopy: insights into diagnosis, management, and prevention. Obstet Gynecol 1990;75:839–843.

31 | Adnexectomy: Preventing Ureteral Damage

Paul D. Silva

Introduction

Techniques for laparoscopic adnexectomy (salpingoophorectomy and oophorectomy) were first devised by Semm in Germany in the 1970s (1, 2). For hemostasis, he reported a modification of the loop that had been developed by Roeder (1866–1918) in the nineteenth century for tonsillectomy. Semm's group did not report any major complications with laparoscopic adnexectomy (1–4). Other groups have studied related techniques (5–12), however, and some have noted significant complication rates (Table 31.1).

A recent review of case reports of laparoscopic ureteral injury indicated that this complication may be most commonly associated with electrocoagulation techniques (13). In addition, the author is aware of a case from the United States in which ureteral injury occurred after laparoscopic adnexectomy involving bipolar electrocoagulation. As electrocoagulation equipment is inexpensive, widely available, and sometimes recommended as the main method for hemostasis during laparoscopic adnexectomy (6, 8), this chapter will review its safe use, as well as other safety considerations for laparoscopic adnexectomy.

In addition to the pelvic surgeon's knowledge of anatomy and experience with avoiding injury to the ureter at laparotomy (14), familiarity with three other areas may help in preventing damage to the ureter at the time of laparoscopic adnexectomy. First, a knowledge of the indications for laparoscopic adnexectomy is important, as the avoidance of unnecessary surgery will obviate complications. Second, considerable information is available about the safety of electrocoagulation and the various other energy sources available for use in laparoscopic adnexectomy. Third, experience is accumulating with the process of dealing with laparoscopic ureteral injuries produced at more common types of laparoscopic procedures, such as treatment of endometriosis and adhesions, sterilization, and diagnostic laparoscopy (13).

Indications

The usual indications for laparoscopic adnexectomy are becoming an even larger subset of the indications for adnexectomy by laparotomy. With further experience, these indications will likely encompass most of the indications involving benign disease. The following list of indications reflects a literature review as well as the author's experience.

1. Chronic lateralizing pelvic pain associated with endometriosis or pelvic adhesive disease that has failed to respond to medical treatment and is not appropriately treated by conservative procedures.
2. Estrogen-receptor-positive advanced metastatic breast carcinoma that has failed to respond to other therapies.
3. Cases of ovarian ectopic pregnancy in which conservation of the ovary is inappropriate or not feasible.
4. Becoming more acceptable are cases of benign cystic neoplasms. A set of criteria proposed by Parker and Berek (9) has included low CA-125 levels and the following ultrasonic features: size less than 10 cm, cystic appearance, distinct borders, no irregular solid parts or thick septa, and no ascites or matted bowel (9). Generally these criteria would apply only to patients who do not desire future fertility, as ovarian cystectomy would be indicated if fertility was desired. Levels of CA-125 are more useful indicators in postmenopausal women, because fewer false positives occur in this group.
5. Benign ovarian cystic teratomas may be treated by laparoscopic adnexectomy or oophorectomy in women who do not desire further fertility. Ultrasound diagnosis has improved to a level that these tumors can be strongly suspected preoperatively.

Table 31.1. Complications reported with laparoscopic adnexectomy in early series.

Source	Number	Complications	Number
Semm and Mettler (3)	37	None	
Reich (6)	24	None	
Goodman et al. (7)	98	Postoperative pyelonephritis	1
		Postoperative ileus	1
		Intraoperative blood loss >100 mL (not requiring laparotomy)	4
		Severe neck pain	1
		Postoperative urinary retention	2
Perry and Upchurch (8)	17	Postoperative bleeding requiring laparotomy (failed loop ligature)	1
			1
		Prolonged postoperative pain (two weeks)	1
		Late urinary retention	1
Parker and Berek (9)	22	Bowel performation during lysis of adhesions requiring laparotomy	1
		Perforation of bladder with trocar	1
Silva et al. (10, 11)	26	Abdominal wall ecchymosis	1
		Postoperative ileus	1
		Ovarian remnant syndrome requiring second laparoscopy	1
Nezhat et al. (12)	76	Abdominal wall ecchymosis	2
		Severe shoulder pain	9
Total	300		28 (9%)

6. Phenotypic females with gonadal dysgenesis with Y chromosomal material or evidence of hyperandrogenism.

Energy sources

The technique of laparoscopic salpingoophorectomy can be divided into three components, not all of which are always necessary (depending on whether the uterus and/or adhesions are present). These steps include lysis of adhesions to isolate the adnexae from pathologic attachments to surrounding organs, separation of the adnexae from its anatomic attachments to the uterus, and separation of the adnexae from the infundibulopelvic ligament.

In the following sections, the main energy sources available for laparoscopic adnexectomy will be discussed in relation to these three aspects of the surgery, with particular attention paid to avoiding ureteral injury during each step. Points relevant to simple laparoscopic oophorectomy are also made.

Lysis of adhesions

Dense adhesions related to endometriosis, chronic pelvic inflammatory disease, or prior surgery are often encountered when adnexectomy is indicated for chronic pelvic pain unresponsive to conservative measures. In such a case, it is generally best to divide the adhesions before the adnexae are separated from their anatomic attachments.

Avoiding damage to the ureter in dissecting the ovary free from pathologic adhesions to the inferior pelvic sidewall is critical. The safest way to perform this step is often analogous to those techniques used at laparotomy—that is, a combination of blunt dissection with a probe and sharp dissection with scissors. In difficult cases, it is useful to open two or three lower quadrant laparoscopic entry sites and operate with the use of a surgical assistant and video screen. A grasping forceps is used to place traction on the ovary for dissection with scissors and probe. While in the vicinity of the ureter, only a few millimeters of tissue should be snipped with the scissors at one time, with the scissors being kept sharp. To help avoid the ovarian remnant syndrome, care should be taken to remove any fragments of ovarian cortex that remain attached to the pelvic side wall.

The carbon dioxide laser and "hydrodissection" (15) represent two other modalities that can aid in dissection around the ureter. The author has found these modalities to be useful but not essential; they do add cost and must be set up for each case by trained personnel. A carbon dioxide laser beam with a small spot size and low power setting in superpulse mode, if available, can aid in sharp dissection around the ureter; this energy source assumes the function of a sharp scissors or knife. Such a beam can vaporize tissue millimeter by millimeter and, in experienced hands, may add precision to critical dissections over the ureter. Other laser wavelengths available for pelviscopic surgery generally penetrate too deeply into tissue to be recommended for use adjacent to the ureter. In addition, electrocoagulation and endocoagulation should not be used close to the ureter because of danger from the spread of heat and electrical energy with the former technology and from heat in the latter. Pressurized irrigation fluids, termed "hydrodissection," may also be employed as an adjunct to blunt dissection; dissection planes may sometimes be produced with little apparent trauma to surrounding tissue.

Although unipolar electrocoagulation should be avoided near the ureter, it need not be totally abandoned, as has been suggested by some authors (16). Provided that the equipment is periodically inspected and replaced before the insulation wears out, it can be used cautiously for lysis of adhesions and treatment of endometriosis away from the bowel and ureter; unipolar electrocoagulation may also be used to perform other adnexal procedures such as salpingostomy for conservative management of ectopic pregnancy (17).

If the ureter cannot be directly seen through the peritoneum of the pelvic side wall at the level of the dissection, its course can often be traced from a more cephalad position. The course of the ureter itself can be dissected with laparoscopic scissors and forceps if necessary; hydrodissection may also be applied. If the operator does not feel confident in separating an adherent ovary from the inferior pelvic sidewall, then conversion to laparotomy is the obvious choice. In general, the standard type of ureteral stent has not proved useful for identifying the course of the ureter in areas of dense scarring; the author has, however, used a lighted ureteral stent in one case where an adnexectomy was being performed on the side of a sole remaining kidney. In this case, dense periadnexal adhesions from previous urinary tract and gynecologic procedures were present, and the lighted stent was able to highlight the course of the ureter and aid in the prevention of injury during adhesiolysis.

Lysis of adhesions is generally not necessary in cases of simple oophorectomy performed for endocrine ablation. If the ovary is located in its normal position in the pelvis, little danger of damage to the ureter ensues. If the utero-ovarian ligament is compliant, three Roeder loops can be placed around the base of the ovary, and then the ovary can be severed with scissors. The ovary can be removed by use of a special sac, by morcellation, by widening the suprapubic trocar site to 2–3 cm, through an open laparoscopy incision, or through the cul-de-sac. Alternatively, an automatic stapling device can be used for oophorectomy, although this option adds considerable cost. If this procedure is performed with bipolar

electrocoagulation and scissors, then the tissue should be carefully pulled away from the vicinity of the ureter before coagulation to avoid damage to the ureter from heat or spread of current.

Dividing the adnexae from the uterus

Semm's original description of adnexectomy incorporated much tissue into the Roeder loops, including the infundibulopelvic ligament, proximal fallopian tube, utero-ovarian ligament, and upper broad ligament. In the patient with an intact uterus, it is often useful to divide the fallopian tube and utero-ovarian ligament prior to placing three endoloops around the adnexa (Fig. 31.1). This technique avoids incorporating large amounts of tissue into the endoloops. Bipolar electrocoagulation may then be applied in this location. The relative safety of this technique in coagulating the proximal fallopian tube is well documented by experience from tubal sterilization. When stretched in a ventral direction, the utero-ovarian ligament generally lies several centimeters away from the ureter at this level, although this positioning should be verified by inspection and dissection if necessary. At this point the ureter runs along the base of the broad ligament under the uterine artery and generally remains protected from injury during the division of the upper broad ligament (Fig. 31.2).

Advice for safely dividing the adnexae from its attachments to the uterus is similar to that recommended for tubal sterilization (18, 19). The structures should be lifted toward the anterior abdominal wall before activating the electrocoagulating current. It is important to avoid inadvertently touching the activated or hot tip of

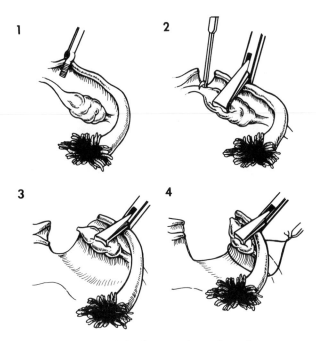

Fig. 31.1 Technique of dividing an adnexa from the uterus.

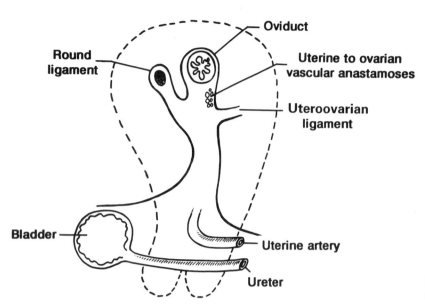

Fig. 31.2 Relationship of the ureter to structures of broad ligament.

the instrument to other intra-abdominal structures. This approach requires intense concentration and good visualization of all relevant structures while the tip of the instrument remains activated. The recently deactivated tip should also not be touched to surrounding structures; although animal studies indicate that touching the recently inactivated tip to the bowel carries little danger of damage to the bowel (20), this effect has not been tested on the urinary tract. The generator should be compatible with the bipolar forceps. Adequate but not excessive cutting current (approximately 25 W against a 100-ohm load) should be applied to cause desiccation and hemostasis of tissues (19); the coagulation mode produces much less power (wattage) if used at an identical setting.

Some surgeons have replaced bipolar electrocoagulation with endocoagulation instruments. Such equipment produces lower temperatures at the level of the tissue and no current spread occurs; as a result, greater safety has been claimed for this approach. Endocoagulation instrumentation is costly, however, and may not be readily available in many operating rooms. It has also been criticized by some as requiring lengthy application times to obtain sufficient coagulation for reliable hemostasis. With bipolar electrocoagulation, obvious desiccation of tissue that produces a parchment-like appearance or the absence of current flow as measured by an ohm meter signals adequate coagulation.

Hemostasis and division of the infundibulopelvic ligament

After the adnexae have been freed from adhesions, and their anatomic attachments lifted from the uterus, three endoloops can be placed around the infundibulopelvic

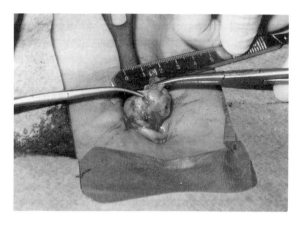

Fig. 31.3 Removing a detached adnexa through an open laparoscopy incision.

ligament and remaining upper broad ligament. The adnexae can then be severed with sharp scissors and removed (Fig. 31.3).

If prior hysterectomy has been performed, lysis of adhesions is followed by only ligation and division of the infundibulopelvic ligament and remnant of the upper broad ligament. After prior hysterectomy most of the risk of damage to the ureter is encountered when dissecting the adnexa free from adhesions to the pelvic side wall and bladder. Techniques similar to those described earlier for lysis of adhesions may be utilized.

Caution should be used if bipolar electrocoagulation is used for hemostasis of the infundibulopelvic ligament rather than endoloops. The ureter should be visualized first, as it often runs within 1–2 cm of the infundibulopelvic ligament at this level (Fig. 31.4). Fortunately,

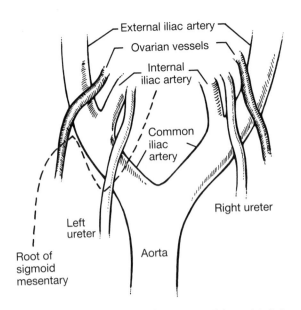

Fig. 31.4 Anatomic structures in the vicinity of the pelvic brim.

the right ureter can almost invariably be visualized at the level of its entrance into the true pelvis as it crosses the external iliac artery just proximal to the point where the infundibulopelvic ligament crosses; peristalsis can be observed spontaneously or stimulated with a blunt probe. On the other hand, the left ureter is often partially obscured by the inverted V-shaped root of the sigmoid mesentery at this level. It descends into the pelvis at a higher level, often actually crossing the left common iliac artery rather than the external iliac artery. If the location of the left ureter at the level of its entrance into the true pelvis cannot be traced back from the lower pelvic side wall, then the application of bipolar electrocoagulation without careful dissection is risky.

Automatic laparoscopic stapling devices that staple, cut, and divide tissues in the same motion can be used for hemostasis of the infundibulopelvic ligament. They do not always provide reliable hemostasis, however, and add significant cost. When this approach is taken, the staple line should be inspected carefully after lowering the intra-abdominal pressure to check for bleeding points. Because of problems of hemostasis with all three techniques applied to the infundibulopelvic ligament (i.e., loops, electrocoagulation, and stapling devices), it is generally wise to observe patients in the recovery area for several hours after laparoscopic adnexectomy. Overnight hospitalization is not unreasonable.

Case reports of laparoscopic ureteral injuries

In 1990, Grainger and coauthors reviewed the eight previously reported cases of laparoscopic ureteral injury and described five new cases from the United States (13). All of the cases except one involved the use of electrocoagulation. The other case was thought to be due to faulty trocar insertion.

The small possibility of trocar injuries to the ureter or bladder (21) can probably be reduced by adhering to the following general caveats in placing trocars. Trocars should be regularly sharpened; although disposable trocars are obviously sharp, they may add too much cost to the procedure to be practical. Ideally, trocars should be palmed during insertion, with the index finger used as a stop at the level of the anterior abdominal wall, thereby preventing sudden advancement of the trocar. Secondary trocars should be placed under laparoscopic visualization and directed away from critical structures. The patient's bladder should be catheterized prior to placement of the secondary trocar on a routine basis for long procedures; this step should also be taken prior to placement of a secondary trocar for a short procedure if the bladder is distended.

Grainger and coauthors (13) felt that some of the electrocoagulation injuries noted in the case reports may have been avoided with the use of a more careful technique. Some of the six injuries to the ureter at the pelvic brim likely occurred when the activated electrodes touched the peritoneum over the surface of the ureter. Because of the potential for damaging the ureter at the pelvic brim, the surgeon should consider three Roeder loops (rather than electrocoagulation) for hemostasis of the infundibulopelvic vessels, if the ureter cannot be distanced from the activated electrodes.

Other injuries may be prevented by avoiding the use of laparoscopic electrocoagulation in the region of the ureterosacral ligaments when the course of the ureter cannot be ascertained. The ureter is not easily seen through the peritoneum at the level at which the uterosacral ligaments are inseted into the cervix, and endometriosis or scarring may distort or obscure its course at this level. It is not always easy to safely dissect the ureter free at this level. In all five cases reviewed by Grainger and coauthors (13) where endometriosis was present, the injury to the ureter was within 2–3 cm from the ureterovesical junction. Methods other than coagulation—including sharp scissors dissection, blunt dissection, and carbon dioxide laser at low power settings, small spot size, and superpulse, if available—are preferred for dissection in such instances. If bleeding is encountered, meticulous isolation of the bleeding vessel prior to applying endocoagulation or electrocoagulation is recommended. Laparoscopically applied individual hemostatic clips may represent a safer alternative to bipolar electrocoagulation for hemostasis in areas adjacent to the ureter. When working close to the ureter, laparoscopic linear stapling devices that take wide tissue bites should be avoided, as ureteral damage can occur even without direct transection (22).

Recognition and treatment of ureteral injury

The most common presentation for laparoscopic ureteral injury is abdominal pain, peritonitis, leukocytosis, and fever approximately 48 to 72 hours postoperatively (13); on rare occasions, symptoms may not develop for several weeks. Because the usual presentation resembles that of bowel perforation, an intravenous pyelogram is recommended to make the diagnosis; typically a urinoma can be identified. In one reported case, the ureteral injury was recognized and treated at the time of laparoscopy by ureteral stenting and laparoscopic suture (23).

Retrograde or percutaneous stenting is being increasingly used for localized ureteral injuries not involving complete ligation or transection of the ureter; these techniques avoid the morbidity of laparotomy (24). If these options are not available or technically feasible, ureteral anastomosis, ureteroneocystostomy, and transureteral ureterostomy may be used to treat these injuries. It is probably wise to stent anastomoses after electrical injury, as necrosis may extend beyond the site of visual damage, and breakdown of the ureteral anastomosis has been reported. In general, urological consultation should be obtained—although ureteral repair techniques are well described in the literature and urologic texts, they require skill and practice for reliable application.

Small trocar injuries (3 or 5 mm) to the dome of the bladder do not necessarily require laparotomy for repair of the bladder (9). Such perforations can be treated by urinary drainage for five to seven days, as the bladder generally heals very rapidly. Unrecognized bladder perforation by the secondary trocar may present with urine drainage through the secondary trocar site rather than with signs of peritonitis.

Conclusion

Although the above discussion may help in avoiding ureteral injuries when performing laparoscopic adnexectomy, it is unlikely that all such injuries can be prevented. Ureteral injury is a rare but recognized complication of pelviscopic surgery and by itself does not imply careless technique or poor judgment. Although the incidence of ureteral injury with laparoscopic adnexectomy is probably low, its seriousness suggests that the possibility of damage to the urinary tract or bowel should be included in the preoperative discussion with the patient. If injury occurs, it is advisable to openly discuss this matter with the patient as well as the recommended interventions for correcting the injury. Early diagnosis and appropriate intervention are the keys to avoiding loss of renal func-

tion. Consequently, urologic consultation should be used when available, rather than having the surgeon attempt unfamiliar reparative techniques.

REFERENCES

1. Semm K. Tissue-puncher and loop-ligation—new aids for surgical-therapeutic pelviscopy. Endoscopy 1978;10:119–124.
2. Semm K. New methods of pelviscopy for myomectomy, ovariectomy, tubectomy and adnexectomy. Endoscopy 1979;2:85–93.
3. Semm K, Mettler L. Technical progress in pelvic surgery via operative laparoscopy. Am J Obstet Gynecol 1980;138:121–127.
4. Semm K, Friedrich ER. Operative manual for endoscopic abdominal surgery. Chicago: Year Book Medical, 1987.
5. Levine RL. Economic impact of pelviscopic surgery. J Reprod Med 1985;30:655–659.
6. Reich H. Laparoscopic oophorectomy and salpingo-oophorectomy in the treatment of benign tubo-ovarian disease. Int J Fertil 1987;32:233–236.
7. Goodman MP, Johns DA, Levine RI, Reich H, Levinson CJ, Murphy AA, Silva PD, Daniell JF, Diamond MP, Cropp CS. Report of the study group: advanced operative laparoscopy (pelviscopy). J Gyn Surg 1989;5:353–360.
8. Perry CP, Upchurch JC. Pelviscopic adnexectomy. Am J Obstet Gynecol 1990;162:79–81.
9. Parker WH, Berek JS. Management of selected cystic adnexal masses in postmenopausal women by operative laparoscopy: a pilot study. Am J Obstet Gynecol 1990;163:1574–1577.
10. Silva PD, Kuffel ME, Beguin EA. Open laparoscopy simplifies instrumentation required for laparoscopic oophorectomy and salpingo-oophorectomy. Obstet Gynecol 1991;77:482–485.
11. Silva PD. Adnexectomy: preventing ureteral damage. In: Corfman RS, Diamond MP, DeCherney A, eds. Complications of laparoscopy and hysterectomy. Boston: Blackwell Science, 1993: 152–159.
12. Nezhat F, Nezhat C, Silfen SL. Video laseroscopy for oophorectomy. Am J Obstet Gynecol 1991;165:1323–1330.
13. Grainger DA, Soderstrom RM, Schiff SF, Glickman MG, DeCherney AH, Diamond MP. Ureteral injuries at laparoscopy: insights into diagnosis, management, and prevention. Obstet Gynecol 1990;75:839–843.
14. Ridley JH. Gynecologic surgery, errors, safeguards, salvage. Baltimore: Williams and Wilkins, 1981.
15. Nezhat C, Nezhat FR. Safe laser endoscopic excision or vaporization of peritoneal endometriosis. Fertil Steril 1989;52:149–151.
16. Baggish MS. Is it necessary to repeat history? J Gyn Surg 1989;5:323.
17. Silva PD. A laparoscopic approach can be applied to most cases of ectopic pregnancy. Obstet Gynecol 1988;944–947.
18. Soderstrom RM, Levy BS. Bipolar systems—do they perform? Obstet Gynecol 1987;69:425–426.
19. Soderstrom RM, Levy BS, Engel T. Reducing bipolar sterilization failures. Obstet Gynecol 1989;74:60–63.
20. DiGiovanni M, Vasilenko P, Belsky D. Laparoscopic tubal sterilization, the potential for thermal bowel injury. J Reprod Med 1990;35:951–954.
21. Yuzpe AA. Pneumoperitoneum needle and trocar injuries in laparoscopy. J Reprod Med 1990;35:485–490.
22. Woodland MB. Ureter injury during laparoscopy-assisted vaginal hysterectomy with the endoscopic linear stapler. Am J Obstet Gynecol 1992;167:756–757.
23. Gomel V, James C. Intraoperative management of ureteral injury during operative laparotomy. Fertil Steril 1991;55:416–419.
24. Mitty HA, Train JS, Dan SJ. Placement of ureteral stents by antegrade and retrograde techniques. Urol Clin North Am 1986;4:587–600.

32 | Complications of Laparoscopic Ovarian Cystectomy

Daniel S. Seidman, Camran Nezhat, Farr Nezhat, and Ceana Nezhat

Laparoscopy is accepted as the preferred approach for removal of ovarian cysts (1–5). The most important step in the prevention of surgical complications, regardless of the technique employed, is avoiding unnecessary procedures. It is recommended to remove persistent ovarian cysts to rule out malignancy, avoid torsion or rupture, and relieve associated symptoms, including pain and infertility. As many ovarian cysts are physiologic, benign-appearing ovarian cysts should typically be evaluated six to eight weeks after their diagnosis. Although hormonal suppressive therapy with oral contraceptives is commonly advocated, its use is not supported by controlled trials (6–8). Although ultrasound-guided aspiration of benign-appearing ovarian cysts represents an alternative to laparoscopic surgery, the high rate of recurrence does not justify this technique (9). Likewise, cyst puncture contributes little to the differential diagnosis of benign ovarian tumors (10). Sclerotherapy of the cysts by injection of alcohol (11, 12) or tetracycline (13) has been investigated as a means of reducing the rate of recurrence, but remains experimental.

Differentiating between malignant and benign ovarian tumors can be accomplished successfully at laparoscopy (14). Furthermore, laparoscopic management of early-stage ovarian cancer has gained acceptance when performed by experienced laparoscopic oncologists (15, 16, 17). In addition, this approach is effective in the initial surgical evaluation of adnexal masses in women with a history of nongynecologic malignancy (18). To date, the exact role of laparoscopy in the management of ovarian cancer has not been definitively determined (19–21). However, all women scheduled to undergo surgery to evaluate an ovarian cyst should be evaluated thoroughly.

Preoperative evaluation

Laparoscopic management of an adnexal mass depends on the patient's age, pelvic examination, sonographic images, and serum markers. A large, solid, fixed or irregular adnexal mass accompanied by ascites is highly suspicious for malignancy. Cul-de-sac nodularity, cystic adnexal structures, and fixed adnexa are noted to occur with endometriosis and ovarian malignancy.

Abdominal or transvaginal ultrasound imaging is the primary evaluation for adnexal masses (22). Cystic unilateral masses less than 10 cm in diameter that are unilocular with regular borders are likely to be benign. Malignant ovarian cysts are associated with irregular borders, size greater than 10 cm, papillae, solid areas, thick septa (>2 mm), ascites, and matted bowel. Using ultrasonographic criteria, accurate prediction of benign masses was made in 96% of patients (22, 23). In a large series of premenopausal women with ovarian cysts managed laparoscopically, preoperative pelvic sonography had a high false-positive predictive value, and none of four malignant cysts met any of the criteria that would indicate malignancy (5).

CA-125 is a tumor-associated antigen used to identify the nature of the ovarian cyst. Levels less than 35 μ/mL are associated with benign tumors. The sensitivity and specificity of this marker varies, however, and the presence of other benign conditions can elevate CA-125 levels. In 80% of premenopausal women, elevated CA-125 levels were associated with pregnancy, endometriosis, fibroids, adenomyosis, cystic teratomas, and acute or chronic salpingitis. More importantly, only 50% of patients with Stage I ovarian cancer had elevated CA-125 levels compared with 90% of patients with Stage II disease (24).

Because the risk of malignancy is relatively low in young women, preoperative evaluation should include a history and physical examination and a pelvic ultrasound to evaluate both ovaries (to rule out bilateral endometriomas or teratomas). The need for hormonal suppressive therapy and the collection of a blood sample for future CA-125 and other tumor markers determination should

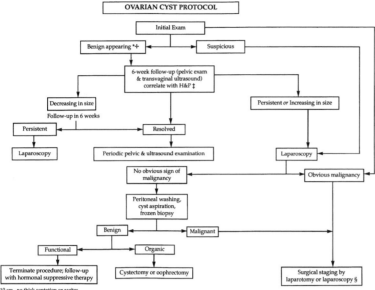

Fig. 32.1 Protocol for the evaluation and management of premenopausal adnexal mass.

*cystic, <10 cm., no thick septation or ascites
+ Hormonal suppressive therapy may or may not be prescribed (see Discussion)
‡ History and Physical
§ Possibly after chemotherapy

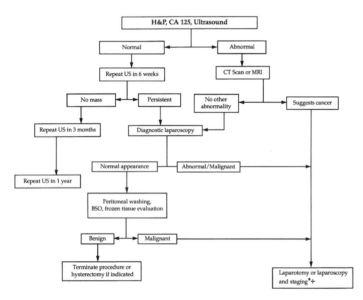

Fig. 32.2 Protocol for the evaluation and management of postmenopausal adnexal mass.

* Depends on the surgeon's experience in managing malignancy by laparoscopy
+ Possibly after chemotherapy

be considered (Fig. 32.1). In postmenopausal women, the preoperative evaluation includes a history, pelvic examination, ultrasound, and measurement of serum CA-125.

If any combination of these tests suggests malignancy, an abdominal and pelvic computerized tomography (CT) scan is performed. If the scan indicates malignancy (e.g., ascites, omental cake), the patient undergoes a staging laparotomy and chemotherapy is administered (Fig. 32.2). If the CT scan is negative, a laparoscopy is planned, and informed consent for possible laparotomy

is obtained. The patient undergoes mechanical and antibiotic bowel preparation, and older women receive a chest X ray.

Intraoperative considerations

Intraoperative evaluation includes cell washings from the pelvis and upper abdomen to be saved for evaluation should a malignancy be found. The upper abdomen and pelvis are explored, and excrescences or suspicious areas are sampled and sent for frozen section. After examination of the pelvis and upper abdomen is complete, the contents of any cystic mass should be aspirated. Once the capsule is opened, the interior of the capsule is examined and suspicious areas biopsied and sent for frozen section. The entire cystic capsule must be removed to search for an early carcinoma that may elude gross detection (5). The decision whether to perform oophorectomy or cystectomy depends on the patient's age and the characteristics of the mass.

Ovarian cystectomy

Three methods are used to manage ovarian cysts: drainage, excision and thermal ablation, and desiccation. By excising cysts, histopathologic examination is more complete and the risk of recurrence is minimized. Aspiration is recommended for functional (follicular or luteal) cysts, which are diagnosed laparoscopically and confirmed by frozen section, followed by postoperative hormonal suppressive therapy. Thermal ablation or desiccation does not destroy the entire cyst wall, and the underlying ovarian cortex can be damaged by the heat. Therefore, excision is preferred. An ovarian cystectomy removes the intact cyst with minimal trauma to the residual ovarian tissue (25). To minimize spillage and facilitate its removal, the cyst's fluid can be drained.

Many cysts are ruptured during manipulation despite careful technique. Removing a cyst of 10 cm or larger intact is difficult laparoscopically. Aspiration before removal of large cysts is practical and can be accomplished using one of two methods. In the first technique, an 18-gauge laparoscopic needle is passed through the suction-irrigator probe while stabilizing the cyst with suction applied over the cyst. The needle is inserted into the cyst and its contents are aspirated. The suction-irrigator system reduces the spillage by applying suction at the cannula, or the suction-irrigator probe can be inserted into the cyst. Alternatively, a 5-mm trocar and sleeve are introduced through a suprapubic port. Both are placed into the cyst, and the trocar is then removed. The suction-irrigator probe is inserted into the cyst through the remaining sleeve. This method works well for endometriomas and cystadenomas but is not advisable for benign teratomas, which contain hair, bone, or fatty tissue that makes removal of the cyst contents very difficult (25). Both of these techniques can be performed while confining the cyst inside of a bag to avoid further spillage of the cyst contents into the abdominal cavity.

Although the aspirate can be sent for cytologic examination, such findings do not have significant clinical value and will not change the course of management, as the entire cyst will still be removed and examined histologically. The ovary is freed from adhesions to the lateral pelvic wall, uterus, or bowel. The cyst and pelvis are irrigated continuously, especially where benign cystic ter-

atomas, mucinous cystadenomas, or endometriomas are present. The most dependent portion of the cyst wall is opened and the internal surface is inspected. If it appears to be a functional cyst (follicular or luteal), a confirmation biopsy specimen is sent for frozen section and the procedure is terminated. Hormonal suppressive therapy to prevent ovulation is administered for the next two months, which should allow spontaneous resolution of the cyst.

If ovarian cystectomy is warranted, hydrodissection is performed by injecting dilute vasopressin between the capsule and ovarian cortex to facilitate cyst removal and to reduce oozing in the capsule. The capsule is stripped from the ovarian stroma using two grasping forceps and the suction-irrigator probe to provide traction and countertraction. It is sent for histologic examination. A low-power energy source, such as the CO_2 laser (10 to 20 W, continuous) or unipolar or bipolar electricity, is used to seal blood vessels at the base of the capsule; administration of the energy source at higher powers is used to vaporize small remnants of the capsule.

If the cyst wall cannot be identified clearly, the edge of the ovarian incision can be "freshened" with scissors; the resulting clean edge will reveal the relevant structures. If this action does not free the capsule, the base of the cyst is grasped, and traction is applied to the cyst with countertraction to the ovary. The entire cyst or portions of the wall may be densely adherent to the ovary, requiring sharp or laser dissection to completely free the cyst wall. Large cysts require partial oophorectomy, using high-power laser or scissors to remove the distorted portion of the ovary. The remaining cyst wall can then be stripped from the ovarian stroma.

If teratomas are mostly solid, they often can be excised intact. Should rupture of a mostly cystic teratoma occur, the resulting contamination is greater than if the cysts were opened and aspirated. Hydrodissection is used to atraumatically develop the plane between the cyst wall and ovarian tissue. An 18- or 20-gauge needle is introduced through an accessory trocar sleeve, or a 7.5-inch spinal needle is inserted through the abdominal wall into the space between the cyst wall and the ovary. The plane is further developed using the suction-irrigator probe for blunt dissection. After the cyst is removed, the base of the capsule is irrigated and hemostasis is achieved with either CO_2 laser or bipolar electrocoagulator. A grasping forceps helps to approximate the ovarian edges. If the ovarian edges overlap, the defect is left to heal. Suture is not used because it is associated with adhesion formation (26). If the edges of the ovarian capsule do not spontaneously approximate, low-power laser applied to the inner surface will invert them. In rare instances, one or two fine, absorbable monofilament sutures are placed inside the ovary to approximate the edges and decrease the risk of adhesion formation. Before terminating the surgical procedure, vigorous washing of the pelvic cavity is performed to remove any remaining cyst content or debris.

Risk of ovarian malignancy

Critics of operative laparoscopy voice concerns over the possibility that an ovarian cyst may be malignant. Even if it is agreed that ovarian cancer should not be managed laparoscopically, most adnexal masses are benign, making most laparotomies unnecessary. Applying protocols that exclude patients with elevated CA-125 levels (in postmenopausal patients) and suspicious cysts containing septations greater than 2 mm thick on ultrasound, solid components within a cyst, multilocular cysts, matted loops of bowel, or ascites has proved successful in selecting appropriate cases (3, 27). The judgment of the surgeon and patient must always prevail, however.

While the effects of intraoperative rupture and spillage of malignant ovarian tumors generate concern, few studies support the idea that accidental rupture specifically worsens the prognosis of patients with early cancer (28, 29). In fact, most studies fail to demonstrate an independent detrimental effect of cyst rupture on long-term outcome (30–37). Other factors such as tumor grade, capsular involvement, presence or absence of ascites, and dense adherence of the tumor to other pelvic organs are more important in determining the spread of the malignant disease. As no prospective study has shown an adverse effect from rupture of the ovarian capsule in Stage I epithelial ovarian cancer, concerns about encountering an ovarian malignancy during laparoscopy appear to be exaggerated.

As noted earlier, when intraoperative rupture of a malignant cyst occurs during laparoscopy, the pelvis and abdomen must be lavaged. Staging and definitive treatment should be performed as soon as possible, preferably under the same anesthesia. The delay in appropriate overall management of this disease appears to be more detrimental than the type of initial surgery (19). Most authorities still call for an immediate conversion to laparotomy when malignancy is suspected—except in cases of an investigational protocol (19).

Large series have demonstrated a reassuringly low incidence of unexpected malignancy at laparoscopy—0.4% (5) and 1.2% (38)—but intraoperative surveillance and generous biopsies are necessary for correct diagnosis of unsuspected cancer. Because cyst fluid cytology used alone is unreliable (39), ruling out ovarian malignancy simply by aspiration without completely removing the cyst wall would provide inadequate management.

In our series of operative laparoscopy for adnexal masses in 1011 women, we encountered four cases of malignancy; three of those cases will illustrate the difficulties of case selection and intraoperative management (5). One woman had a recurrent mucinous cystadenoma, confirmed by histology, but because of dense adhesions on the contralateral ovary, hysterectomy and bilateral salpingo-oophorectomy were suggested. At laparotomy the tumor was found to be a mucinous cystadenocarcinoma. Recurrent epithelial tumors should be approached more aggressively than an initial occurrence, and oophorectomy considered in these cases. In a second case, bilateral endometriomas were drained and removed; histology reported that the smaller lesion was an endometrioid low-malignant potential tumor. Because assumptions based on "typical appearance" and size of lesion can be misleading, such a histology confirmation is always necessary. In the third case, a translucent cyst was opened. A thickening lesion on the wall was biopsied and sent for frozen section, which revealed necrotic tissue of inconclusive significance. Oophorectomy rather than cystectomy was carried out, and permanent histology was clear cell carcinoma. In this case, a high index of suspicion led to the correct diagnosis.

Abdominal wall tumor implantation

Metastatic tumors have been reported at trocar sites on the anterior abdominal wall, following biopsy of ovarian cancer (40–43). It has been suggested that the process of incision implantation is not related to the surgical approach, however, but rather to the invasive properties, or biologic virulence, of the tumor (44, 45). Furthermore, preliminary surveys of laparoscopy for gynecologic (44, 46) and colon (47) cancer suggest that port-site recurrence is infrequent. Because endometriosis can also be implanted at incisional sites, suspicious ovarian tissue should be removed from the abdomen while avoiding direct contact with the abdominal incision. Small lesions can be removed through the 5- or 10-mm trocar sleeve without contamination of the abdominal wall. For large lesions, several options are available. A laparoscopic bag can be used to contain the mass (48); the bag is then removed from the abdominal cavity via a minilaparotomy, posterior colpotomy, or an 18- or 33-mm trocar sleeve.

Ovarian remnant syndrome

Ovarian remnant syndrome, a late complication of oophorectomy, is defined as pelvic pain in the presence of persistent ovarian tissue. This condition can result from incomplete excision of the ovaries and infundibulopelvic ligament or the reimplantation of functioning ovarian fragments on peritoneal surfaces. In a recent study with rat models, 75% of such devascularized tissue revascularized and resumed functioning (49). Similar findings were noted in cats after suturing devascularized ovarian tissue to the peritoneum (50). Implantation of a small ovarian remnant on the bladder has been reported following laparoscopic adnexectomy (51). The authors have encountered a benign tumor on the surface of the bowel containing a corpus luteum and other ovarian tissue. A fragment of excised ovary was apparently inadvertently left in the peritoneal cavity after laparoscopic oophorectomy, and subsequently adhered to the bowel surface. To avoid this problem, the operative laparoscopist should be careful to remove all ovarian fragments from the peritoneal cavity.

Laparoscopy for oophorectomy, with or without hysterectomy, is rapidly becoming the standard of care, raising concerns that the prevalence of ovarian remnant syndrome will increase (49). This risk has been attributed to two sources: the technical difficulty associated with laparoscopic surgery, and the greater numbers of patients with severe adhesions and endometriosis undergoing laparoscopy. We recently reported on nine women who developed ovarian remnant syndrome after laparoscopic oophorectomy (52). All patients had undergone multiple previous pelvic surgeries for pelvic endometriosis, adhesions, or both. Endoloop suture ligation was used in four patients and bipolar electrodesiccation in five. At subsequent laparoscopy, ovarian remnants were found and removed from the lateral pelvic side wall (broad ligament) in five patients, the ureter in four women, the rectum and/or rectosigmoid colon in six women, the posterior uterus in one patient, and a residual uterosacral ligament in one patient (52).

If an endoloop is applied, the suture must be placed carefully below the ovary to avoid trapping ovarian tissue in the pedicle. Electrodesiccation and transection of the infundibulopelvic ligament allows the surgeon to follow anatomic planes, thereby increasing the likelihood that the entire ovary will be removed and eliminating the chance of foreign-body reaction. When the ovaries are tightly attached to the broad ligament by endometriosis and adhesions, removal of the attached peritoneum will decrease the possibility of leaving ovarian tissue behind.

Spillage of benign cysts

Spilling material in cases of benign cystic teratoma, mucinous cystadenoma, or endometrioma has been suspected of causing chemical peritonitis or disseminated intraperitoneal disease. Endometrial cysts mainly consist of old blood and only rarely contain endometrial glands and stroma; thus the overall risk of spreading endometriosis by rupturing the cyst and spilling its contents is low. Spontaneous leakage of endometriomas apparently is not uncommon. In many women with ovarian endometriomas, laparoscopy will reveal hemosiderin deposition on different parts of the abdominal and pelvic peritoneal cavity without endometrial implants.

Chemical peritonitis and pseudomyxoma peritonei caused by the rupture and spillage of a dermoid cyst and mucinous cyst, respectively, have been seen when a cyst ruptured and its contents remained in the peritoneal cavity for some time before surgical removal. During laparoscopic excision, every effort should be made to avoid such spillage. If it does occur, these complications can be prevented by copious irrigation using several liters of Ringer's lactate and is performed with the patient in reverse Trendelenburg position. Our experience and that of others (1, 14) indicate that these precautions minimize the risk of such complications.

Recurrence

Recurrence of ovarian cysts represents a contraindication for simple aspiration. Although others have suggested fenestration of the ovarian cyst to limit recurrence, only complete wall excision can reduce the risk of recurrence for endometriomas (53) or benign epithelial tumors. Follow-up with ultrasound will help identify any recurrence at an early stage. The authors have encountered a high rate of recurrence following only aspiration of endometrioma (54).

Overtreatment

Overtreatment can result in the loss of ovarian function. Generally, overly aggressive vaporization, electrodesiccation or resection of the ovarian cortex or aggressive coagulation of bleeding at the cyst base causes ovarian destruction. Dilute vasopressin injection or low-power CO_2 laser may be used for hemostasis in this area.

Vascular injury

Ovarian vascular injuries can occur during dissection of the infundibulopelvic ligament, mesovarium, or lateral pelvic wall. If a major vessel is injured, the area should be suctioned vigorously, allowing the surgeon to identify, isolate, grasp with Kleppinger forceps, and desiccate the vessel. If adnexal preservation is desired, aggressive overdesiccation should be avoided to prevent compromise of ovarian function. Occasionally, injecting fluid around a very small vessel that has retracted in the mesovarium will aid in achieving hemostasis. If the surgeon remains calm and the assistant is attentive, laparotomy should rarely be necessary to repair an injured ovarian vessel. Ovaries may appear devascularized, but should be left in place because the ovarian tissue remains viable in most cases.

After achieving hemostasis in the ovarian pedicle, the pneumoperitoneum is decreased under continued observation. The pedicle occasionally begins actively bleeding after this deflation. Once pneumoperitoneum is restored, the bleeding may stop. The pressure of the pneumoperitoneum apparently prevents pumping of smaller vessels that are actually still patent. The ovarian pedicle or other surgical sites should be reinspected after decreasing the pneumoperitoneum in every case, before hemostasis is considered adequate (25).

Adhesions

Adhesions form in most women after reproductive pelvic surgery, and usually involve the ovary. These formations may have severe clinical consequences, including infertility, bowel obstruction, and chronic pelvic pain (55). Prevention of their development requires attention to proper surgical technique (26). Meticulous hemostasis, and careful suture selection and application, are essential for minimizing adhesions (55).

Animal studies have shown that closing peritoneal surfaces increases tissue necrosis and foreign body reactions that may slow healing and result in adhesion formation (56). Avoiding peritoneal closure may mitigate the inflammatory reaction and allow prompter reperitonealization. Rinsing the powder from the surgical gloves or using powder-free gloves may also be important for adhesion prevention (57), although this problem represents a minor issue for laparoscopic operations.

Barriers that separate tissues during mesothelial healing hinder the development of fibrin bands that connect pelvic structures. Clinically approved barriers include absorbable regenerated oxidized cellulose (Interceed) (58–60) and permanent polytetrafluoroethylene (Gore-Tex Surgical Membrane) (61, 62). Both materials can be applied laparoscopically (63–65). Because the ovary is small and often associated with adhesion formation, Interceed or Gore-Tex application is recommended after laparoscopic cyst removal, particularly if sutures were used to approximate the ovarian capsule.

Conclusion

Because laparoscopy is so widely used, many residents have limited exposure to the treatment of benign adnexal masses by laparotomy. Proper patient selection, meticulous technique, and adequate experience are essential, however, when performing laparoscopic cystectomy to minimize trauma to the ovary and associated complications.

REFERENCES

1. Nezhat C, Winer W, Nezhat F. Laparoscopic removal of dermoid cysts. Obstet Gynecol 1989;73:278–281.
2. Mettler L, Caesar G, Neunzling S, Semm K. Value of endoscopic ovarian surgery—critical analysis of 626 pelviscopically operated ovarian cysts at the Kiel University Gynecologic Clinic 1990–1991. Geburts Frauennh 1993;53:253–257.
3. Parker WH, Berek JS. Management of selected cystic adnexal masses in postmenopausal women by operative laparoscopy: a pilot study. Am J Obstet Gynecol 1990;163:1574–1577.
4. Nezhat F, Nezhat C, Allan CJ, Metzger DA, Sears DL. A clinical and histologic classification of endometriomas: implications for a mechanism of pathogenesis. J Reprod Med 1992;37:771–776.
5. Nezhat C, Nezhat F, Welander CE, et al. Four ovarian cancers diagnosed during laparoscopic management of 1,011 adnexal masses. Am J Obstet Gynecol 1992;167:790.
6. Steinkampf MP, Hammond KR, Blackwell RE. Hormonal treatment of functional ovarian cysts: a randomized, prospective study. Fertil Steril 1990;54:775–777.
7. Ben-Ami M, Geslevich Y, Ba S, Matilsky M, Shalev E. Management of functional ovarian cysts after induction of ovulation: a randomized prospective stud. Acta Obstet Gynecol Scand 1993;72:396–397.
8. Nezhat CH, Nezhat F, Borhan S, Seidman DS, Nezhat CR. Is hormonal treatment efficacious in the management of ovarian cysts in women with endometriosis? Hum Reprod 1996 (accepted for publication).
9. Lipitz S, Seidman DS, Menczer J, Bider D, Oelsner G, Moran O, Shalev J. Recurrence after fluid aspiration from sonographically benign-appearing ovarian cysts. J Reprod Med 1992;37:845–848.
10. Vercellini P, Oldani S, Felicetta I, Bramante T, Rognoni MT, Crosignani PG. The value of cyst puncture in the differential diagnosis of benign ovarian tumors. Hum Reprod 1995;10:1465–1469.
11. Bret PM, Atri M, Guiband L, Gillett P, Syemore RJ, Senterman MK. Ovarian cysts in postmenopausal women: preliminary results with transvaginal alcohol sclerosis. Radiol 1992;184:661–663.
12. Lipitz S, Seidman DS, Schiff E, Achiron R, Manczer J. Treatment of pelvic peritoneal cysts by drainage and ethanol instillation. Obstet Gynecol 1995;86:297–299.
13. AbdRabbo S, Atta A. Aspiration and tetracycline sclerotherapy for management of simple ovarian cysts. Int J Gyn Obstet 1995;50:171–174.
14. Canis M, Mage G, Pouly JL, Wattiez A, Manhes H, Bruhat MA. Laparoscopic diagnosis of adnexal cystic masses: a 12-year experience with long-term follow-up. Obstet Gynecol 1994;85:707–712.
15. Amara DD, Nezhat CR, Teng NT, et al. Operative laparoscopy and management of ovarian cancer. Surg Laparosc Endosc 1996;61:38–45.
16. Pomel C, Provencher D, Dauplat J, Gauthier P, LeBouedec G, Drouin P, Audet-Lointe P, Dubic-Lissoir J. Laparoscopic staging of an early ovarian cancer. Gynecol Oncol 1995;58:301–306.
17. Childers JM, Nasseri A, Surwit EA. Laparoscopic management of suspicious adnexal masses. Am J Obstet Gynecol 1996;175(6):1451–1457; discussion 1457–1459.
18. Chi DS, Curtin JP, Barakat RR. Laparoscopic management of adnexal masses in women with a history of non-gynecologic malignancy. Obstet Gynecol 1995;86:964–968.
19. Childers JM, Masseri A. Minimal access surgery in gynecologic cancers: we can, but should we? Curr Opin Obstet Gynecol 1995;7:57–62.
20. Crawford RA, Gore ME, Sheperd JH. Ovarian cancers related to minimal access surgery. Br J Obstet Gynaecol 1995;102:726–730.
21. Nezhat C, Seidman DS, Nezhat F, Nezhat CH. Laparoscopic surgery for gynecologic cancer. In: Szabo Z, Lewis JE, Fantini GA, eds. Surgical technology international IV. San Francisco: Universal Medical Press, 1995:235–241.
22. Herrmann U, Locher G, Goldhirsch A. Sonographic patterns of malignancy: prediction of malignancy. Obstet Gynecol 1987;69:777.
23. Granberg S, Norstrom A, Wikland M. Comparison of endovaginal ultrasound and cytological evaluations of cystic ovarian tumors. J Ultrasound Med 1991;10:9.
24. Jacobs I, Bast R. The CA-125 tumor associated antigen: a review of the literature. Hum Reprod 1989;4:1.
25. Nezhat CR, Nezhat F, Luciano AA, Siegler AM, Metzger DA, Nezhat CH. Ovarian cysts. In: Nezhat CR, Nezhat F, Luciano AA, Siegler AM, Metzger DA, Nezhat CH, eds. Operative gynecologic laparoscopy: principles and techniques. New York: McGraw-Hill, 1995:149–165.
26. Nezhat C, Nezhat F. Postoperative adhesion formation after ovarian cystectomy with and without ovarian reconstruction. Presented at the 47th annual meeting of the American Fertility Society, Orlando, Florida, October 21–24, 1991.
27. Goldstein SR, Subramanyam B, Snyder JR, Beller U, Raghavendra BN, Bechman EM. The post-menopausal cystic adnexal mass: the

potential role of ultrasound in conservative management. Obstet Gynecol 1989;73:8–10.

28. Webb MJ, Decker DG, Mussey E, Williams TJ. Factors influencing survival in stage I ovarian cancer. Am J Obstet Gynecol 1973;116:222–228.

29. Sainz de la Cuesta R, Goff BA, Fuller AF, Nikrui N, Eichhorn JH, Rice LW. Prognostic importance of intraoperative rupture of malignant ovarian epithelial neoplasms. Obstet Gynecol 1994;84:1–7.

30. Dembo AJ, Davy M, Stenwig AE, Berle EJ, Bush RS, Kjorstad K. Prognostic factors in patients with stage I epithelial ovarian cancer. Obstet Gynecol 1990;75:263–273.

31. Sevelda P, Dittrich C, Salzer H. Prognostic value of the rupture of the capsule in stage I epithelial ovarian carcinoma 1989;35:321–322.

32. Finn CB, Luesley DM, Buxton EJ, et al. Is stage I epithelial ovarian cancer ever treated both surgically and systemically? Results of a five year cancer registry review. Br J Obstet Gynaecol 1992;99:54–58.

33. Vergote IB, Kaern J, Abeler VM, Pettersen EO, De Vos LN, Trope CG. Analysis of prognostic factors in stage I epithelial ovarian carcinoma: importance of degree of differentiation and deoxyribonucleic acid ploidy in predicting relapse. Am J Obstet Gynecol 1993;169:40–52.

34. Sjovall K, Nilsson B, Einhorn N. Different types of rupture of the tumor capsule and the impact on survival in early ovarian carcinoma. Int J Gynecol Cancer 1994;4:333–336.

35. Smith JP, Day TG. Review of ovarian cancer at the University of Texas Systems Cancer Center, M. D. Anderson Hospital and Tumor Institute. Am J Obstet Gynecol 1979;135:984–993.

36. Sigurdsson K, Alm P, Gullberg B. Prognostic factors in malignant epithelial ovarian tumors. Gynecol Oncol 1983;15:370–380.

37. Monga M, Carmichael JA, Shelley WE, et al. Surgery without adjuvant chemotherapy for early epithelial ovarian carcinoma after comprehensive surgical staging. Gynecol Oncol 1991;43:195–197.

38. Mage G, Canis M, Manhes H, Pouly JL, Wettiez A, Bruhat MA. Laparoscopic management of adnexal cystic masses. J Gynecol Surg 1990;6:71–79.

39. DeCrespigny LC, Robinson HP, Davoren RA, Fortune D. The "simple" ovarian cysts: aspirate or operate? Br J Obstet Gynaecol 1989;96:1035–1039.

40. Hsiu JG, Given FT, Kemp GM. Tumor implantation after diagnostic laparoscopy of serous ovarian tumors of low malignant potential. Obstet Gynecol 1986;68:902–903.

41. Miralles RM, Petit J, Gine L, Balquero L. Metastatic cancer spread at laparoscopic puncture site. Eur J Gynaecol Oncol 1980;IX:442–444.

42. Gleeson NC, Nicosia SV, Mar JE, et al. Abdominal-wall metastases from ovarian carcinoma after laparoscopy. Am J Obstet Gynecol 1993;169:522–523.

43. Shepherd JG, Carter PG, Lowe DG. Wound recurrence by implantation of a borderline ovarian tumor following laparoscopic removal. Br J Obstet Gynaecol 1994;101:265–266.

44. Childers JM, Aqua KA, Surwit EA, et al. Abdominal-wall tumor implantation after laparoscopy for malignant conditions. Obstet Gynecol 1994;84:765–769.

45. Berek JS. Ovarian cancer spread: is laparoscopy to blame? Lancet 1995;346:200.

46. Walsh DC, Wattchow DA, Wilson TG. Subcutaneous metastases after laparoscopic resection of malignancy. Aust NZ J Surg 1993;63:563–565.

47. Ramos JM, Gupta S, Anthone GJ, et al. Laparoscopy and colon cancer: is the port site at risk? A preliminary report. Arch Surg 1994;129:897–899.

48. Amos NN, Broadbent JAM, Hill HCW, et al. Laparoscopic "oophorectomy-in-a-bag" for removal of ovarian tumors of uncertain origin. Gynaecol Endoscopy 1992;1:85–89.

49. Minke T, DePond W, Winkelmann T, Blythe J. Ovarian remnant syndrome: study in laboratory rats. Am J Obstet Gynecol 1994;171:1440–1444.

50. Shemwell R, Weed J. Ovarian remnant syndrome. Obstet Gynecol 1970;36:299–303.

51. Wood C, Hill D, Maher P, Lolatgis N. Laparoscopic adnexectomy—indication, technique and results. Aust NZ J Obstet Gynecol 1992;32:362–366.

52. Nezhat F, Nezhat C, Nezhat CH, Seidman DS. Ovarian remnant syndrome following laparoscopic oophorectomy. Presented at the Society of Gynecologic Surgeons annual meeting, Albuquerque, New Mexico, March 4, 1996.

53. Hasson HM. Laparoscopic management of ovarian cysts. J Reprod Med 1990;35:863–867.

54. Nezhat C, Winer WK, Nezhat F. Is endoscopic treatment of endometriosis and endometrioma associated with better results than laparotomy? Am J Obstet Gynecol Health 1988;2:78–85.

55. Thompson JN, Whawell SA. Pathogenesis and prevention of adhesion formation. Br J Surg 1995;82:3–5.

56. Elkins TE, Stovall TG, Warren J, Ling F, Meyer NL. A histologic evaluation of peritoneal injury and repair: implications for adhesion formation. Obstet Gynecol 1987;70:225.

57. Kamffer WJ, Jooste EVW, Nel JT, DeWet JI. Surgical glove powder and intraperitoneal adhesion formation. S Afr Med J 1992;81:158.

58. Franklin RR. Ovarian Adhesion Study Group. Reduction of ovarian adhesions by the use of Interceed. Obstet Gynecol 1995;86:335–340.

59. Nordic Adhesion Prevention Study Group. The efficacy of Interceed (TC7) for prevention of reformation of postoperative adhesions on ovaries, fallopian tubes, and fimbriae in microsurgical operations for fertility: a multicenter study. Fertil Steril 1995;63:709–714.

60. Mais V, Ajossa S, Marongilu D, Peiretti RF, Guerriero S, Melis GB. Reduction of adhesion formation after laparoscopic endometriosis surgery: a randomized trial with an oxidized regenerated cellulose absorbable barrier. Obstet Gynecol 1995;86:512–515.

61. Surgical Membrane Study Group. Prophylaxis of pelvic sidewall adhesions with Gore-Tex Surgical Membrane: a multicenter clinical investigation. Fertil Steril 1992;57:921–923.

62. Myomectomy Adhesion Multicenter Study Group. An expanded polytetrafluoroethylene barrier (Gore-Tex Surgical Membrane) reduces post-myomectomy adhesion formation. Fertil Steril 1995;63:491–493.

63. Pados G, Camus M, De Munck L, Devroey P. Laparoscopic application of Interceed (TC7). Human Reprod 1992;7:1–3.

64. Azziz R, Murphy AA, Rosenberg SM, Patton GW Jr. Use of an oxidized, regenerated cellulose absorbable adhesion barrier at laparoscopy. J Reprod Med 1991;36:479–482.

65. Crain J, Curole D, Hill G, Hurst B, Metzger D, Murphy A, Perloe M, Reich H, Rowe G, Sanfillipo J, Schlaff W, Taylor S, Wing R. Laparoscopic implant of Gore-Tex Surgical Membrane. J Am Assoc Gynecol Laparosc 1995;2:417–420.

Laparoscopic Uterine Myomectomy: Hemorrhagic Complications | 33

Joseph S. Sanfilippo and Stephen R. Lincoln

Introduction

The frontiers of minimally invasive surgery (operative laparoscopy) continue to expand rapidly—even in logarithmic proportions. Recent advances in pelviscopic surgical techniques have enabled the endoscopic surgeon to perform a vast array of challenging procedures once reserved for laparotomy.

Laparoscopic uterine myomectomy is a reliable alternative for incision of uterine leiomyomata when preservation of reproductive function is the desired objective. The incidence of complications, including hemorrhagic and adhesion formation, arising from this procedure is difficult to ascertain with exactness, either separately or compared with a laparotomy approach to myomectomy. The most recent American Association of Gynecologic Laparoscopists' (AAGL) survey of endoscopic surgeons (1993 survey) was published in 1995 (1). When 45,042 procedures were evaluated, the rate of unintended laparotomy for hemorrhage and bowel or urinary tract injury increased in comparison with previous surveys; however, the overall complication and death rates remained essentially unchanged. In the survey, 1968 myomectomies were evaluated. When statistics were noted for this procedure in association with all other operative laparoscopic procedures (e.g., ectopic pregnancy, lysis of extensive adhesions, laparoscopic-assisted vaginal hysterectomy), the complication rates given in Table 33.1 were found.

This chapter discusses the prevention, recognition, and management of problems associated with laparoscopic myomectomy, with primary emphasis on prevention and intraoperative correction of hemorrhage. The operative technique of myomectomy also will be reviewed, with special emphasis on how and where hemorrhage may occur during laparoscopy.

Prevention

A preoperative discussion regarding the planned procedure, its risks and benefits, and alternatives should be undertaken with the patient. In addition, accurate documentation of this conference is of the utmost importance.

The optimal methods for minimizing the risk of hemorrhage in any surgical procedure apply to laparoscopic myomectomy as well. A preoperative evaluation for underlying bleeding diathesis, anemia, pelvic inflammatory disease, and pregnancy should be carried out, including a thorough history, physical examination, and appropriate baseline laboratory assessment. Hemorrhagic complications have been reported at myomectomy when degenerating leiomyomas and pregnancy are present (2).

A thorough understanding of uterine vasculature is imperative for the surgeon performing laparoscopic myomectomy. The location of uterine leiomyomas appears to be integrally related to the potential for bleeding. In particular, arterial hemorrhage from the branches of the uterine and ovarian arteries is more likely to occur when a myomectomy covers the lateral and lower posterior aspects of the uterus.

When one considers the implications of recurrent second-trimester spontaneous abortions, it becomes evident that myomas have an adverse effect on the uterine-endometrial blood supply. Evidence reported by Buttram and Reiter indicates that blood vessel obstruction can produce venule ectasia with resultant abnormal implantation (3). Their research used radiographic evidence to identify where submucosal, intramural, and subserosal leiomyomas cause congestion and dilatation of these subadjacent endometrial venous plexuses. The enlarging "tumor" impinges on the venous plexus of the

Table 33.1. Myomectomy complication rates.

	Rate (%)
Hospitalization >24 hr	39.6
Hospital readmission	4.6
Unintended laparotomy	10.7
Hemorrhage	10.4
Transfusion for hemorrhage	4.5
Bowel or urinary tract injury	4.1
Nerve injury	0.5
Death	6.7*

*Rate per 100,000 procedures. (Reproduced with permission from Hulka J, Peterson HB, Phillips JM, Surrey MW. Operative laparoscopy: American Association Gynecologic Laparoscopists' 1993 membership survey. J Amer Assn Gyn Lapar 1995;2:133–136.)

inner myometrium or the arcuate and radial veins as they course through the intramural and subserosal regions of the myometrium. The obstruction resulting in venule ectasia probably plays an important role in the production of abnormal uterine bleeding in patients with leiomyomata.

Numerous research endeavors have provided strong support for the use of gonadotropin-releasing hormone agonists (GnRH-a) in reducing the size of the uterine leiomyomata and blood loss at the time of surgery (4). A 40% reduction in mean uterine volume has been noted, with maximal reduction being achieved by 12 weeks of therapy and little additional change observed after 24 weeks of treatment (4). It is important for the surgery to be performed after the patient has received such therapy for at least four weeks and for the physician to remain aware that leiomyomata can revert quickly to their original size upon discontinuation of therapy (5). In addition, GnRH-a therapy can restore normal hemoglobin concentration prior to surgical intervention in patients with severe menorrhagia secondary to uterine leiomyomas (6).

In a study by Dubuisson and co-workers, prophylactic antibiotics were administered for one week preoperatively in addition to GnRH-a therapy. In this series of 147 laparoscopic myomectomies, no complications were noted that required laparotomy or blood transfusion for "significant bleeding." At follow-up laparoscopy (six weeks) in seven patients, no adhesions were noted in six cases; one patient had a severe bowel adhesion to the myomectomy scar, localized to the posterior wall (7).

Prevention of hemorrhagic complications may best be accomplished by recognition of contraindications to the laparoscopic approach. Many authors (8, 9, 10) believe myomas invading the uterine cavity should not be removed laparoscopically. Not only is blood loss

greater in these examples, but uterine rupture in the pregnant state is a greater risk with a laparoscopic uterine closure.

Recognition

Definition of a hemorrhagic complication at the time of myomectomy is of paramount importance. Placing the patient in the Trendelenburg position and creating adequate number of second puncture sites to place instruments for retraction and dissection are mandatory to enable the laparoscopist to have a clear view of the operative site. A properly functioning and efficient suction-irrigation system must be available at all times. The surgeon must know his or her limitations with advanced pelviscopic surgical procedures, so that when a laparotomy can be performed promptly severe hemorrhage cannot be controlled safely and efficiently.

Indications and technique of laparoscopic myomectomy

The surgical procedure for myomectomy has a number of indications, with the primary ones being excessive menometrorrhagia in the patient desiring preservation of her child-bearing potential, habitual abortion during the second trimester, and infertility when the remainder of the work-up is normal. The latter two indications are often secondary to distortion of the endometrial cavity, which may be noted on hysterosalpingogram or screening hysteroscopy. Excessive menometrorrhagia in the reproductive age group often presents with failure to respond to medical therapy, and further investigation reveals the presence of uterine leiomyomas. In addition, removal of subserosal leiomyomas larger than 2 cm has been recommended when evidence of obstruction of the fallopian tube exists, as demonstrated at hysterosalpingogram or previous laparoscopic investigation (11). Myomectomy for recurrent early fetal wastage remains controversial. The evidence supporting subsequent successful pregnancy is sparse at best (11). Pedunculated leiomyomas may undergo torsion with resultant infarction and associated pelvic pain, and may have either a subserosal attachment or lie directly within the uterine cavity.

When the patient is adequately anesthetized, she is placed in a lithotomy position. Following examination under anesthesia, the patient is prepped. Depending on the surgeon's preference, a Foley catheter may be inserted. It is helpful to stain the endometrium prior to embarking upon the laparoscopic surgical procedure. Methylene blue or indigo carmine (undiluted) can be applied by means of a uterine cannula (manipulator). In addition, the placement of a uterine cannula can facilitate the laparoscopic myomectomy procedure. Ideally, tubal patency can be assessed intraoperatively.

Concern persists regarding for adhesion formation after myomectomy (12). A number of adhesion prevention approaches have been utilized, including use of carboxymethylcellulose (TC-7, Interceed, Johnson & Johnson, Arlington, Texas). Polytetrafluoroethylene (Gore-Tex Surgical Membrane, W.L. Gore & Associates, Inc., Flagstaff, Arizona) has been utilized as well. These agents have been compared with instillation of Ringer's lactate with respect to adhesion prevention, although these studies have not been specific for laparoscopic myomectomy. Controversy remains regarding which entity is most efficacious (13, 14).

One must always be concerned with the potential for sarcomatous change, although this conditions appears to be rare (incidence 0.1%–1%) in evaluations of patients with uterine cavity enlargement (15). This concern is especially important if rapid enlargement has occurred and a histology of surgical specimens is required.

The actual surgical procedure of operative laparoscopy requires an electronic (high-flow) insufflator to maintain an adequate pneumoperitoneum. The blood supply to the myoma must be identified and secured. This step is often accomplished initially with injection of dilute vasopressin (1:200) solution (with normal saline or a similar combination) injected directly over the leiomyoma, followed by coagulation with cutting techniques for incision over the leiomyoma. Alternative methods of securing hemostasis include a defocused-mode laser, endocoagulator, unipolar-point coagulator, or bipolar systems with Kleppinger forceps. In addition, the myoma may be shelled out; use of the myoenucleator with the endocoagulator (WISAP, Tomball, Texas), for example, appears to provide appropriate dissection and coagulation simultaneously. The stump should also be coagulated prior to completion of excision. In many cases, endoscopic scissors are necessary to accomplish complete removal. Point coagulation can be used to control any bleeding areas during this process. Irrigation suctioning systems are also instrumental in identifying bleeding points.

An alternative method of achieving hemostasis incorporates the use of Endoloop ligatures (Ethicon, Somerville, New Jersey). Each ligature is loaded into a 3-mm applicator, which is then inserted through a 5-mm port. The Endoloop is placed over the stalk. After the ligatures are appropriately positioned, the stalk is resected with scissors.

The size of the leiomyoma may serve as a limiting factor in myomectomy, although technologic advances to enhance removal from the peritoneal cavity continue to be developed. Myomas can be sectioned further with blended currents for unipolar coagulation systems as well as endoscopic scissors or laser. In addition, morcellators can be employed to further fragment the leiomyoma. A myoma screw may be used for manipulation of the leiomyoma as it is being extracted. A colpotomy incision may be necessary under direct laparoscopic view to remove large fibroids. After the leiomyoma is completely removed from the peritoneal cavity, copious irrigation is administered to remove any remaining segment of the leiomyoma.

Significant advancement has been made with respect to laparoscopic suturing. Introduction of curved needles now complements the original "straight needle" array of suture ligature materials. With the advent of extracorporeal and intracorporeal knot-tying, appropriate reapproximation of the uterine musculature and serosa can be accomplished endoscopically.

Myolysis

Recently a modified technique of myoma coagulation has been described as an alternative to myomectomy or hysterectomy patients with leiomyoma (16, 17). Both Nd:YAG laser and bipolar needles have been used to coagulate leiomyomas. Multiple punctures are drilled at different angles; approximately 50 to 75 such punctures are needed to thoroughly coagulate a typical 5-cm fibroid. Fluid is applied continuously to cool either the fiber tip or the electrode needles to minimize complications during this process. The uterine grasper is often helpful in elevating the fibroid away from other organs such as the rectum, bladder, bowel, and uterine blood vessels.

More than 150 cases of myoma coagulation have been reported with the Nd:YAG laser with no hemorrhagic complications noted (17). A similar number of patients with the bipolar needle also had no hemorrhagic complications.

The use of GnRH-a may prove helpful in reducing the tumor size prior to coagulation necrosis. It is generally recommended that this procedure be performed on fibroids ranging between 3 and 10 cm. The patient must be informed of the potential for adhesion formation.

Management of intraoperative bleeding

Several methods of controlling intraoperative hemorrhage should always be available during a laparoscopic myomectomy. As mentioned earlier, complete visualization with adequate suctioning and irrigation is necessary for exposure. Use of an electrocautery technique is the most efficient and time-saving method of controlling hemorrhage. The endocoagulator may be placed in the bed of the defect in the uterine wall to halt bleeding. Alternatively, use of the Kleppinger bipolar forceps may provide better hemostasis when the arterial bleeding site can be visualized. The surgeon should always be cognizant of the potential for thermal injuries to the bowel, particularly at this point in the procedure.

If hemorrhage is not controlled successfully with these techniques, use of endoscopic sutures becomes necessary.

Both straight and curved needles have become available for laparoscopic suturing and can be used successfully for ligation of arterial bleeding. Endoscopic suturing can be time-consuming and frustrating for the novice laparoscopist; therefore, one should be well versed in these techniques before attempting laparoscopic myomectomy. With the expansion of gynecological and surgical laparoscopy, newer and more efficient methods for controlling hemorrhage will undoubtedly become available.

In a series of 56 patients who underwent laparoscopic myomectomy for the indication of persistent abnormal uterine bleeding, pelvic pain and/or pressure symptoms, or a specific pelvic mass, blood loss varied from 100 to 400 mL with a mean of 75 mL [18]. In this group of patients, none required transfusion. Twenty-four of the patients eventually underwent second-look laparoscopic procedures; adhesions were noted in 66% of this group. Among those patients desiring fertility, 71% achieved a pregnancy.

The debate: leave open or close the uterine incision?

Many investigators have debated the need to close the uterine defect after laparoscopic myomectomy. The authors believe that if a significant uterine defect is present it should be closed at least with a single layer of sutures. Currently, the endoscopic stapler may be used as a research tool to accomplish reapproximation in a far less time-consuming manner.

The incidence of uterine rupture during pregnancy after myomectomy is extremely rare [19]. One should be cognizant of the risk of uterine rupture while attempting vaginal delivery after cesarean section, however, as this event's incidence has been reported to range from 0.5% to 5% [20]. The authors feel the surgeon should make a decision at the time of laparoscopic myomectomy as to the extent of muscular wall damage as well as the need for cesarean section versus vaginal delivery (ideally at the onset of labor).

Adhesion formation

As previously noted, one specific concern with myomectomy is the potential for formation of adhesions. A direct correlation between the presence of sutures to reapproximate myometrium and increased incidence of adhesion formation has been reported by Nezhat and co-workers [21]. Specifically, 154 women underwent laparoscopic myomectomy, and second-look procedures were performed "when clinically indicated." In such cases, adhesion formation was classified and scored, with the results ranging from 0 (none) to 3 (thick and vascular or the presence of bowel adhesions). Larger leiomyomata (i.e., >3 cm) were associated with increased adhesion forma-

tion, implying a need for suture reapproximation of myometrium. Furthermore, adhesion formation was noted when the myoma was located posteriorly compared with the presence of fundal-anterior portion of the uterus. To minimize this complication, it remains of paramount importance that every effort at hemostasis be provided, including appropriate use of sutures and use of less reactive suture material when possible.

Summary

The role of laparoscopic uterine myomectomy in the management of leiomyomata continues to increase. The prerequisite to surgical extirpation includes treatment with GnRH-a in an effort to decrease the size of the leiomyoma and normalize hemoglobin concentrations, facilitating the surgical procedure. Hemorrhagic complications can be minimized with appropriate preoperative evaluation. When complications do occur, recognition and acceptance are of utmost importance. Appropriate coagulation or suture techniques should achieve hemostasis, but one should always be prepared to undertake laparotomy in a timely and efficient manner. At this time, closure of the myometrial defect is recommended unless minimal intramural damage is apparent.

REFERENCES

1. Hulka J, Peterson HB, Phillips JM, Surrey MW. Operative laparoscopy: American Association Gynecologic Laparoscopists' 1993 membership survey. J Am Assn Gyn Lapar 1995;2:133–136.
2. Hasan F, Arumugan K, Sivanesaratnam V. Uterine leiomyomata in pregnancy. Int J Gynecol Obstet 1991;34:45–48.
3. Buttram VC Jr, Reiter RC. Uterine leiomyomata: etiology, symptomatology, and management. Fertil Steril 1981;36:433–445.
4. Friedman A, Rein M, Harrison-Atlas D, Garfield J, Doubilet P. A randomized, placebo-controlled, double-blind study evaluating leuprolide acetate depot treatment before myomectomy. Fertil Steril 1989;52:728–733.
5. Letterie G, Coddington C, Winkel C, Shawker T, Loriaux D, Collins R. Efficacy of a gonadotropin-releasing hormone agonist in the treatment of uterine leiomyomata: long-term follow-up. Fertil Steril 1989;51:951–956.
6. Fedele L, Bianchi S, Baglioni A, Arcaini L, Marchini M, Bocciolone L. Intranasal buserelin versus surgery in the treatment of uterine leiomyomata: long-term follow-up. Eur J Obstet Gynecol Reprod Biol 1991;38:53–77.
7. Dubuisson JB, Lecuru F, Foulot H, Mandelbrot L, de la Joliniere JB, Aubriot FX. Gonadotropin-releasing hormone agonist and laparoscopic myomectomy. Clin Therap 1992;14(suppl A):51–56.
8. Nezhat F, Seidman DS, Nezhat C, Nezhat CH. Laparoscopic myomectomy today, why, when and whom? Hum Reprod 1996;11:933.
9. Dubuisson JB, Chapron C. A good technique when correctly indicated. Hum Reprod 1996;11:934.
10. Dicker D, Dekel A, Orvieto R, et al. The controversy of laparoscopic myomectomy. Hum Reprod 1996;11:935.
11. Levine RL. Myomectomy. In: Sanfilippo J, Levine R, eds. Operative gynecologic endoscopy. New York: Springer-Verlag 1989;133–139.
12 Operative laparoscopy Study Group. Postopeative adhesion development after operative laparoscopy: evaluation at early second-look procedures. Fertil Steril 1991;55:700–704.

13. Pagidas K, Tulandi T. Effects of Ringer's lactate, Interceed (TC7) and Gore-Tex Surgical Membrane on postsurgical adhesion formation. Fertil Steril 1992;57:199–201.
14. Haney AF, Doty E. Murine peritoneal injury and de novo adhesion formation caused by oxidized-regenerated cellulose (Interceed [TC7]) but not expanded polytetrafluoroethylene (Gore-Tex Surgical Membrane). Fertil Steril 1992;57:202–208.
15. Leibsohn S, d'Ablaing G, Mishell D Jr, Schlaerth J. Leiomyosarcoma in a series of hysterectomies performed for presumed uterine leiomyomas. Am J Obstet Gynecol 1990;162:968–976.
16. Goldfarb HA. Nd:YAG laser laparoscopic coagulation of symptomatic myomas. J Reprod Med 1992;37:636.
17. Nisolle M, Smets M, Malvaux V, *et al.* Laparoscopic myolysis with the Nd:YAG laser. J Gynecol Surg 1993;9:95.
18. Hasson HM, Rotman C, Rana FN, Sistos F, Dmowski WP. Laparoscopic myomectomy. Obstet Gynecol 1992;80:884–888.
19. Golan D, Aharoni A, Gonen R, Boss Y, Sharf M. Early spontaneous rupture of the postmyomectomy gravid uterus. Int J Gynecol Obstet 1990;31:167–170.
20. Precis IV. An update in obstetrics and gynecology. Washington, DC: American College of Obstetrics and Gynecology, 1990: 150.
21. Nezhat C, Nezhat F, Silfen SL, Schaffer N, Evans D. Laparoscopic myomectomy. Int J Fertil 1991;36:275–280.

34 | Difficulties in Removing Specimen from the Abdominal Cavity at Laparoscopy

Togas Tulandi

Advances in laparoscopic techniques have allowed detachment of almost any intra-abdominal organs from their original sites. Small organs or specimen can be removed easily via the trocar. Any specimen larger than the diameter of the conventionally used trocar can, however, prove difficult to remove and needs a special method for its removal. In this chapter, several techniques to remove specimens from the abdominal cavity are discussed.

Laparoscopic approach

Most laparoscopic procedures require the use of a primary trocar of 10 mm and two secondary trocars of 5 mm. If removal of a large specimen is anticipated, one of the ancillary trocars should be at least 10 mm. Alternatively, the surgeon may begin with two secondary trocars of 5 mm, replacing one with a larger trocar when needed.

Although some surgeons remove specimens via an enlarged subumbilical incision (1), removal via the site of a secondary trocar is preferable. In this technique, removal is performed under direct laparoscopic control. If the specimen is dropped, it will be immediately seen and can be grasped again. Because of concerns over intraperitoneal spillage of malignant cells, ovarian cysts are best removed intact and puncture should be avoided (2). The unruptured cyst is placed in a laparoscopic pouch inserted via a 10-mm secondary trocar. Several types of these pouches are currently available. The most practical is a laparoscopic pouch that automatically opens after introduction into the abdominal cavity, allowing easy insertion of the specimen. Other types must be opened within the abdominal cavity, which may require extra time. The pouch is then retracted from the abdominal cavity and the trocar removed.

In this procedure, the pouch is held tightly against the abdominal wall and then opened. The cyst wall seen just under the abdominal wall is incised using a regular scalpel, a suction irrigator probe is immediately inserted into the cyst, and the cyst contents are aspirated. Once the cyst collapses, the pouch—with the cyst wall inside—slides out of the abdominal cavity.

Sometimes the cyst's content is very thick and the cyst must be irrigated repeatedly with solution of Ringer's lactate. In the case of dermoid cyst, hair and sometimes tooth or bone can be extracted using a regular Kelly forceps inside the pouch. Not uncommonly, a portion of the cyst can be delivered out of the abdomen, but the bulk of the cyst remains inside the abdomen (Fig. 34.1). In such a case, the extracorporeal site of the cyst is opened and its content removed. With the techniques described, not only is intraperitoneal spillage avoided, but the potential of implanting possible cancer cells in the trocar site is also eliminated.

Attempts should be made not to spill the contents of the cyst during surgery. Because endometriomas tend to have thin walls, however, spillage often occurs. This event does not seem to be associated with adverse outcome, nor does spillage of the contents of a dermoid cyst (3). Extensive irrigation of the peritoneal cavity at the completion of the procedure appears to mitigate any potential damage. In addition, spillage of the contents of a benign mucinous cyst does not appear to cause pseudomyxoma peritonei (4).

If spillage occurs, a cystoscopy to examine the inner surface of the cyst should be undertaken. If vegetations are found, a frozen-section examination should be immediately performed. Any findings of cancer cells should be followed by immediate laparotomy for staging and treatment. Otherwise, a laparoscopic ovarian cystectomy or oophorectomy is performed, with the choice of procedure being based upon the patient's menopausal and clinical status. Several studies have suggested that the prognosis is not influenced by spillage of a malignant tumor if treatment begins immediately (5–8). Other studies suggest that intraoperative spillage of a malignant

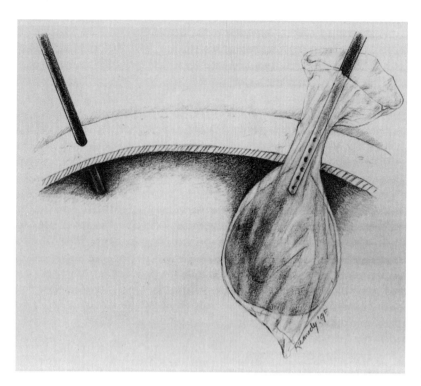

Fig. 34.1 Removal of an ovarian cyst. The contents of the cyst are aspirated extracorporeally. A laparoscopic pouch prevents spillage.

tumor may worsen the prognosis (9, 10). In any event, the prognosis is certainly impaired if the treatment is delayed for several weeks (8, 11).

Removal of solid specimens such as a myoma or uterine corpus requires morcellation. The best manual morcellator consists of a cylinder with a circular coning saw at the end (Fig. 34.2). A 20-mm tool enables rapid morcellation and removal of the tissue. In this procedure, one of the secondary trocars is replaced with a 20-mm trocar and the morcellator is inserted into the abdominal cavity. The solid specimen is grasped with a 10-mm-long jaw forceps inserted into the morcellator and is retracted against its end. The morcellator is rotated while the tissue is pulled against it until no more resistance is felt, suggesting that a portion of the tumor has been detached. When the morcellator and the forceps are withdrawn, the cylinder-like tissue found inside the morcellator can be removed. This procedure is repeated until the entire specimen is removed from the abdominal cavity.

It is crucial that morcellation be performed under laparoscopic control because the sharp end of the morcellating cylinder could potentially damage other intra-abdominal organs. The surgeon should ensure that the forceps is grasping only the tissue to be removed; otherwise injury to intra-abdominal organs such as intestines might ensue. To prevent an incisional hernia, the fascia of an abdominal incision of 10 mm or larger should be properly sutured.

A laparoscopic myoma screw can also be used inside the morcellator to stabilize the solid specimen for morcellation (see Fig. 34.2). In addition, an

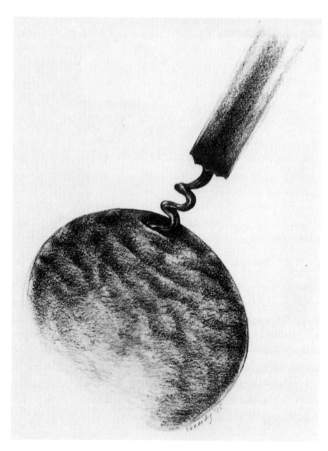

Fig. 34.2 A myoma screw inside a morcellator stabilizing the myoma. Note the sharp serrated edge of the coning saw at the end of the morcellator. (Reproduced by permission from Tulandi T. Operative laparoscopy. Telinde operative gynecology updates, vol. 2, no. 3, pp. 1–3.)

electrical morcellator has recently been developed that may allow faster removal of a large solid specimen by laparoscopy.

Vaginal approach

Specimens can also be removed via a culdotomy opening, although contamination of the abdominal cavity with the vaginal flora is a possibility with this technique. The anatomical relationship between the posterior wall of the vagina and the rectum is first confirmed. This examination is facilitated by inserting a rectal probe or a sponge stick (a sponge on a ring forceps) into the rectum, with another inserted into the posterior vaginal fornix. A culdotomy opening is made using a laser or a unipolar needle electrode, a unipolar spatula, or unipolar scissors. If the posterior cul-de-sac is obliterated, the rectum must be dissected off the posterior vaginal wall. This dissection involves creating a plane under the peritoneum between the rectum and the vagina and then pushing the rectum posteriorly. The posterior vaginal fornix is distended using a wet sponge stick, and a transverse incision is made between the rectum and the vagina. The sponge then becomes visible and, when wet, will reduce leakage of CO_2 gas from the vagina.

Small specimens can be delivered through the culdotomy opening. A large cyst must first be evacuated by pushing it into the culdotomy opening. The lower pole of the cyst is incised using a scalpel or a scissors vaginally. After the contents of the cyst leak out of the vagina, the cyst collapses and can be easily removed. Solid material inside can be removed using a forceps before complete removal of the cyst. This technique prevents spillage of the cyst's contents into the peritoneal cavity. Similarly, a myoma can be pushed into the culdotomy opening and then grasped with a tenaculum via the vagina. If the CO_2 gas escapes despite the presence of specimen in the culdotomy opening, a wet sponge should be inserted into the vagina around the tenaculum. To prevent injury to the intestines with a tenaculum or a forceps, it is important to apply the instrument under laparoscopic control. Maintenance of the pneumoperitoneum is therefore crucial.

A specifically designed vaginal extractor consisting of a trocar fitted with a ball-shaped head at the upper extremity allows removal of specimens as large as 7 cm without loss of CO_2 gas. The round surface of the ball adapts well to the vaginal fornix; a midline horizontal groove on one side guides the surgeon to perform the culdotomy opening by laparoscopy. A grasping forceps can then be introduced into the trocar to extract the specimen.

A large myoma must be morcellated either using a morcellator or a scissors vaginally. The culdotomy opening can be closed vaginally or laparoscopically.

Mini-laparotomy approach

Because of possible contamination with vaginal flora, some surgeons prefer to use a mini-laparotomy technique instead of the vaginal approach for removing specimens. This approach is particularly useful for removing a large uterine myoma (i.e., laparoscopically-assisted myomectomy). Multiple myomectomies require multiple incisions. At laparotomy, the author chooses a uterine incision that allows removal of as many myomas as possible—a feat that laparoscopy has difficulty in matching.

In addition, because laparoscopic suturing is time-consuming and requires special training and expertise, the standard multilayered closure of a uterine defect may be neglected in the laparoscopic procedure. This choice has led to uterine defects, indentations, and fistula that might represent a structural defect (12). Uterine dehiscence after laparoscopic myomectomy has also been reported (13). This problem can be overcome if multilayered laparoscopic suturing is performed much like that undertaken at laparotomy. Otherwise, a laparoscopically-assisted myomectomy should be done. It facilitates removal of the specimen and allows multilayered closure of the uterine defect.

In this procedure, the myoma is partially enucleated. A 10- to 15-mm trocar is inserted suprapubically on the midline, and a grasping forceps or a myoma screw is used to grasp the enucleated myoma. The abdominal opening is enlarged with a mini-Pfannenstiel incision until it can accommodate the myoma and the myoma is delivered out of the abdominal cavity. Sometimes a regular myoma screw must be used to secure the myoma. The enucleation is completed extracorporeally and the uterine defect is sutured in a standard manner. To decrease the likelihood of adhesion formation, an adhesion barrier, such as expanded polytetrafluoroethylene, can be used to cover the uterine incisions (14, 15). The mini-laparotomy incision is then closed and laparoscopic examination is repeated to ascertain hemostasis, undertake peritoneal lavage, and instill irrigating solution. Because manipulation of the intestine is limited and an intra-abdominal pack is not used, this technique provides a rapid return of intestinal function.

Conclusion

Specimens can be extracted from the abdominal cavity by laparoscopy, vaginal, or mini-laparotomy approach. The availability of a morcellator permits removal of large specimens in small pieces via the laparoscope. For removal of an ovarian cyst, the use of a laparoscopic pouch is recommended to mitigate concerns about intraperitoneal spillage of possible malignant cells and implantation of the cells in the trocar sites.

Specimens can also be removed by a culdotomy or

mini-laparotomy opening. The latter technique is especially helpful when large and multiple leiomyomata must be removed.

REFERENCES

1. Pelosi MA, Pelosi MA III. Laparoscopic appendectomy using a single umbilical puncture (minilaparoscopy). J Reprod Med 1992;37:588–594.
2. Tulandi T. Laparoscopic management of ovarian cyst in perimenopausal women. Gynaecol Endos 1996;5:1–4.
3. Lin P, Falcone T, Tulandi T. Excision of ovarian dermoid cyst by laparoscopy and by laparotomy. Am J Obstet Gynecol 1995; 173:769–771.
4. Parker WH, Berek JS. Management of selected cystic adnexal masses in postmenopausal women by operative laparoscopy: a pilot study. Am J Obstet Gynecol 1990;163:1574–1577.
5. Kliman L, Rome RM, Fortune DW. Low malignant potential tumors of the ovary: a study of 76 cases. Obstet Gynecol 1986;68:338–344.
6. Hopkins MP, Kumar NB, Morley GW. An assessment of the pathologic features and treatment modalities in ovarian tumors of low malignant potential. Obstet Gynecol 1987;70:923–929.
7. Sevelda P, Vavra N, Schemper M, Salzer H. Prognostic factors for survival in stage I epithelial ovarian carcinoma. Cancer 1990;65:2349–2352.
8. Dembo AJ, Davy M, Stenwig AE, Berle RS, Bush RS, Kjorstad K. Prognostic factors in patients with stage I epithelial ovarian cancer. Obstet Gynecol 1990;75:263–273.
9. Sainz de la Cuesta R, Goff BA, Fuller AF, Nikrui N, Eichhorn JH, Rice LW. Prognostic importance of intraoperative rupture of malignant ovarian epithelial neoplasms. Obstet Gynecol 1994;84:1–7.
10. Finn CB, Luesley DM, Buxton EJ, Blackledge GR, Kelly K, Dunn JA, Wilson S. Is stage I epithelial ovarian cancer overtreated both surgically and systemically? Results of a five year cancer registry review. Br J Obstet Gynaecol 1992;99:54–58.
11. Maiman M, Seltzer V, Boyce J. Laparoscopic excision of ovarian neoplasms subsequently found to be malignant. Obstet Gynecol 1991;77:563–565.
12. Nezhat C, Nezhat F, Silfen SL, Schaffer N, Evans D. Laparoscopic myomectomy. Int J Fertil 1991;36:275–280.
13. Harris WJ. Uterine dehiscence following laparoscopic myomectomy. Obstet Gynecol 1992;80:545–546.
14. Myomectomy Adhesion Study Group. An expanded-polytetrafluoroethylene barrier (Gore-Tex surgical membrane) reduces post-myomectomy adhesion formation. Fertil Steril 1995; 63:491–493.
15. Murray C, Tulandi T. Prevention of post-myomectomy adhesions. Infertility Reprod Med North America 1996;7:169–177.

35 | Complications of Laparoscopic Hysterectomy: Prevention, Recognition, and Management

C. Y. Liu

The first laparoscopic hysterectomy was performed in the United States in January 1988. Published literature regarding this procedure remains limited, however. Although the reported surgeries were performed by experienced laparoscopic surgeons, nonetheless they were associated with some serious complications. The term "laparoscopic-assisted vaginal hysterectomy" can be confusing, as it is used to describe a number of procedures ranging from a minimum amount of surgery performed laparoscopically with a fairly standard vaginal hysterectomy, to most or all of the hysterectomy being performed laparoscopically with minimal vaginal surgery. To conduct a statistically significant series-to-series comparison of the results and complication rates, a generally accepted definition and classification of the laparoscopically assisted hysterectomy must be standardized and used by the gynecologist.

The author is part of a group that has proposed the following classification system. Securing and dividing the uterine artery is regarded as the most critical step in the procedure. If the laparoscopic component of the operation is completed above the uterine artery and the uterine arteries are subsequently ligated vaginally, we suggest that such a procedure be called "laparoscopic-assisted vaginal hysterectomy" (LAVH). If the uterine arteries are secured laparoscopically and the remaining cardinal and uterosacral ligaments are secured vaginally, we suggest the procedure be termed "laparoscopic hysterectomy" (LH). If the uterosacral and cardinal ligaments are also secured laparoscopically and the cervix is completely freed from the vagina by laparoscopic technique, the procedure is analogous to a total abdominal hysterectomy and should be called a "total laparoscopic hysterectomy" (TLH). The complete descriptive classification of laparoscopic-assisted hysterectomy is as follows:

1. Diagnostic laparoscopy with vaginal hysterectomy.
2. Laparoscopc-assisted vaginal hysterectomy (LAVH).
3. Laparoscopic hysterectomy (LH).
4. Total laparoscopic hysterectomy (TLH).
5. Laparoscopic supracervical hysterectomy (LSH or CASH).
6. Laparoscopic hysterectomy with lymphadenectomy (LHL).
7. Laparoscopic hysterectomy with lymphadenectomy and omentectomy (LHL + O).
8. Radical laparoscopic hysterectomy (RLH).

The complications of laparoscopic-assisted vaginal hysterectomy are essentially the same as those encountered with traditional laparoscopic surgery plus vaginal hysterectomy. However, laparoscopic hysterectomy (LH), total laparoscopic hysterectomy (TLH), laparoscopic hysterectomy with lymphadenectomy (LHL), and radical laparoscopic hysterectomy (RLH) pose additional risk of injury to the large pelvic vessels, ureters, bladder, rectum, and sigmoid colon. Complications of operative laparoscopy most commonly mentioned in literature include anesthesia problems, bleeding at the abdominal-wall puncture site, injury to the major vessels or viscera by trocars or Veress needle, and thermal injury to the bowel or ureters by electrosurgery or laser. As these complications are addressed elsewhere in this book, this chapter will concentrate on the complications specific to laparoscopic hysterectomy (LH) and total laparoscopic hysterectomy (TLH).

In our (Liu and Reich) series of 518 cases of laparoscopic hysterectomy and total laparoscopic hysterectomy, we found a complication rate of 5.7%. These complications included febrile morbidity (2.1%), injury to the urinary tract system (1.3%), injury to the bowel (1.1%), delayed postoperative vaginal cuff bleedings (0.5%), unanticipated blood transfusion (0.3%), and pulmonary embolism (0.2%) (Table 35.1). As a rule, the more complex the pelvic pathology and the more technically difficult the procedure, the more likely that serious complications will occur. The chapter will address the possible sites of complications, precautionary measures for avoiding intraoperative complications, and the management of the complications should they arise.

Standard procedure for total laparoscopic hysterectomy

As with any type of surgery, a thorough knowledge of anatomy is of paramount importance when undertaking laparoscopic hysterectomy. A surgeon who is familiar with all structures to be met at operation is best able to appreciate distortions produced by disease and to take advantage of the natural planes of cleavage when present. This benefit is especially evident with the laparoscopic surgeon who has a precise knowledge of the different fascial planes. A neat, effortless operation is performed, with minimal bleeding and intraoperative complications.

As with any other surgery, the operative techniques for total laparoscopic hysterectomy may vary from case to case, but the following description outlines the standard procedure.

Step 1: Both pelvic ureters are identified and dissected to at least the level of the ureteric canal, where the uterine artery crosses above the ureter and the dense cardinal ligament lies below the ureter. This step is accomplished by opening the peritoneum covering the ureter with CO_2 laser or scissors. If pelvic side-wall pathology is observed, such as ovarian endometrioma, dense tubo-ovarian-pelvic side-wall adhesion, or ovarian tumor, the ureters should be identified and dissected cephalad to the pathology. In many cases, the dissection of the ureter will begin at or above the pelvic brim. Working under direct visualization of the ureter, the adnexal organs are then dissected and freed from the pelvic side wall. Dissection of the ureter continues downward to the deep pelvis. The uterosacral ligaments, at this point, are dissected away

Table 35.1. Complications observed during 518 laparoscopic hysterectomies and concomitant surgeries.

Complication	No. of Patients	Rate (%)	Rate per 100 Women[a]
Febrile mobility	11		2.12
Pneumonia[b]	1	0.19	
Pelvic hematomas[c]	4	0.77	
Dehydration	1	0.19	
Transient febrile episodes	5	0.96	
Urinary tract system	7		1.35
Bladder injury	5	0.96	
Vesicovaginal fistula	1	0.19	
Ureterovaginal fistula	1	0.19	
Intestinal complications	6		1.15
Small bowel enterotomy	2	0.38	
Thermal injury of sigmoid colon	1	0.19	
Partial bowel obstruction	1	0.19	
Richter's hernia[d]	2	0.38	
Vaginal cuff bleeding	3		0.57
Unanticipated blood transfusion	2		0.38
Pulmonary embolism	1		0.19
Total	30		5.76

[a] Rate per 100 women who underwent hysterectomy and concomitant surgery.
[b] This patient later developed adult respiratory distress syndrome and died.
[c] Two of the patients had second-look laparoscopy and the hematomas were evacuated.
[d] Richter's hernia occurred at the 12-mm trocar puncture sites.
Reproduced with permission of Blackwell Science Publishing Company from Liu CY, Reich H. Complications of total laparoscopic hysterectomy in 518 cases. Gynecol Endoscopy 1994;3:203–208.

from the ureters, coagulated with bipolar electrosurgery, and divided under direct visualization of ureters.

Step 2: In this step, the bladder is reflected to the upper part of the vagina. First, both round ligaments are coagulated with bipolar Kleppinger forceps and divided with scissors. A transverse incision is made on the vesico-uterine peritoneal fold and the vesico-cervical ligaments and bladder pillars are identified. The vesico-cervical ligament is cut in the middle. The bladder pillars, which hold the bladder to the cervix and contain blood vessels from the cervix, are then coagulated and divided. The bladder can then be dissected down easily all the way to the upper part of vagina. This process also pulls the ureters laterally and away from the cervix. If the cul-de-sac is obliterated partially or completely because of endometriosis or previous pelvic inflammatory disease, the rectosigmoid colon is dissected away from the cervix, and the endometriosis nodules in that area are resected.

The hysterectomy should *not* start until both ureters are identified and dissected, and the bladder and rectosigmoid colon are reflected all the way to the upper vagina.

Step 3: The anterior leaf of the broad ligaments is opened downward and toward the cervix, and the uterine artery is identified. An opening is usually made on the avascular portion of the posterior leaf of the broad ligament above the uterine vessels.

Step 4: If removal of the tube and ovary is planned, the infundibulopelvic ligament is first mobilized. Next, Kleppinger bipolar forceps are used to compress and desiccate the vessels, which are divided with the scissors or laser under direct visualization of the ureter. This step is followed by desiccation and division of the mesosalpinx and meso-ovarian. If the ovary is to be preserved, the utero-ovarian junction, which includes the proximal part of the fallopian tube, utero-ovarian ligament, and mesosalpinx (the round ligament divided in step 3), is desiccated with Kleppinger bipolar forceps and then divided. An automatic laparoscopic stapling device (Multi-Fire Endo GIA-30 or Lineal Cutter-35) may save time during this portion of the procedure. In addition, this step can be accomplished by using ligatures through an opening in the broad ligament and tying the infundibulopelvic ligament or the utero-ovarian junction with the extracorporal knot tying technique, using the Clark knot pusher.

Step 5: At this point the posterior leaf of the broad ligament is divided to the uterine artery, which is skeletonized laterally to the ureteric canal where the uterine artery crosses above the ureter. With the ureter in direct view, the uterine artery is desiccated with Kleppinger bipolar forceps and divided. A suture technique with

0-Vicryl on a CT-B needle may also be employed. The suture can include both uterine artery and cardinal ligament. The uterine artery can also be suture-ligated before it crosses over the ureter at the area of the ureteric canal. An automatic laparoscopic stapling device can be used effectively in this step. Before firing the stapling device, both the ureter and the bladder must be carefully monitored, ensuring that the jaws of the stapling device encompass only the uterine artery and the cardinal ligament.

Step 6: With direct visualization of both ureters, the remaining cardino-uterosacral ligaments are desiccated with bipolar forceps and divided with scissors or laser.

Step 7: The surgical assistant puts a wet 4×4 sponge on the tip of a sponge forceps and places it in the anterior vaginal fornix, tenting the vagina from below. The anterior culdotomy is performed laparoscopically via a high-power-density CO_2 laser or monopolar scissors. Using the sponge in the vagina as a guide and the suction-irrigator probe as the backstop for the CO_2 laser, circumferential culdotomy is performed and the cervix completely detached from the vagina. This step requires careful coordination between the surgeon and the assistants, because the CO_2 gas leaks rapidly as soon as the anterior cul-de-sac is opened. To facilitate this procedure, the uterine manipulator should be removed from the cervix as soon as the anterior culdotomy is complete. A small sponge pad in a sugical glove, with its opening tied and placed inside the vagina, will maintain positive pneumoperitoneum. The anterior lip of the cervix and the anterior vaginal wall are then grasped laparoscopically with toothed grasping forceps, and the circumferential culdotomy is performed with scissors or monopolar needle electrode. The uterus is then pulled or pushed into the vagina to maintain the pneumoperitoneum. For the large fibroid uterus, morcellation of the uterus intraperitoneally through the vagina is possible.

Step 8: The vagina is closed either transversely or vertically, with special emphasis on suturing both uterosacro-cardinal ligaments to the vaginal vault to ensure adequate vaginal support. Four interrupted figure-of-eight or continuous sutures with 0-Vicryl are used to close the vaginal cuff laparoscopically. Under direct visualization of the left ureter, a suture is placed deeply through the left uterosacro-cardinal ligament and into the vagina; it exits the vagina through the anterior vaginal wall, including the pubocervical fascia. The same steps are taken again, to make figure-of-eight stitches to ensure closure of the vaginal corner. The suture is tied with an extracorporal knot-tying technique using a knot pusher. The procedure is repeated on the right side of the vaginal corner, which includes the right uterosacro-cardinal ligament and the posterior and anterior vaginal walls. Two additional figure-of-eight or continuous sutures are placed between these two lateral sutures to close the middle portion of the vagina.

Step 9: The entire pelvic cavity is carefully inspected laparoscopically and irrigated with copious amounts of Ringer's lactate solution. All debris and blood clots are removed and the pelvis is viewed underwater to ensure satisfactory hemostasis. Both ureters are inspected carefully. If ureteral injury is suspected, 5 mL of indigo-carmine dye and 20 mg of furosemide (Laxis) are injected intravenously, and a cystoscopic examination is performed. Visualization of the normal peristalsis of the intramural portion of the ureters and ejection of the Indigocarmine dye from the ureteral orifices provides assurance that the integrity of ureters has not been compromised.

Urinary tract system injury

Injury to the pelvic ureters

The incidence of ureteral injury in laparoscopic hysterectomy is unknown at present. In our (Liu and Reich) series of 518 laparoscopic hysterectomies, only one ureteral injury occurred. However, our private correspondences with gynecological laparoscopists from around the world lead us to believe that the incidence of ureteral injury in laparoscopic-assisted hysterectomy is higher than that in traditional abdominal or vaginal hysterectomies, which is reported to vary from 0.4% to 1.5%.

Most ureteral injuries during laparoscopic hysterectomy occur in the area between the ureteric canal and the bladder base. Patients at risk for ureteral injury should be identified prior to surgery. Women with a history of extensive pelvic inflammatory disease or endometriosis, preoperative pelvic findings of large pelvic mass, intraligamentary leiomyomata, obliterated cul-de-sac, and induration in the paracervical area should arouse suspicion of ureteral involvement. Preoperative evaluation with IVP is helpful in patients with these conditions.

Prevention of the ureteral injury

The best way to prevent ureteral injury during laparoscopic hysterectomy is to be certain of the ureters' location at all times during the procedure. With laparoscopic surgery, one loses the ability to palpate the pelvic organs, but gains a much improved visibility of the pelvic structures. For this reason, we do not advocate preoperative ureteral catheterization in high-risk patients. Potentially the transillumination of the ureter through recently developed lighted ureteral catheters could make the course of the ureter obvious during the laparoscopy. The currently available lighted ureteral catheters are all rather rigid and large in caliber, however, and the mucosa of the ureter can be easily damaged by the heat emitted from the lighted catheter and from intraoperative manipulation of the catheter against the ureter.

Ureteral injury can be especially severe in cases of pre-existing periureteral fibrosis and scarring, which may be secondary to previous infection or endometriosis. We recommend routine identification and dissection of the pelvic ureters at the beginning of the hysterectomy; the ureteral locations will then remain clear throughout the entire surgical procedure. We have not had any ureteral injury since following the practice of ureteral identification and dissection as the first step of any laparoscopic hysterectomy. Every pelvic surgeon must be skilled in identifying and, if necessary, dissecting the entire pelvic ureter. Identification and dissection of the ureter is an acquired skill; as with any other type of surgery, this skill is obtained by practice. By routinely identifying the ureter in all laparoscopic hysterectomies, the surgeon will gain the confidence and experience that is required to deal with difficult situations as they arise.

Recognition of the ureteral injury

Intraoperative recognition

Ureteral injuries have the best prognosis when they are recognized and repaired intraoperatively. Only one-third of ureteral injuries are detected during surgery, however. Intraoperative recognition and treatment of ureteral injury is critical to prevent compromising renal function. As many as 25% of unrecognized ureteral injuries result in eventual loss of the affected kidney.

Whenever ureteral injury is suspected or pelvic surgery proves especially difficult, we routinely perform a cystoscopic examination. Five milliliters of indigo-carmine dye and 10 to 20 mg of furosemide (Laxis) are administered intravenously prior to cystoscopic examination. Within 5 to 10 minutes, the indigo-carmine dye can be seen spurting out of ureteral orifices, confirming the patency of the ureter or ureters. Ureteral obstruction or injury is suspected if no dye effuses from the ureteral orifice after 15 minutes of indigo-carmine dye injection.

A 6- or 8-French pediatric feeding tube or a small 4- or 5-French whistle-tip ureteral catheter can be used to pass up the ureter in retrograde fashion. If the catheter can be passed to the renal pelvis and free drainage of urine from the catheter occurs, obstruction has been ruled out. It is crucial that urine comes out of the catheter, for it is possible to pass a catheter without resistance through a defect in the ureteral wall and into the retroperitoneal space. If the indigo-carmine dye or the ureteral catheter emerges from a pelvic side wall, a lacerated or transected ureter is diagnosed. If resistance is met or if the location of the catheter is uncertain, a retrograde pyelogram can be performed by injecting the contrast medium dye through the catheter; an X ray is taken to determine the exact location of the obstruction. Laparoscopically, a dilated and bluish ureter can usually be seen proximal to the site of obstruction a few minutes after the injection of dye.

Postoperative recognition

Patients with undetected ureteral injuries will present with various signs and symptoms, such as flank pain, costvertebral angle tenderness, unexplained fever and chills, abdominal distention, and ileus. High suspicion of ureteral injury and prompt investigation with IVP are crucial for diagnosis of the postoperative ureteral injury. Cystoscopy and retrograde pyelography are often needed to determine the exact location of the lesion or obstruction.

Treatment for the ureteral injury

As soon as intraoperative ureteral injury is detected, immediate laparotomy with ureteral repair is recommended. Although a few gynecologists can effectively repair ureteral injury laparoscopically, the surgeon must consider his or her own experience and skills and maintain a cautionary stance, especially when laparoscopic repair of ureteral injury is intended. Consultation with colleagues experienced in ureteral repair is highly recommended.

The timing of repair of postoperatively recognized ureteral injuries is more complicated; the patient's general condition, the degree of edema, and any associated local inflammation should be carefully evaluated, as the surgery for this type of ureteral reconstruction is usually more difficult and lengthy. Some authors suggest that early intervention—as soon as diagnosis of ureteral injury is made—does not increase postoperative complications or sequelae. However, we recommend that, in the presence of edema, local inflammation, and poor general condition of the patient, surgery for the ureteral reconstruction should be postponed for four to six weeks. The exception arises when a percutaneous nephrostomy cannot be done or evidence indicates a progressively deteriorating renal function despite intensive conservative treatments.

Surgical considerations

Regardless of whether the injury is recognized intraoperatively or detected postoperatively, the surgery for ureteral reconstruction should adhere to the following principles:

1. Have adequate debridement, and use only the healthy part of the ureter for reanastomosis.
2. Avoid using too many sutures.
3. Avoid any tension at the anastomotic site.
4. Obtain complete hemostasis if possible.

5. Insert an indwelling ureteral catheter and place retroperitoneal drainage.

Three options are available for ureteral repair: end-to-end reanastomosis, uretero-neocystostomy, and transuretero-ureterostomy.

End-to-end reanastomosis: If the site of ureteral injury lies above the midpelvis, and the injury is not very extensive, then end-to-end anastomosis of the ureter can be performed easily. First, the injured portion is debrided. Next, the ureter is mobilized to avoid undue tension on the anastomotic site. A double-J ureteral catheter is inserted and some type of extraperitoneal suction drainage, such as a Jackson-Pratt drain, is placed close to the anastomotic site. The bladder is then drained with a urethral or suprapubic catheter.

Uretero-neocystostomy: Most ureteral injuries in laparoscopic hysterectomies occur near one of the ureteric canals or along the site of the cardinal ligament between the ureteric canal and the base of the bladder. These areas are located deep in the pelvis. After resection of the damaged section of the ureter, the continuity of the urinary tract can best be restored by performing a uretero-neocystostomy rather than an end-to-end uretero-ureterostomy. To avoid any tension in the anastomotic site, the bladder must be mobilized from the back of the pubis. An anterior cystostomy is performed, and the ureter is brought through the wall of the bladder by means of a submucosal tunnel. An end-to-side mucosa-to-mucosa anastomosis between the end of the ureter and the side wall of the bladder is then performed. A double-J ureteral catheter is inserted and a Jackson-Pratt drain is placed retroperitoneally close to the anastomotic site but not touching it. If adequate mobilization of the bladder proves difficult, a bladder hitch can be carried out by simply displacing the bladder upward and attaching it to the fascia of the iliopsoas muscle. Similarly, the upper segment of the ureter can be further mobilized to reduce the tension on the anastomotic site.

Transuretero-ureterostomy: If a large segment of the ureter has been damaged and a uretero-neocystostomy is not possible, a transuretero-ureterostomy by an experienced urologist is advised.

Bladder injury

Bladder injury occurs in approximately 0.5% to 1% of all major pelvic surgeries. Laparoscopic hysterectomy should be associated with approximately the same incidence as other major pelvic surgery. In our series of 518 laparoscopic hysterectomies, however, six (1.5%) bladder injuries occurred—a slightly higher rate than reported in abdominal hysterectomy.

Two types of bladder injuries may arise during laparoscopic hysterectomy: intraperitoneal and extraperitoneal bladder injuries. Intraperitoneal bladder injury involves perforation of the bladder and its covering peritoneum, resulting with urine leakage into the peritoneal cavity. In extraperitoneal bladder injury, the peritoneum remains intact, and the urine leaks into the space of Retzius. Bladder injury during laparoscopic hysterectomy is always caused either mechanically by instruments (e.g., improperly placed trocar and scissors) or thermally by electrosurgery and/or laser.

Recognition of bladder injury

Intraoperative recognition

An intraperitoneal bladder injury can be easily recognized by leakage of the indigocarmine dye. On rare occasions with small trocar injury, no leakage of dye may be observed. High suspicion is needed to make the proper diagnosis. If the trocar tip appears to push through the muscular organ, bladder injury should be ruled out by performing cystoscopic examination. Cystoscopic examination is also necessary in cases in which excessive electrosurgery has been performed around the bladder.

Postoperative recognition

Unexplained hematuria found in postoperative catheterization, decreased urine output, anuria, suprapubic swelling and pain, and abdominal distention with elevated blood urea nitrogen (BUN) level may be indicative of bladder injury. A cystogram and a cystoscopic examination should be performed to make the proper diagnosis. Thermal injury to the bladder wall usually does not manifest itself immediately after the surgery. Instead, sudden hematuria or a vesicovaginal fistula 7 to 14 days postoperatively may be the first sign of such a thermal injury. Cystoscopic examination should be performed to confirm the diagnosis.

Prevention of bladder injury

We find the following steps very helpful for preventing injury to the bladder during laparoscopic hysterectomy.

Step 1: The bladder should be emptied prior to surgery. We routinely instill 15 to 20 mL of concentrated indigocarmine dye into the empty bladder to facilitate the early recognition of the bladder injury during the surgery. The Foley catheter need not be left in the bladder during prolonged complicated laparoscopic procedures, which usually require extensive uterine or vaginal manipulation from below by the assistant. The catheter may inadvertently be pulled and tucked by the assistant while manipulating the uterus or vagina, thereby bruising the trigon area of the bladder with the balloon tip of the catheter. If the bladder becomes distended during the surgery, it can be emptied with straight catheter.

Step 2: Insert all secondary trocars under direct visualization. This principle is especially important when the anatomy is distorted due to infection, extensive endometriosis, or previous surgery.

Step 3: Separate the bladder from the low uterine segment by using sharp dissection. Never dissect the bladder bluntly. This consideration is especially important when the patient has experienced a previous cesarean section, infection, or endometriosis.

Step 4: If an automatic multifire stapling device is to be used during the hysterectomy, make sure that the bladder is not inside the jaws of the laparoscopic stapling device before firing it.

Step 5: Avoid using electrosurgery extensively around the bladder, especially with monopolar electrosurgery in a coagulation mode. Brisk bleeding around the bladder usually indicates injury to the muscular layer of the bladder wall. Hemostatic suture, rather than electrocoagulation, will reduce the possibility of whole thickness bladder wall thermal injury, which will result in fistula formation if unrecognized and untreated.

Management of the bladder injury

Any bladder injury must be evaluated cystoscopically; the integrity of both ureters needs to be confirmed. For a small extraperitoneal bladder injury, catheterization with a Foley catheter for 10 to 14 days should be adequate. For a larger injury, a mini-laparotomy with standard two-layer repair using absorbable sutures should be performed, followed by 10 to 14 days catheterization.

For intraperitoneal bladder lacerations of less than 1 cm, a two-layer purse-string suture with 2-0 absorbable sutures can be used. The first purse-string suture includes the muscular and mucosal portion, and the second purse-string includes the serosa and muscular layer.

If the laceration of the bladder exceeds 1 cm, the bladder is mobilized to ensure that the suture site is free from tension. A standard two-layer closure is then undertaken. We recommend using a 3-0 delayed absorbable suture with SH needle for the first-layer closure, which includes the muscular and mucosal portion of the bladder, with continuous nonlocking running stitches. After the first layer is closed, 250 to 300 mL of indigocarmine dye or sterile infant formula should be instilled into the bladder to ensure that the repair is watertight. If any leakage is observed from the suture line, the bladder is deflated and a figure-of-eight suture is placed at the leaking site. The bladder is reinflated with 250 to 300 mL of dye or infant's formula and checked for leakage. If no leak appears, the bladder is deflated and a second layer of either interrupted or continuous stitches, to include the serosa and muscular portion of the bladder, is placed with 2-0 delayed absorbable sutures. The bladder is then drained with a Foley catheter for 10 to 14 days.

A cystoscopic examination should be performed at the end of any bladder repair to confirm that the injury is repaired and to ensure the integrity of the ureters is not compromised. The intraperitoneal bladder injury can always be performed laparoscopically without any difficulty. If the injury is caused by through-and-through thermal burn, the devitalized tissue of the thermal injury of the bladder wall needs to be excised. The defect can then be repaired with the two-layer technique as described above.

Other postoperative urinary complications

In our series of 518 cases of laparoscopic hysterectomies, one patient developed a vesicovaginal fistula, and another patient had a ureterovaginal fistula. Both fistulas occurred between 5 and 10 days after the hysterectomy. A genitourinary fistula, especially vesicovaginal in nature, may occur any time postoperatively. A very small one may not become evident until weeks or even months after surgery. Such fistulas usually develop as a result of unrecognized or inadequately repaired site of trauma. To avoid vesicovaginal and ureterovaginal fistula formation, immediate recognition and repair of bladder and ureteral injury are of paramount importance. Preoperative instillation of 15 mL of concentrated indigo-carmine dye is especially helpful. Blue-stained urine in the operative field provides evidence of unwanted bladder penetration. When a fistula is detected, the possibility of multiple fistulas must be ruled out, and differentiation between a vesicovaginal and a ureterovaginal fistula must be made by retrograde pyelogram. A careful preoperative evaluation with cystoscopic examination is carried out, paying particular attention to the relationship of the fistula to the ureteral orifices, bladder neck, and trigone.

Several types of surgical repair may be applied to vesicovaginal fistula: transvaginal, transabdominal, and transvesical. The principles of surgery include the following:

1. Surgery should not be performed when acute inflammation is present—wait until infection and inflammation have subsided.
2. The bladder should be mobilized from the vaginal and fistula tracts, and vaginal scar tissue needs to be excised.
3. The surgical site should be closed without tension.
4. The bladder should be drained adequately postoperatively, and either a urethral or a suprapubic catheter left in place for about two weeks.

The ureterovaginal fistula should be approached abdominally with uretero-neocystostomy or transureteroureterostomy as described earlier.

Bowel injury

Bowel injury during laparoscopic hysterectomy is rare; when it occurs, it is usually associated with trocar insertion, extensive intraperitoneal adhesions, or endometriosis. In our series of 518 cases of laparoscopic hysterectomies, two small bowel injuries occurred during enterolysis due to extensive adhesions. One superficial thermal injury affected the anterior wall of the sigmoid colon. Two intentional anterior rectal-wall resections for full-thickness endometriosis were performed. Two patients developed Richter's hernia in the 12-mm trochar sites postoperatively. Early recognition of the bowel injury is crucial (preferably detected during surgery), as immediate implementation of appropriate treatment can reduce the morbidity.

Small bowel injury

Most small bowel injuries observed during laparoscopic hysterectomies are caused by trocar insertion and enterolysis secondary to extensive adhesions. Patients with a history of multiple laparotomies, prior ruptured appendix, inflammatory bowel disease, previous pelvic inflammatory disease, and extensive endometriosis are particularly at risk for bowel adhesions. Trocar injury of the small bowel usually occurs in cases involving bowel adhesions to the anterior abdominal wall, especially around the umbilical area.

Recognition of the small bowel injury

Three different sources of small bowel injuries are noted during laparoscopic hysterectomy.

Trocar injury: If the umbilical trocar has made a large laceration in the small bowel, the surgeon may be able to laparoscopically view the mucosal surface of the small bowel. In addition, small bowel contents may be seen leaking from the laceration or a hematoma may be observed on the small bowel surface. If adhesions are detected around the umbilical area but no evidence of bowel injury is found, inspection of the umbilical trocar in its entirety, with a 5-mm laparoscope through a secondary trocar sleeve, must be performed to rule out occult or through-and-through small bowel laceration. If a trocar or laparoscope is detected to be inside the small bowel lumen, do not remove it before the laparotomy or laparoscopic repair of the injury, as it will seal the puncture and serve to identify the site of laceration.

Injury secondary to enterolysis or electrosurgery: When dense adhesions exist and require extensive enterolysis and electrosurgery for hemostasis, small bowel injury is usually obvious. Monopolar electrosurgical energy should not be used around the small bowel unless the surgeon possesses the highest level of expertise. Another drawback to electrosurgery is that discharge of static electric energy from the trocar sleeve or instruments can produce bowel injury. In such cases, electrical burns can prove difficult to detect and to evaluate because the injury usually lies outside the laparoscopic viewing field. Furthermore, monopolar electrical injury of the small bowel often appears smaller than it actually is.

Richter's hernia: Manipulation of the trocar sleeve during the operative laparoscopy can enlarge fascia and peritoneal defects, often allowing a loop of small intestine to herniate into this defect and become incarcerated. Therefore, any fascia defect of the puncture site for any trocar greater than 10 mm should be closed to prevent the formation of Richter's hernia. Various instruments are available commercially for this purpose. Richter's hernia usually manifests as signs and symptoms of the small bowel obstruction within 48 hours of the surgery.

Avoiding small bowel injury

Most small bowel injuries occur during the insertion of the Veress needle to establish a pneumoperitoneum or during the insertion of the initial trocar. Unintentional preperitoneal insufflation can complicate the initial trocar insertion, although this effect is more common with the obese patient. Do not attempt to reinsert the trocar in the face of preperitoneal insufflation. The risk of injuring the intraabdominal organs will be much higher because the ballooned-out peritoneum is in much closer proximity to the abdominal organs, and the tip of the trocar can easily injure the small bowel. Preperitoneal gas should be emptied through the trocar sleeve, after which pneumoperitoneum can be reestablished.

Factors that may cause an uncontrolled sudden trocar entry into the abdominal cavity include an inadequate umbilical incision, scar tissue from a prior laparoscopy or laparotomy, and a dull trocar. These risk factors become important in the absence of intra-abdominal adhesions or other predisposing pelvic pathology.

Treatment for the small bowel injury

The small bowel injury caused by the Veress needle usually remains innocuous as long as no leakage of bowel contents is observed and the laceration does not involve the mesenteric vessels. Superficial bowel injury caused by the trocar seals readily and requires no further treatment. When the lacerations involve the muscularis or mucosa, repair with sutures becomes necessary. Small lacerations can be repaired laparoscopically or through laparotomy. If the laceration exceeds one-half the diameter of the lumen, or if the mesenteric blood supply is interrupted or damaged, a segmental resection and anastomosis should be performed through laparotomy.

For small lacerations that do not compromise the mesenteric blood supply, we recommend a two-layer closure. The first layer involves 3-0 absorbable sutures, to include the muscularis and the mucosa, applied in either interrupted or continuous running nonlocking stitches. A second layer of reinforcing sutures of 3-0 silk Lembert stitches is used to approximate the muscularis and serosal edges. All lacerations should be closed transversely to prevent narrowing of the bowel lumen. After completion of the bowel repair, thorough lavage of the entire abdomen and pelvis with copious amounts of Ringer's lactate solution is essential to eliminate the possibility of peritonitis. A nasogastric tube should be placed and postoperatively removed when the patient starts to pass flatus.

Our experience shows that the postoperative recovery for patients who undergo laparoscopic small bowel repair is short. Their bowel function resumes rather quickly, and all of our patients were able to have the nasogastric tube removed within 24 hours of surgery.

When the patient presents with signs and symptoms of possible small bowel obstruction or peritonitis after discharge from hospital, a second-look laparoscopy or laparotomy should be done as soon as the patient is stablized. This procedure will rule out unrecognized intestinal perforation or Richter's hernia. The prognosis is usually favorable if the intervention occurs before the incarcerated bowel is damaged or extensive peritonitis has developed (in the case of undetected bowel perforation). For Richter's hernia, the trapped loop of the small bowel can usually be pulled out of the previous trocar puncture site and abdominal wall defect sutured, either laparoscopically or through laparotomy.

Wheeless presented a seven-point plan for the management of patients with peritonitis secondary to unrecognized bowel perforation:

1. Preoperative stablization with fluids, electrolytes, and nasogastric suction.
2. Exploratory laparotomy with repair or resection of the injured bowel.
3. Resection of all necrotic tissue.
4. Copious and repeated lavage with saline of the abdomen.
5. Pelvic drainage through the vagina using a closed drainage system.
6. Aggressive antibiotic therapy.
7. Starting mini-dose Heparin (5000 units every eight hours) for embolus prophylaxis.

Large intestine injury

Injury to the colon during laparoscopic surgery arises only rarely. Its actual incidence is unknown at present. In our series of 518 cases of laparoscopic hysterectomies, one case of superficial thermal injury of the sigmoid colon was encountered and two cases of intentional resection of the anterior rectal wall occurred because of the full-thickness bowel-wall infiltration of the endometriosis. We do not consider these two cases of intentional resection of the rectal wall in our series to be complications, but rather part of the therapeutic process.

Recognition and prevention of injuries to the large intestine

Colon injury due to trocar insertion

Most injuries to the large intestine occur during trocar insertions. The incidence of trocar injury to the large intestine is estimated to be approximately 0.1%. The transverse colon and sigmoid colon are most commonly traumatized by the trocar insertion, with the damage usually happening during blind insertion of the umbilical trocar. The diagnosis of colon injury is obvious when fecal material appears on the tip of trocar or in the abdomen during the procedure. If the injury to the bowel is not a full-thickness perforation or if the colon is empty, however, the only sign may be a rent and bleeding from the site of injury. Therefore, a systematic and thorough inspection of the abdominal organs should be conducted during the initial viewing through the laparoscope to rule out injury during the trocar insertion. A distended stomach and anterior omental adhesions should draw special attention to the possibility of colon injury.

To prevent trocar injury to the large intestine during laparoscopic hysterectomy, the patient's history should be carefully reviewed to reveal any special risk. The risk of bowel injury increases in patients with previous abdominal surgery, including bowel resection, colostomy, appendectomy for ruptured appendix, or a history of intestinal obstruction or inflammatory bowel disease. A nasogastric tube should always be used in patients known to have difficulty with endotracheal intubation at the initial stage of anethesia. Routine use of this tube is even better, as it will prevent the gastric distention and subsequent inferior displacement of the transverse colon. The importance of having an adequate umbilical incision and sharp trocar to forestall injury to the bowel has already been described in the section on avoiding small bowel injury in this chapter.

Colon injury secondary to electrosurgery and laser

Laparoscopic hysterectomy requires extensive use of electrosurgical devices for hemostasis and tissue division; these instruments, however, can produce thermal injury to the bowel. The rectosigmoid colon is especially vulnerable because of its close proximity to the uterus and ovaries. The inherent risk of burn injury to bowel, ureter, and skin necessitates the use of bipolar rather than unipolar electrosurgical devices. Burn injury to the rectosigmoid colon from bipolar forceps is almost always caused by poor exposure—that is, the surgeon did not see the prong tips of the forceps touch the rectosigmoid colon when he or she stepped on the pedal. Therefore, the surgeon must first ensure that both prongs are in clear view and away from the bowel before stepping on

the pedal. Viewing the magnified operative field on the video monitor is not only less fatiguing for the surgeon, but also reduces the incidence of bowel injury. Colon injury caused by bipolar electrocoagulation can be readily identified by viewing the blanched area on the surface of the bowel.

Colon injury caused by unipolar electrosurgery can be difficult to detect and evaluate. This type of injury usually results from a direct burn or discharge of static electricity built up in the trocar sleeve. According to Thompson and Wheeless, signs and symptoms of electric bowel burns appear between three and seven days postoperatively. Wheeless also reported that only two out of 33 known bowel burn patients developed perforation. With the exception of the cecum, the wall of the colon is much thicker than the wall of the small bowel, which renders large intestines more resistant to thermal injury than the small bowel.

Although laser energy can theoretically cause colon injury, the actual risk is extremely low, especially in the hands of a well-trained laser surgeon. The only laser that may potentially inflict significant trauma to the colon is Nd:YAG laser delivered through the bare fiber tip. Fortunately, gynecologists using the Nd:YAG laser to perform laparoscopic hysterectomies employ sapphire tips, which practically eliminate the risk of colon injury by laser if used judiciously.

Colon injury related to the obliterated cul-de-sac

Cul-de-sac obliteration, caused by either endometriosis or previous pelvic inflammatory disease, presents a difficult challenge for the gynecological surgeon. The sigmoid colon and rectum are at risk with this condition. Accidental entry into the rectum or sigmoid colon during their separation from the posterior wall of the uterus and cervix or during excision of infiltrating endometriosis on the rectal wall, can cause a serious major complication if the bowel goes unrepaired or is repaired improperly. Intentional bowel entry for adequate excision of full-thickness infiltrating endometriosis of the bowel wall seldom results in any complication—probably reflecting the expertise of the surgeon who performs this difficult surgery.

After extensive dissection of the cul-de-sac, a careful inspection for complete hemostasis and evidence of possible bowel injury should be carried out. It is prudent also to perform a thorough rectovaginal examination to ensure that all infiltrating endometriosis has been excised and that no rectal injury has occurred during the dissection.

Management of colon injury

Early recognition of large bowel injury, preferably before the patient leaves the operating room, is crucial to avoid catastrophic consequences. Patients at risk for large bowel injury are those who have experienced previous bowel surgery, such as bowel resections and colostomies. Also at risk are patients who have the following conditions: a history of bowel obstruction and extensive intra-abdominal adhesions; a history of bowel inflammatory disease; a history of, or by examination, obliterated cul-de-sac with rectal nodules. These at-risk patients should be identified preoperatively, and standard bowel preparation should be implemented prior to surgery. The author's standard bowel preparation includes the following:

1. Neomycin 1 g every four hours and erythromycin 500 mg every six hours by mouth, starting 48 hours before surgery.
2. Clear liquid diet, starting 36 hours before surgery.
3. GoLytely 4 liters by mouth, beginning the afternoon before surgery.

This bowel preparation regimen has worked well in both open laparotomy and laparoscopic surgery.

Repair of colon injury can be performed via either laparoscopy or laparotomy. Copious irrigation and suction are necessary to wash off and dilute the intraperitoneal contamination. Adequate debridement of the wound is followed by primary closure of the defect in two layers; we use 2-0 delayed absorbable sutures to include muscular and mucosal as the first layer, applied in either interrupted or continuous nonlocking stitches. The second layer is closed with interrupted stitches to include the serosal and muscular layer without undue tension. Although most surgeons use a permanent suture for the second-layer closure, we prefer to use 2-0 delayed absorbable suture for fear of fistula formation when permanent suture material is incorporated in a potentially contaminated area. The closure must be airtight or watertight. This characteristic can be tested by filling the pelvis with irrigation solution, reducing the pneumoperitoneal pressure, and performing laparoscopic underwater examination while pumping the air. Alternatively, 300 mL of indigo-carmine dye or diluted Betadine solution may be injected through the anus by a rectal tube or large Foley catheter with a 30-mL inflated balloon tip inside the anus. Intravenous antibiotics with broad coverage should be administered immediately after detection of the colon injury. Gastric decompression to reduce the intestinal peristalsis with a nasogastric tube is crucial for the smooth healing of the repaired site. Do not feed the patient too early, as food will stimulate intestinal peristalsis and increase the intraluminal pressure of the bowel. The patient should remain on a low residual diet until the repaired site heals adequately, which usually takes about two weeks.

Bleeding complications

The recognition and management of bleeding complications from trocar injury to the abdominal wall vessels and life-threatening hemorrhage from injury to the major abdominal vessels are addressed elsewhere in this book.

In our 518 laparoscopic hysterectomies, four patients developed postoperative pelvic hematomas (0.77%) and three patients had delayed cuff bleedings (0.57%). In each of the four patients who had a pelvic hematoma, an automatic laparoscopic stapling device was used in the original surgery. This instrument supposedly included a built-in mechanism to preserve the microcirculation and thus to promote healing of the stapling sites. When an automatic stapling device is used, careful underwater examination of the stapler line for complete hemostasis at the end of surgery after discontinuation of the pneumoperitoneal pressure is important for hematoma prevention. Any bleeding, including oozing, detected at this time requires bipolar coagulation behind the stapler line. No hematoma formation occurred in either group using electrosurgery or sutures for large-vessel hemostasis.

Intraoperative hemorrhage

Massive and troublesome intraoperative hemorrhage can occur with slipped ligature ties or hemoclips, large ovarian or uterine artery injury, or premature division before the vessels are completely desiccated. The principles to follow in dealing with massive bleeding laparoscopically are the same as those in open laparotomy: compression, suction and irrigation of the bleeding site, and clear identification of the bleeder.

After the bleeder is identified, it can be controlled by suture ligation, electrodesiccation, or hemoclip application. Most bleeding can be controlled by bipolar desiccation alone; however, the surrounding anatomy should be checked before initiating electrodesiccation to avoid thermal injury to vital structures such as the ureter, bladder, or bowels. Suture ligation or application of the hemoclips is more appropriate when the bleeder is close to the vital structures.

The key to preventing premature division before the large vessels are completely desiccated is to have the assistant or circulating nurse carefully observe the ammeter on the generator of the electrosurgery unit to ensure that the flow of the electric current has completely ceased between the prongs of bipolar forceps. If the vessels are not completely desiccated and occluded, the electric current will continue to flow between the tips of the forceps, and the needle of the ammeter will not return to the 0 position. If a large vessel cannot be desiccated after the bipolar forceps is applied for 8 to 10 seconds, the two prongs of the forceps must not have completely grasped it. In such a case, the forceps must be reapplied. Injuries to external iliac vessels, aorta, or vena cava require immediate laparotomy and intraoperative consultation with a vascular surgeon.

Early postoperative complications

The usual early postoperative complications of abdominal and vaginal hysterectomies (e.g., postoperative fever, ileus, pelvic cellulitis, thrombophlebitis, atalectasis of the lungs, and dehiscence of the wound) are extremely rare with laparoscopic hysterectomy. This situation probably reflects the fact that the patient experiences much less discomfort after laparoscopic hysterectomy and is able to ambulate much sooner.

Another factor contributing to the low incidence of early postoperative complications is the fact that removal of the uterus and closure of the vagina are followed by careful inspection of the pelvis and irrigation with copious amounts of Ringer's lactate solution; underwater examination of the vascular pedicles is then performed to ensure complete hemostasis.

As with vaginal hysterectomy, however, dehiscence of the apex of the vagina with extrusion of the intestines of omentum must be considered, although such complications are rare. Vaginal eviscerations are mostly associated with significant Valsava maneuvers, such as violent coughing, retching, or heavy lifting, which result in sudden massive increase in intra-abdominal pressure. Prevention, then, aims to reduce and contain those factors that would rapidly inflate intra-abdominal pressure. Most eviscerations through the vagina are associated with injury of the mesentery of the small bowel. Because the viability and integrity of the small bowel are at stake, appropriate treatment involves immediate laparotomy through a midline incision. A complete inspection of the entire intestine and its mesentery from the ligament of Treitz to the cecum is mandatory. The pelvic defect is repaired abdominally, with special attention to obliterating the cul-de-sac and enterocele, if present. If the viability of the intestine is questionable, bowel resection is performed.

Conclusion

In reviewing the literature and from our own experience in performing laparoscopic hysterectomies, we conclude that, even with experience, laparoscopic hysterectomy is not an innocuous procedure. Gynecologists who are interested in performing laparoscopic hysterectomy must know their limits and select patients accordingly. The transition from open surgery to video-guided surgery requires considerable adjustment. Knowledge of laparoscopic instrumentation, suturing techniques, physics and clinical applications of electrosurgery and laser, and avoidance and management of laparoscopic complications are required. Assisting and precepting with surgeons proficient in laparoscopic hysterectomy are critical, for no one can learn the operation outside the operating room. "Primum non nocere" (above all, do no harm) is our first and ultimate duty as physicians. Conversion to abdominal hysterectomy should never be considered a complication; rather it is a prudent surgical decision when the surgeon becomes uncomfortable with the laparoscopic approach.

RECOMMENDED READINGS

1. Penfield AJ. Trocar and needle injury. In: Phillips JM, ed. Laparoscopy. Baltimore: Williams & Wilkins, 1977:236–241.
2. Hurd WW, Pear ML, DeLancey JOL. Laparoscopic injury of abdominal wall blood vessels: a report of three cases. Obstet Gynecol 1993;82:673–676.
3. Hulka JF. Major vessel injury during laparoscopy. Am J Obstet Gynecol 1980;138:590.
4. Corson SL. Major vessel injury during laparoscopy. Am J Obstet Gynecol 1980;138:589.
5. Shin CS. Vascular injury secondary to laparoscopy. NY State J Med 1982;82:935–936.
6. Yuzpe AA. Pneumoperitoneum needle and trocar injuries in laparoscopy. A survey on possible contrubuting factors and prevention. J Reprod Med 1990;35:485–490.
7. Phillips JM, Hulka JF, Peterson HB. American Association of Gynecologic Laparoscopists' 1982 membership survey. J Reprod Med 1984;29:592–594.
8. Liu CY, Kadar N. Identification and dissection of the pelvic ureter. In: Liu CY, ed. Laparoscopic hysterectomy and pelvic floor reconstruction. Boston: Blackwell Science, 1996:126–145.
9. Moore JG, Hibbard LT, Growdon WA, et al. Urinary tract endometriosis: enigmas in diagnosis and management. Am J Obstet Gynecol 1979;134:162–172.
10. St Lezin MA, Stoller ML. Surgical ureteral injuries. Urology 1991;38:497–506.
11. Case AS. Diagnostic studies in bladder rupture. Urol Clin North Am 1989;16:267–273.
12. Reich H, McGlynn F. Laparoscopic repair of bladder injury. Obstet Gynecol 1990;76:909–910.
13. Shah PM, Kim K, Ramirez-Schon G, et al. Elevated blood urea nitrogen: an aid to the diagnosis of intraperitoneal rupture of the bladder. J Urol 1979;122:741–743.
14. Peters PC. Intraperitoneal rupture of the bladder. Urol Clin North Am 1989;16:279–282.
15. Corriere JN Jr, Sandler CM. Management of the extraperitoneal bladder rupture. Urol Clin North Am 1989;16:275–277.
16. Grainger DA, Soderstrom RM, Schiff SF, et al. Ureteral injury at laparoscopy: insights into diagnosis, management, and prevention. Obstet Gynecol 1990;75:839–843.
17. Gomel V, James C. Intraoperative management of ureteral injury during operative laparoscopy. Fertil Steril 1991;55:416–419.
18. Ball TL, Platt MA. Urological complications of endometriosis. Am J Obstet Gynecol 1962;84:1516–1518.
19. Neto WA, Lopes RN, Cury M, et al. Vesical endometriosis. Urology 1984;24:271–274.
20. Bradford JA, Ireland EW, Warwick BG. Ureteric endometriosis: three cases reports and a review of the literature. Aust NZ J Gynecol 1989;29:421–424.
21. Zinman LM, Libertino JA, Roth RA. Management of operative ureteral injury. Urology 1978;12:290–303.
22. Mann WJ, Arato M, Pastiner B, et al. Ureteral injuries in an obstetric and gynecology training program: etiology and management. Obstet Gynecol 1988;72:82–85.
23. Hoch WH, Kursh ED, Persky L. Early aggressive management of intraoperative ureteral injuries. J Urol 1975;114:530–532.
24. Tarkington MA, Dejter SW Jr, Bresette JF. Early surgical management of extensive gynecologic ureteral injuries. Surgery 1991;173:17–21.
25. Symmonds RE. Ureteral injuries associated with gynecologic surgery: prevention and management. Clin Obstet Gynecol 1976;19:623–644.
26. Harrow BR. A neglected maneuver for ureterovesical implantation following injury at gynecological operations. J Urol 1968;100:280–287.

27. Fry DE, Milholen L, Harbrecht PJ. Iatrogenic ureteral injury. Options in management. Arch Surg 1983;118:454–457.

28. Winslow PH, Kreger R, Ebbesson B, Oster E. Conservative management of electrical injury of ureter secondary to laparoscopy. Urology 1986;27:60–62.

29. Witters S, Cornelissen J, Vereecken R. Iatrogenic ureteral injury: aggressive or conservative treatment. Am J Obstet Gynecol 1986;155:582.

30. Zinman LM, Libertino JA, Roth RA. Management of operative ureteral injury. Urology 1978;12:290–303.

31. Gambee LP, Garnjobst W, Hardwick CE. Ten years' experience with a single layer anastomosis in colon surgery. Am J Surg 1956;92:222–227.

32. Montz FJ, Holschneider CH, Munro MG. Incisional hernia following laparoscopy: a survey of the American Association of Gynecologic Laparoscopists. Obstet Gynecol 1994;84:881–884.

33. Barnhill D, Doering D, Remmenga S, et al. Intestinal surgery performed on gynecologic cancer patients. Gynecol Oncol 1991;40:38–41.

34. Thompson BH, Wheeless CR Jr. Gastrointestinal complications of laparoscopic sterilization. Obstet Gynecol 1973;41:669–676.

35. Wheeless CR Jr. Gastrointestinal injuries associated with laparoscopy. In: Phillips JM, ed. Endoscopy in gynecology. Downey, CA: American Association of Gynecologic Laparoscopists, 1978:317–324.

36 | Complications of Laparoscopic Subtotal Hysterectomy

Christopher Sutton

When E. L. Richardson introduced the concept of the total abdominal hysterectomy in 1929, he was mainly concerned with the risk of cervical carcinoma developing in the residual cervical stump. The risk at that time—long before the introduction of cytological screening for cervical intraepithelial neoplasia (CIN)—was found to be only 0.4% in 6600 cases (1). The subtotal hysterectomy, which had hitherto been the only method of abdominal hysterectomy since its introduction by Charles Clay in 1853 (2), was inherently even safer because of the decreased likelihood of ascending infection and ureteric injury.

The total laparoscopic hysterectomy was first introduced by Harry Reich in 1988 (3), who demonstrated his technique in all five populated continents. It became immediately obvious to observers that the length of the procedure and the technical skills required rendered it inappropriate in countries where surgical workloads were heavy. The concept of employing laparoscopic surgery to convert an abdominal hysterectomy into a vaginal one (LAVH), whereby the surgeon dealt with pelvic pathology and secured the upper pedicles, did little to make the vaginal surgery any easier. Vaginal access was, by definition, impaired in such cases; otherwise a vaginal hysterectomy would have been performed at the outset. Thus it became clear that LAVH had a potential for inappropriate use and that vaginal removal of the uterus was extremely difficult. Not surprisingly, reports of prolonged operating time and ureteric injury began to surface when it was attempted with greater frequency.

In response, several laparoscopic surgeons turned their attention to reevaluating the supracervical hysterectomy on the grounds that, with the development of more-sophisticated tissue morcellating equipment, it has become a "purer" laparoscopic procedure. That is, because it is necessary to ligate only the ascending branches of the uterine artery, the ureter stays well clear of the operating field and thus appears less likely to suffer damage. The complications of the procedure are therefore less during the actual operative procedure, although experience has taught us that they tend to be related to retention of the cervical stump.

Operative complications

Complications from subtotal hysterectomy are essentially those that occur in any laparoscopy, especially during the insertion of the Veress needle and the first trocar, which are essentially blind procedures. They occur in less than one per 10,000 cases (0.1%) (4). No published evidence indicates that the use of the open technique attributed to Hassan results in less bowel injury, although it may be easier to recognize any damage immediately and effect the necessary surgical repair.

The ureter must be carefully identified and positively distinguished from other lateral pelvic side-wall structures by its characteristic peristalsis. In any event, the incision lines for the desiccation and dividing or stapling of the ovarian vessels, round ligaments, and ascending branches of the uterine artery should remain well clear of this vital structure. Care must, however, be taken with the use of bipolar diathermy, especially if the parametrium is very vascular, because prolonged use of this technique can result in extensive lateral thermal damage. The employment of irrigation to limit this problem is a wise precaution, as is the use of an electrosurgical generator that automatically cuts out when no further current flows due to tissue desiccation. The operator must also be aware that the blanched white area represents irreversible tissue damage and must switch off the current if it approaches a vital structure such as bowel or ureter.

Immediate postoperative problems

In the author's experience, although the operating time for subtotal laparoscopic hysterectomy (SLH) is longer than for total abdominal hysterectomy (TAH), the SLH hospital stay is usually half that associated with TAH. All patients are given prophylactic antibiotics in the form of 750 mg Cephazolin preoperatively. This precaution is taken because the surgeon must operate through a potentially infected field, especially if an attempt is made to remove the transformation zone, either by electrosurgical wire loop excision or by morcellation using the serrated edged macro-morcellator developed by Semm (5). Apart from the occasional patient who incurs bruising of the abdominal wall, most women make a remarkably quick recovery and are back to full activity within 21 days (6).

Complications following discharge from hospital

If the patient has undergone excision of the central part of the cervix, she should be warned about the possibility of heavy bleeding or an offensive discharge during the secondary healing phase. If this complication occurs, the patient should report to her family doctor and receive a broad-spectrum antibiotic and Metronidazole by mouth. Essentially these patients have had the same operation on the cervix as a cone biopsy and could experience problems with infection during the secondary healing phase. Although this complication probably affects only about one in 30 cases and the risk is decreased by giving prophylactic antibiotics during surgery, patients should be warned about this possibility so that they can take appropriate action.

Late complications (more than six weeks after surgery)

In the past when the cervix was routinely retained at the time of hysterectomy, some patients complained of a serosanguineous discharge that they found troublesome. After performing an initial series of laparoscopic subtotal hysterectomies, we became uncomfortably aware that a certain number of patients were requiring late surgery to the cervical stump; in contrast, secondary surgery was extremely unusual following TAH, vaginal hysterectomy, or LAVH. This secondary surgery took the form of laparoscopic adhesiolysis, laparoscopic vaporization of endometriosis on the cervical stump, and in one instance laparoscopic drainage of a mucocele. Several other patients required a laser trachelorrhaphy, and one required laparoscopic oophorectomy for recurrent endometriosis. In addition, some patients required removal of the stump because of persistent pain, bleeding, or both.

To examine this issue, we performed an audit of 52 supracervical laparoscopic hysterectomies compared with a similar number of abdominal hysterectomies (7)

conducted during the same time frame. Our analysis of the data showed that the patients who were having secondary surgery had a history of endometriosis and, in most cases, the hysterectomy was performed to alleviate recurrent endometriosis. In the abdominal hysterectomy group, even though a similar number had received a hysterectomy for reasons of recurrent endometriosis, the patients did not have a similar history of secondary surgery related to problems with the retained stump. Although other surgeons performing laparoscopic subtotal hysterectomy have not yet reported the same problems, we do not advise retention of the cervix if hysterectomy is being undertaken for endometriosis.

Conclusion

Laparoscopic supracervical hysterectomy appears to offer a safe way of performing laparoscopic hysterectomy, with less likelihood of injury to the ureter and fewer problems with subsequent bladder dysfunction. Most patients experience a quick and uncomplicated recovery. Although some concern has been raised about the risk of development of cervical carcinoma if the stump is retained, the actual risk of stump carcinoma is 0.1% to 0.4% (8). This risk is, in reality, no greater than the risk of vaginal cancer following total abdominal hysterectomy, and no one would seriously advocate the removal of the vagina as a prevention against subsequent neoplasia (9).

This operation appears to represent a purer form of laparoscopic hysterectomy that is more suitable for universal adoption. At this time, however, it probably should not be offered to patients who have had a history of abnormal cervical smears or if the hysterectomy is being performed for endometriosis.

REFERENCES

1. Cutler EC, Zollinger RM. Atlas of surgical operations. New York: Macmillan, 1949.
2. Sutton CJG. One hundred and fifty years of hysterectomy from Charles Clay to the laparoscopic hysterectomy. RCOG historical lecture. In: Studd JWW, ed. Year book of the Royal College of Obstetricians and Gynaecologists. London: RCOG Publishers, 1995.
3. Reich H, Decaprio J, McGlynn F. Laparoscopic hysterectomy. J Gynaecol Surg 1989;5:213–216.
4. Wheeler J. Major vascular injury at laparoscopy. In: Corfman RS, Diamond MP, DeCherney A. Complications of laparoscopy and hysteroscopy. Cambridge, Mass.: Blackwell Scientific Publications, 1993.
5. Semm K. Hysterectomy by pelviscopy: an alternative approach without colpotomy (CASH). In: Garry R, Reich H, eds. Laparoscopic hysterectomy. Oxford, UK: Blackwell Scientific Publications, 1993:118–132.
6. Ewen SP, Sutton CJG. Initial experience with supracervical laparoscopic hysterectomy and removal of the cervical transformation zone. Br J Obstet Gynaecol 1994;101:225–228.

7. Jacobs S, Sutton CJG, Pooley A, Ewen SE. Consecutive case series of supracervical laparoscopic hysterectomy compared with total abdominal hysterectomy—short- and long-term follow-up. Audit Department, Royal Surrey County Hospital Publications, Guildford, UK, pp 1–15, 1996.

8. Storm HA, Clemmenson IH, Manders T, Brinton LA. Supravaginal uterine amputation in Denmark 1978–1988 and risk of cancer. Gynaecol Oncol 1992;45:198–201.

9. Lyons TL. Laparoscopic supracervical hysterectomy using the contact Nd:YAG laser. Gynaecol Endoscopy 1993;2:79–81.

Laparoscopic Appendectomy: Avoiding Complications | 37

Chau-Su Ou, Edward M. Beadle, and James B. Presthus

Introduction

Appendectomy is one of the most frequently performed surgical procedures in the western world (1). Consequently, conventional appendectomy is one of the first major operations mastered by general surgeons. This procedure is performed quickly through a small muscle-splitting incision, with minimal perioperative morbidity (2). Although laparoscopic appendectomy is a less commonly used approach, it has been shown by numerous authors to have advantages over conventional appendectomy (3–5).

In particular, laparoscopic appendectomy offers the following benefits:

- It allows for more thorough exploration of the abdominal cavity and thereby improves the surgeon's ability to accurately diagnose normal appendices (2, 6). Typically 20% to 30% of open appendectomies prove histologically normal (7, 8).

- It results in decreased postoperative morbidity and improved cosmesis, particularly in obese patients for whom conventional appendectomy requires a larger-than-normal incision (2, 5, 9, 10).

- It yields significantly reduced (from 80% to 20%) postoperative adhesion formation (11). The authors have also observed this pattern.

- It reduces hospital stay because recovery times are shorter (2). Even though the conventional appendectomy incision is smaller than the cumulative length of the laparoscopic trocar incisions, those made for laparoscopic trocar placement split the muscle rather than dividing it, producing less tissue injury and lower postoperative morbidity (9, 10).

- It should be more cost-effective overall than conventional appendectomy even though it incurs higher hospital charges (6).

Although laparoscopic appendectomy has not gained the widespread acceptance of laparoscopic cholecystectomy, it is becoming increasingly recognized as a viable alternative to conventional appendectomy. As a result, this technique is now offered in many advanced laparoscopy courses.

Method

The surgeon who is comfortable with other laparoscopic procedures possesses nearly all of the skills needed for laparoscopic appendectomy. Unfortunately, the surgical literature presents a sometimes confusing array of positions and techniques (2, 5, 6). It is important that the surgeon choose a position that works well for him or her.

As most appendectomies are performed in acute stages, the surgeon must pay attention to the distended and fixed bowel.

Once the pneumoperitoneal is obtained, the trocar can be established. The appendix must be visualized so that the tip can be grasped with an instrument. If the appendix is markedly swollen, a pretied loop may be placed over the tip and used for retraction (2). Specialized atraumatic bowel-grasping forceps have recently become available that may be used to secure the tip of the appendix (2).

Once the appendix is identified and freed from adhesion, several tactics may be employed to perform the appendectomy, depending on the degree of inflammation (12–14).

In cases of acute inflamed appendix, including perforated appendix, the mesoappendix can be bipolar-cauterized or stapled. After freeing the appendix from the mesoappendix, transect the appendix with staples before cutting to prevent spillage of its contents.

In cases where the appendix is less inflamed or in cases of a non-inflamed incidental appendectomy, the mesoappendix is thinner. Part of it is transilluminated, allowing the formation of a small "window." The mesoappendix can then be bipolar-cauterized. Milk the base of the appendix with atraumatic forceps and bipolar-cauterize it. Next, tie the proximal end of the appendix with two pretied loops and the distal end with one pretied loop. The appendix can then be transected and removed.

Complications

Complications associated with laparoscopic procedures in general, such as needle trocar injuries, are discussed more thoroughly elsewhere in this book. The most common complications specifically associated with laparoscopic appendectomy are bleeding and infection (15).

Bleeding

Bleeding can occur during both laparoscopic and conventional appendectomy, especially in cases involving acute inflammation. Oozing can also result from adhesion or from sharp dissection. In most cases, bleeding can be controlled using bipolar cautery. Occasionally the bleeding may require sutures with pretied loops (16). To avoid bowel injury, bleeding—particularly around the mesoappendix, close to the cecum—must be cauterized carefully. Irrigation and underwater examination are required after hemostasis. The following points require special attention:

- The majority of patients operated on for acute appendicitis show strong evidence of peritoneal irritation. The small and large bowel may be distended or fixed in position, making injury from a blind sufflation needle more likely. In this case, conventional appendectomy is suggested.
- Acute inflammation indicates that the appendix probably has significant adhesion or is less mobile. In such cases the mesoappendix can be thick, leaving little or no transluminal window visible. Atraumatic forceps should be used during blunt dissection to avoid bowel serosa injury. Particular care should be taken when skeletonizing the appendix and handling the bowel.
- When the appendix is less mobile, especially in the case of retroceal appendix, the lateral attachment to the right colon and pelvic floor should be carefully divided. To avoid injuring the right ureter and iliac vessels, these structures should be identified early.

Infection

The risk of infection due to leakage of appendiceal contents can be minimized by following these precautions:

- If the appendix has ruptured before or during surgery, carefully tie the tip of the inflamed appendix with a pretied loop and cut the loop for traction instead of continually grasping with forceps.

- Use endoscopic staples and a cutting device when transecting the appendix, especially if it is abscessed or severely inflamed.
- When transecting a less inflamed or non-inflamed appendix, thermal sterilization can be achieved by using bipolar cautery. Milk the appendix before cauterizing. After cauterizing, attach two pretied loops—one on the proximal end of the appendix and another below the cauterization. Each tie must be separated from the others by 2 to 3 mm. Tie the loop on the distal end of the appendix above the cautery, and then transect the appendix through the middle of the cauterization. If spillage occurs, the periceal area should be irrigated copiously.
- When appendiceal leakage is suspected, one to three doses of a broad-spectrum antibiotic is recommended.
- Spillage can be drained by placing a closed suction drain through the puncture sites.
- Use a sterilized bag or condom to remove the appendix. This step should be performed under laparoscopic observation using dull instruments.

Even with these precautions, contamination may still occur. The patient should therefore be monitored for postoperative complications due to infection.

Controversies

Complications during laparoscopic appendectomy have been reported to occur more frequently among surgeons who are less familiar with the laparoscopic approach (2). These complications tend to arise more often in cases with severely inflamed appendices or extensive peritonitis. Because experience can significantly reduce the incidence of complications, we highly recommend that the surgeon work with an experienced preceptor until becoming thoroughly familiar with the procedure.

In addition, laparoscopic appendectomy, like other laparoscopic procedures, requires informed patient consent. The discussion with the patient should cover any potential backup procedures, such as laparotomy.

Conclusion

Laparoscopic appendectomy offers some immediate advantages over conventional appendectomy. In recent years marked improvements in the instruments and techniques used to perform this surgery have appeared (17, 18). When performed by a trained surgeon, the laparoscopic method can be used to treat almost any kind of appendicitis with minimal probability of complications. The ease with which this procedure can be carried out and the advantages of the laparoscopic approach will soon make this the technique of choice for treatment of appendicitis.

REFERENCES

1. National Inpatient Profile. Health Care Knowledge Systems, 1989.
2. Oreilly MJ, Reddick EJ, Miller WD, Saye WB. Surgical Laparoscopic Textbook. 1993;9:301–326.
3. Semm K. Endoscopic appendectomy. Endosc 1993;15:59–64.
4. Pier A, Gotz F, Bacher C. Laparoscopic appendectomy in 625 cases: from innovation to routine. Surg Laparosc Endosc 1991;I:8–13.
5. Bryant T. Laparoscopic appendectomy, a simplified technique. J Lap Surg 1992;2:6.
6. Cohen M, Dangleis K. The cost effectiveness of laparoscopic appendectomy. J Lap Surg 1993;3:2.
7. Lewis FR, Holcroft JW, Boey J, Dunphy JE. Appendicitis: a critical review of diagnosis and treatment in 1000 cases. Arch Surg 1975;110:677–684.
8. Berry J, Malt R. Appendicitis near its centenary. Ann Surg 1984;20:567–575.
9. Sosa JL, Sleeman D, McKenney MG, Dygert J, Yarish D, Martin L. A comparison of laparoscopic and traditional appendectomy. J Lap Surg 1993;3:2.
10. Vallina VL, Velasco MV, McCulloch CS. Laparoscopic versus conventional appendectomy. Ann Surg 1993;218:685–692.
11. DeWilde RL. Goodbye to late bowel obstruction after appendectomy (letter). Lancet 1991;338:1012.
12. Gangal HT, Gangal MH. Laparoscopic appendectomy. Endosc 1987;19:127–129.
13. Leahy PF. Technique of laparoscopic appendectomy. Br J Surg 1989;76:616.
14. McKernan JB, Saye WB. Laparoscopic technique and appendectomy with argon laser. South Med J 1990;83:1019–1020.
15. Daniell J, Gurly L. Appendectomy: avoiding complications. Laparosopic Appendectomy Textbook. 1991;46:246–249.
16. Hay DL, Levine RL, et al. Chromic gut pelviscopic loop ligature: effect of the number of pulls on the tensile strength. J Reprod 1990;35:260–262.
17. Schreiber JH. Early experience with laparoscopic appendectomy in women. Surg Endosc 1987;1:211–216.
18. Gotz F, Pier A, Bacher C. Modified laparoscopic appendectomy in surgery. Surg Endosc 1990;4:6–9.

38 | Complications of Laparoscopic Biliary Surgery

Jeffrey E. Everett and William G. Gamble

Introduction

Few technical advances in surgery have rivaled that of laparoscopic cholecystectomy (LC), which dates back only to 1986, when Muhe reported its use at a surgical meeting in Germany. Muhe performed the first clinical procedure in September 1985 and had completed a small series by early 1986 (1). Despite this revolutionary technical achievement, laparoscopic cholecystectomy did not gain widespread enthusiasm until late 1986, when Phillipe Mouret, a general surgeon with extensive experience in gynecological laparoscopy, proposed a slightly modified technique (1–4). Two years later, Reddick and Olsen from Nashville, Tennessee, were credited with popularizing the procedure in the United States (1, 5).

The movement that unfolded over the next few years has dramatically altered the approach to biliary calculus disease. Despite lacking clinical trials, laparoscopic cholecystectomy has undergone widespread clinical application, partly driven by competition, patient demand, and rapid dissemination of technology by instrument manufacturers. Shorter hospital stays, improved cosmesis, decreased pain, and reduced disability have challenged the open technique, which represented the gold standard for 110 years (1, 2, 6, 7). As might be expected for a technique that has existed for less than a decade, this surgical approach has been faulted for a higher complication rate and a well-described learning curve (2, 6, 8). This chapter describes the common complications specific to laparoscopic biliary surgery and suggests ways to avoid these common pitfalls.

Complications

Overview

The overall incidence of complications following laparoscopic cholecystectomy is essentially the same as that seen with the traditional open technique. The reported mortality rate is 0.15% and the morbidity approximately 2.5% (9). The outcome of LC is clearly influenced by the experience and level of training of the operating surgeon. A defined learning curve has been established for this new technology (2, 8). Adequate experience is gained somewhere between 30 and 35 cases, a time frame in which most complications occur. The overall complication rate ranges from 4.5% to 1.7% after the first 30 cases (2). Likewise, common bile duct injuries follow a learning curve in which 90% of complications occur within the first 30 cases.

Multivariate analysis has revealed that the only significant factor associated with an adverse outcome is the surgeon's experience. A regression model based on 8839 procedures predicts a 1.7% chance of bile duct injury on the first case—a risk that drops to 0.17% after 50 cases are handled (8). Based on these findings, it has been recommended that surgeons perform their first 30 procedures in conjunction with an experienced laparoscopic surgeon.

Bile duct injury and bile leak

Injury to the common bile duct is a well-described complication of cholecystectomy. It is a serious, potentially life-threatening complication, with associated morbidity, prolonged hospitalization, high cost, and litigation. Such injuries occur in 0.1% to 0.3% of patients undergoing open cholecystectomy, compared with 0.6% incidence during laparoscopic cholecystectomy reported in review of 21 series involving more than 87,000 procedures (1). Although the higher rate is cause for concern, further analysis reveals that such complications typically arise early in the surgeon's practice. The reported incidence is as high as 2.2% for a surgeon's first 30 cases, but then drops sharply to 0.1% thereafter. In fact, a single institution has reported a series of 1525 consecutive cases without biliary injury (10). Excluding the learning curve, it would appear that laparoscopic cholecystectomy may be performed safely with an incidence of biliary complication equal to or less than the rate for the open technique.

Laparoscopic biliary injuries generally result from misidentification of the biliary ducts or technical failure. The lack of three-dimensional orientation and anatomic variability are well-recognized dangers of LC. Misidentification of the bile duct as the cystic duct produces the most severe injury. Typically the common hepatic duct is clipped or divided, resulting in complete obstruction or leak. This injury is frequently associated with division of the right hepatic artery. Even when recognized, extensive mobilization of the common duct leads to devascularization that may appear as a late stricture. Injury to an aberrant right hepatic duct follows a similar pattern when it is mistaken for the cystic duct.

Biliary injury may also follow from technical errors including failure to securely clip the cystic duct, improper plane of dissection of the gallbladder off the liver bed, and thermal injuries. Because clips may not be as secure as ligatures, dislodgment may occur during further dissection of the gallbladder. Furthermore, metallic clips serve as a thermal conductor for electrical cautery in the area, resulting in cystic stump necrosis or adjacent bile duct injury. In addition, an improperly deep plane of dissection may be entered during gallbladder removal, especially if acute inflammation is present. This penetration may damage accessory ducts in the liver bed, with consequent bile leak. Cautery may also produce significant biliary injury as a result of too-high settings and injudicious use to control bleeding (7).

A modification of the Bismuth classification of bile duct injuries has been recently reported to be more inclusive of those injuries seen with LC (7). This system defines five types of injury.

Type A injury refers to bile leaks occurring from minor ducts of the biliary tree, in which the main ductal anatomy remains in continuity. These complications include failure of cystic duct clip occlusion and leaks from accessory cystic ducts or the liver bed. They are treated by maneuvers that reduce intrabiliary pressure, such as sphincterotomy or stenting. Percutaneous placement of a subhepatic drain may also be necessary.

Type B injury denotes occlusion of a segment of the biliary tree. It most often refers to ligation or division of an aberrant right hepatic duct into which the cystic duct drains. When this duct is ligated, it is classified as type B; if transected without occlusion, it is considered a type C injury. Patients with type B injury may often remain asymptomatic, with hepatic atrophy proximal to the level of occlusion. Others may experience cholangitis, jaundice, or pain from the occluded segments. Treatment of asymptomatic injuries that are remote or that involve a small hepatic segment focuses on expectant observation. Patients with a large section of liver occluded (i.e., the right lobe) and symptomatic patients may be managed by Roux-en-Y hepaticojejunostomy. Hepatic resection may be necessary in some cases.

Type C injuries are likewise managed according to size of ductal disruption. If the duct is less than 2 mm, then ligation of the transected duct combined with drainage of the bile collection is preferred. Larger ducts are usually repaired with biliary-enteric anastamosis.

Type D injuries are lateral injuries to the extrahepatic ducts, with continuity otherwise intact. If recognized at the time of injury or shortly thereafter, suture repair over a T-tube may prove sufficient. Successful treatment with endoscopic sphincterotomy and stent placement has been reported. Small injuries may be managed by external drainage and biliary cannulation or by simple suture closure.

Lastly, type E injury is a circumferential injury of a major bile duct. When continuity is intact, as with strictures or clip occlusions, nonoperative treatment with balloon dilation and stent placement is often successful. Operation is indicated for failure of conservative therapy or when a disruption of continuity occurs. The goal of operative intervention is a tension-free mucosa-to-mucosa anastamosis. Roux-en-Y hepaticojejunostomy is used in almost all instances.

Gallbladder perforation and stone spillage

Gallbladder perforation resulting in stone spillage has been reported as occurring in as many as 30% to 40% of LC procedures (11). With greater surgeon experience, the incidence of gallbladder disruption and stone spillage declines. Traditional management involves aspiration of bile, copious irrigation, and often painstaking retrieval of stones. Several reports have indicated no adverse sequelae from follow-up on patients with retained stones, although one case of a chronic draining trocar wound was found to be the result of a stone within the tract (12–14). Experimental data support these clinical findings, with free intraperitoneal stones becoming adherent to omentum within eight weeks and causing no increase in adhesion formation (11). Based on these findings, it is proposed that easily removed stones be extracted but that meticulous removal may not be necessary.

Hemorrhage

Bleeding may be first encountered during removal of omental adhesions. Adhesion to the gallbladder may be taken down bluntly and bleeding points controlled with electrocautery. On the other hand, adhesions to the liver must be dissected sharply because blunt dissection will result in capsular tear. The areolar tissue within the triangle of Calot is relatively avascular. Minor bleeding should be controlled with direct pressure. Should a small vessel be encountered, compression is usually sufficient. Bleeding from a larger vessel requires judgment of its magnitude and etiology, with suction and irrigation assisting in this assessment. If blood pools with no identifiable site, pressure is applied and the area irrigated to clear it. An additional cannula may be added to facilitate exposure. After pressure is released, an attempt is made to control the bleeder with fine graspers. If this effort proves unsuccessful or the procedure becomes significantly prolonged, conversion to the open technique is advisable.

Rare complications

In addition to aforementioned major complications, a plethora of individual case reports have noted complications following LC. These problems include cystic artery pseudoaneurysm, cutaneous seeding of gallbladder carcinoma, abdominal wall tuberculosis, subcapsular hematoma, hepatic infarction from inadvertent ligation of the right hepatic artery, perforation of a Meckel's diverticulum, and hemobilia (15–21). Undoubtedly, numerous others exist as well.

Prevention

Prevention is the key to management of LC complications. As previously noted, inadequate experience is the only factor that predicts adverse outcome. Difficult cases should not be undertaken early in one's training, and supervision is recommended for the first 30 cases.

Anatomic variants occur in 15% of patients and must be correctly recognized. Most importantly, the cystic duct and artery must be clearly identified. This goal is achieved by careful removal of all adjacent fat and fibroareolar tissue within the triangle of Calot. This dissection is facilitated by lateral traction on Hartmann's pouch, which splays open the triangle (Fig. 38.1). Vertical traction alone must be avoided as it will cause the cystic duct to lie parallel to the common bile duct, allowing the common duct to be mistaken for a segment of the cystic duct (Fig. 38.2). In addition, the lower end of the gallbladder is dissected off the liver bed to prevent injury

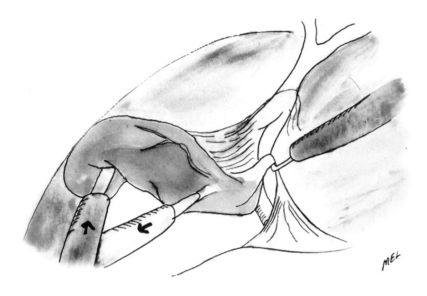

Fig. 38.1 Posterolateral traction on the infundibulum of the gallbladder so as to place the cystic duct at right angles to the common duct, adding greater safety to the dissection.

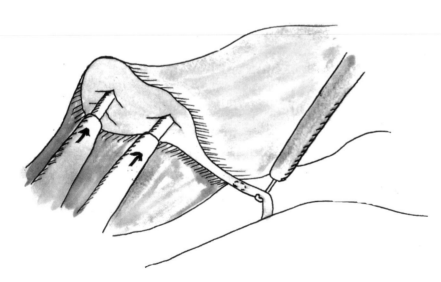

Fig. 38.2 Vertical traction on the infundibulum of the gallbladder causes the cystic duct to lie parallel to the common duct, increasing the potential for injury.

to structures located posteriorly. This technique isolates the two structures entering the gallbladder. Only then may they be safely clipped and divided.

Several modifications have been recommended for use of LC in acute cholecystitis (12). They include use of additional cannulas, use of angled or side-viewing telescopes, early gallbladder decompression, liberal use of ligatures for cystic artery and duct control, and selective use of cholangiography and sterile collection bags to remove infected tissues.

Hemostasis must be achieved in a well-controlled fashion. Blind cautery or clip application should never be performed. To control bleeding, direct pressure should be applied via a pledget or oxycellulose pad. When using cautery, a low setting must be maintained at all times, and instruments must be properly shielded to limit application to a defined area.

The use of routine intraoperative cholangiogram (IOC) during LC has been touted as a means to reduce complication, although its application remains controversial (22–28). Proponents argue that IOC can identify biliary anatomic variants, yet no data support a reduction in bile duct injury. In fact, this technique may identify an injury only after it has already occurred. Typical symptomatology, ultrasonography, and liver function tests will identify 95% of patients with common duct stones. For the majority of patients who do not have stones, routine IOC will merely increase operative time and expense. In addition, the 5% of patients with false-positive cholangiograms will undergo unnecessary common duct exploration.

REFERENCES

1. Kerin MJ, Gorey TF. Biliary injuries in the laparoscopic era. Eur J Surg 1994;160:195–201.
2. Cagir B, Rangraj M, Maffuci L, Ostrander LE, Herz BL. A retrospective analysis of laparoscopic and open cholecystectomies. J Laparoendosc Surg 1994;4:89–100.
3. Bezzi M, Silecchia G, Orsi F, Materia A, Salvatori FM, Fiocca F, Fantini A, Basso N, Rossi P. Complications after laparoscopic cholecystectomy. Coordinated radiologic, endoscopic, and surgical treatment. Surg Endosc 1995;9:29–36.
4. Dubois F, Icard P, Berthelot G, Levard H. Coelioscopic cholecystectomy: preliminary report of 36 cases. Ann Surg 1990;211:60–62.
5. Reddick E. Laparoscopic laser cholecystectomy; short hospital stay, minimal scarring. Laser Pract Rep 1988;Dec:15.
6. Woods MS, Traverso LW, Kozarek RA, Tsao J, Rossi RL, Gough D, Donohue JH. Characteristics of biliary tract complications during laparoscopic cholecystectomy: a multi-institutional study. Am J Surg 1994;167:27–33.
7. Strasberg SM, Hertl M, Soper NJ. An analysis of the problem of biliary injury during laparoscopic cholecystectomy. J Am Coll Surg 1995;180:101–125.
8. Moore MJ, Bennett CL. The learning curve for laparoscopic cholecystectomy. The Southern Surgeons Club. Am J Surg 1995;170:55–59.
9. Ponsky JL. The incidence and management of complications of laparoscopic cholecystectomy. Adv Surg 1994;27:21–41.
10. Newman CL, Wilson RA, Newman L, Eubanks S, Duncan TD, Mason EM, Wilson JP, Lucas GW. 1525 laparoscopic cholecystectomies without biliary injury: a single institution's experience. Am Surg 1995;61:226–228.
11. Cline RW, Poulos E, Clifford EJ. An assessment of potential complications caused by intraperitoneal gallstones. Am Surg 1994;60:303–305.
12. Zucker K, Bailey R, Flowers J. Laparoscopic management of acute and chronic cholecystitis. Surg Clinics N Am 1992;72:1045–1067.
13. Welch N, Hinder R, Fitzgibbons R, Rouse J. Gallstones in the peritoneal cavity: a clinical and experimental study. Dallas Med J 1991;1:246–247.
14. Soper N, Dunnegan D. Does intraoperative gallbladder perforation influence the early outcome of laparoscopic cholecystectomy? Surg Laparosc Endosc 1991;1:156–161.
15. Bergey E, Einstein D, Herts B. Cystic artery pseudoaneurysm as a complication of laparoscopic cholecystectomy. Abdom Imaging 1995;20:75–77.
16. Westcott CJ, Westcott RJ, Kerstein MD. Perforation of a Meckel's diverticulum during laparoscopic cholecystectomy. South Med J 1995;88:661.
17. Wachsberg RH, Cho KC, Raina S. Liver infarction following unrecognized right hepatic artery ligation at laparoscopic cholecystectomy. Abdom Imaging 1994;19:53–54.
18. Kim H, Roy T. Unexpected gallbladder cancer with cutaneous seeding after laparoscopic cholecystectomy. South Med J 1994;87:817–820.
19. Jindal D, Pandya R, Sharma SS. Abdominal wall tuberculosis following laparoscopic cholecystectomy. Br J Surg 1994;81:719.
20. Erstad BL, Rappaport WD. Subcapsular hematoma after laparoscopic cholecystectomy, associated with ketorolac administration. Pharmacotherapy 1994;14:613–615.
21. Bloch P, Modiano P, Foster D, Bouhot F, Gompel H. Recurrent hemobilia after laparoscopic cholecystectomy. Surg Laparosc Endosc 1994;4:375–377.
22. Bruhn E, Miller F, Hunter J. Routine fluoroscopic cholangiography during laparoscopic cholecystectomy, an argument. Surg Endo 1991;8:111–115.
23. Cronan J. Operative cholangiography. JAMA 1994;271:1210.
24. Flowers J, Zucker K, Graham S, Scovill W, Imbembo A, Bailey R. Laparoscopic cholangiography, results and indications. Ann Surg 1992;215:209–216.
25. Gerber A, Apt M. The case against routine operative cholangiography. Am J Surg 1992;143:734–736.
26. Lorimer JW, Fairfull SR. Intraoperative cholangiography is not essential to avoid duct injuries during laparoscopic cholecystectomy. Am J Surg 1995;169:344–347.
27. Pace B, Cosgrove J, Breur B, Margolis I. Intraoperative cholangiography revisited. Arch Surg 1992;127:448–450.
28. Soper NJ, Brunt LM. The case for routine operative cholangiography during laparoscopic cholecystectomy. Surg Clin North Am 1994;74:953–959.

39 | Intra-Abdominal Complications Associated with Extra-Peritoneal Dissection of the Lymphatic Nodes

Jacques Salvat, Alain Vincent-Genod, and Muguette Guilbert

Introduction

Recognizing the extent of pelvic lymph node invasion is vital for accurate prognosis in the case of gynecological cancers. Despite the innocuousness of noninvasive techniques, their anatomical insufficiency (e.g., lymphangiography investigates only the external iliac areas) or methodological insufficiency (e.g., the scanner does not recognize adenopathies of normal diameter) lowers their sensitivity or specificity, even when the examination is completed by simultaneous cytological exploration. Surgical methods, on the other hand, permit a very complete analysis and are the reference. Using surgery in cases of small tumors with little lymphatic invasion still carries the same risks of morbidity and even mortality, however. For example, a small T1b tumor is associated with a 15% chance of lymphatic invasion, and 85 patients out of 100 experience complications of and sequelae to surgical lymphadenectomy. Radiotherapy has the same drawbacks, in that patients with localized lesions must undergo the same widespread preventive irradiation as those with lesions at more remote locations.

Do endoscopic techniques, such as panoramic retroperitoneal pelviscopy (1), have their own disadvantages when applied to lymphatic investigation? How can these shortcomings be remedied? As we will see, more technical difficulties than accidents occur with the application of this surgical approach.

Technical difficulties of panoramic retroperitoneal pelviscopy

In approximately 10% of cases, the terrain, type of tumor, operator inexperience, and lack of appreciation of certain technical artifices will render laparoscopic exploration laborious. The authors have carried out complete examinations in 51 cases of panoramic retroperitoneal pelviscopy undertaken from January 24,

1987, to December 31, 1995, and report their findings below.

The terrain

Serious obesity is always an obstacle to successful laparoscopic treatment. Access is laborious because penetration must be deep. In addition, visualization is imperfect because of fatty deposits on the optical instrument, and dissection may become hemorrhagic because of obstruction by fatty tissues. For these reasons, the inexperienced operator should avoid such cases.

Parietal scars on the abdomen

Parietal scars on the abdomen are not an absolute contraindication for this technique, but do call for care if a suprapubic incision is made. In the case of a median laparotomy, a transverse incision is made two fingers' width above the pubis, and two (not one) lateral detachments are carried out with the index finger, going through the retropubic area of Retzius from one area to another.

If a transverse scar exists, an incision of one finger's width is made under the scar. This approach is taken in an attempt to avoid any adhesions.

For some operations access is particularly complicated. For example, Marshall Marchetti Burch's operation is especially taxing when the fixing on the Cooper ligament is very lateral. Likewise, Doleris Pellanda ligamentopexy with fixing to the aponeurosis of the round ligaments can be very challenging. In these difficult cases, a double lateral incision is preferable to a single median access when carrying out a bilateral inguinaloscopy.

The tumor

We have experienced four cases in which surgery has been hindered by large tumors that obstructed the manipulation and lateral dissection because they occupied the entire pelvis. A large uterus would probably cause the same problems during dissection. It is preferable to avoid endoscopy in such cases.

Inexperience of the operator

Inexperience with endoscopy is a fundamental contraindication to carrying out this procedure. A perfect knowledge of anatomy is necessary as well as experience in surgical dissection of the area during a lymphadenectomy. The surgeon should understand and be able to use video-endoscopic and endoscopic operation techniques and have adequate familiarity with cancer surgery. He or she will then be able to avoid prolonging the operation time and, in particular, will be prepared to cope with any vascular incidents.

Technical considerations

Problems with pneumostasis

Leakage of carbon dioxide prevents the inter-iliac area being properly inflated. To ensure that the pneumoperitoneum is maintained, the surgeon should employ a double pursestring suture: one on the aponeurosis, and a second to make the drain around the optical tube airtight. This strategy prevents leaks and ensures that the cavity can be inflated correctly and without delay.

Loosening the peritoneal sac

As during a sympathectomy, the vesico-peritoneal sac is loosened along the posterior face of the rectus abdomini from where it is attached to the pubis. If any resistance is encountered, this movement should not be forced because the sac has vascular attachments—for example, the epigastric artery and its vein or the anastomosis of the obturator vein (found under the external iliac vein).

The sliding movement may be facilitated by wetting the finger with antiseptic soap. The finger is then moved sideways toward the external iliac vessels passing under the round ligament, creating a para-vascular cavity for exploration of the lymphatic nodes situated in the area between the iliac artery and vein on one side, the obturator pedicle on the other, and finally the inside umbilical artery (Figs. 39.1 and 39.2). Palpation will allow the consistency of the tissue and any adenopathic adhesions on a vascular level to be felt. The movement should remain gentle so as to avoid tearing, which is a source of hemorrhage. Through this exploration, the surgeon may discern hard lumps that indicate the presence of adenopathies and then determine whether these masses are attached to the vessels.

If the peritoneal sac is pierced, the breach should be closed with forceps or by using Trendelenburg's position so that the pneumoperitoneum remains intact. Three breaches have occurred during our operations, each one so small that it did not interrupt the operation itself or hamper the continuation of the dissection.

Passing the instruments through the abdominal wall

The index finger, having created two lateral spaces toward the right and left external pedicles, loosens the peritoneal sac and moves it toward the navel. Next, the finger makes the muscle and skin stand out. Any incision is made at the top, approximately 2 cm from the navel, on the parietal swelling. The 5-mm trocar and its shaft are directed through this incision toward the pad of the index finger. After moving the instrument safely through the parietal area, the finger then accompanies the end of the tube into the interparietal area.

The same technique is employed to place two lateral trocars on the inside of the epigastric vessels, after tracking the course of the pedicles so as to avoid them. When the loosening operation is finished, the three 5-mm tubes are in place. Next, the 10-mm trocar with its rubber covering is positioned above the pubis.

The pneumoperitoneum is inflated, with the air pres-

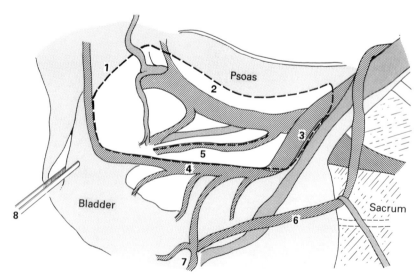

Fig. 39.1 Landmarks of the "interiliac area." 1 Pelvic brim, 2 external iliac artery, 3 internal iliac artery, 4 umbilical artery, 5 obturator vein, 6 ureter, 7 uterine artery, and 8 forceps.

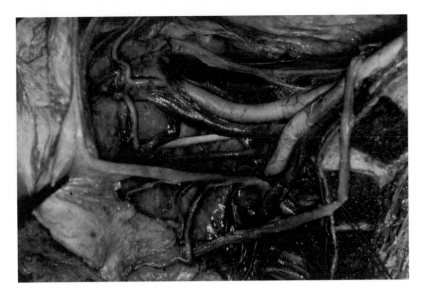

Fig. 39.2 The "interiliac area" (sagittal section).

sure being controlled as during a laparoscopy. The sac is pushed back when the carbon dioxide is injected and clears the field of vision. This step can be accomplished by use of the Trendelenburg position or by rolling the table.

We have not yet experienced any problems from spreading of the pneumoperitoneum into the neighboring spaces above.

Vision problems

Clear vision may be prevented by fatty deposits becoming stuck to the optical tube. To remedy this problem, a tepid wetting solution (37°) should be applied to prevent condensation.

Incorrect anatomical reference marking

Misidentification of anatomical landmarks can give rise to mistaken investigation. On one occasion, we probed too far on the outside toward the anterior face of the psoas and searched for the external iliac vessels too high. Looking for these vessels below the obturator pedicle also hinders the procedure. To avoid these problems, reference should be taken on the iliac arterial pulsations on discovering the round ligament or the external iliac vein (blue) and possibly on the obturator nerve (white). Once these elements have been marked out, dissection can begin.

Difficulties with dissection

Dissection should be carried out slowly and carefully. When the authors first carried out these operations, we used smooth instruments initially and then gradually introduced the use of scissors, but always with extreme care (see Fig. 39.2). As already indicated, the dissection is begun by creating the neo-cavity with the index finger. The vein must be followed to avoid harming

the tributary vessels. Once the tributary vessels have been identified (especially the superficial circumflex iliac vein, in front of and under the external anastomotic obturator iliac tributary), the ganglionic network can be pinpointed. It will be dissected with two forceps, one used as traction and the other holding the pedicle against the wall to avoid vascular tearing and to complete hemostasis if necessary. At the end, these landmarks must be clear.

Difficulties with hemostasis

Vascular hemorrhage is extremely rare during panoramic retroperitoneal pelviscopy. It has only occurred during our operations, and involved very small blood vessels. If this complication does occur, the vessels should be held and then coagulated either with a bipolar forceps or a unipolar forceps via correct isolated instrumentation. Endoclips are rarely necessary.

Lavage with warm serum safely completes the baro-hemostasis already begun by the pneumohemostasis of the area. Washing out should not be undertaken too soon, however, as it wastes time because of the aspiration phenomena of the pneumoperitoneum.

Difficulties with extraction

It is very important to avoid the nodes breaking up. The authors use a "Dargent coelio-extractor" (Lépine; Lyon, France) to protect lymphatic nodes during extraction through the parietal wall. Whenever possible, it is preferable to enlarge the parietal incisions at the end of the operation if the node is too large, rather than to force a node through and risk contaminating surrounding areas. In the same way, the surgeon should avoid exerting pressure on the nodes that could cause seepage of lymphatic fluid that contains cells that could graft onto structures in situ.

Problems with drainage

When the authors initially performed this procedure, we drained systematically. This technique did not prevent a nonserious hematoma, which was found during a secondary operation without consequences.

Need for laparotomy or operation

If a laparotomy or follow-up operation becomes necessary, it is preferable not to wait too long. On several occasions the authors carried out two operations—pelviscopy followed by a laparotomy—separated by an interval of more than one week. The area involved in the first operation was noted to have an extremely dense postoperatory sclerosis that made the subsequent dissection difficult. We now prefer to carry out the follow-up operation immediately after the pelviscopy with an immediate lymphatic node examination.

Anesthesia problems

We have not experienced any anesthesia problems. Indeed, tolerance appears good with elderly women.

Complications

Pelvic abscess

During inter-iliac exploration in a patient who appeared negative, a minute adenopathy fragment was lost in the loosened area that could not be recovered despite our best efforts. While waiting for the results (at this time no immediate pathologic examination of the lymphatic nodes was carried out) on the eighth postoperative day, the patient experienced fever and pelvic pain, and a laparotomy had to be performed earlier than intended. A $4\,cm^3$ volume of pus was found. The bacteriologic test indicated the presence of a *Staphylococcus* epidermitis, and a hysterectomy was therefore carried out. The follow-up was straightforward. This complication could have resulted from contamination from the wall, but was believed to arise from the cutaneous opening made during a lymphography carried out 48 hours prior to the pelviscopy.

Since that time, we have avoided lymphographies and now systematically undertake abdominopelvic scanning instead to explore the aorto-iliac axes. Our patients also receive prophylactic antibiotics in the form of an antistaphylococcal agent at the induction of the anesthesia.

Parietal grafts

On three occasions, neoplastic grafts have been noted on the walls of patients who had undergone a retroperitoneal pelviscopy. Two of these grafts occurred when this surgical method was first used; they probably arose when lymph node fragments became grafted during their extraction through the parietal wall, as we did not use a coelio-extractor at that time. The Dargent system we now employ acts like a sugar forceps of 1 cm diameter, with a trocar protecting the extraction through parietal wall. In the first case, a pathologic fragment probably remained intraparietally while the extracted fragment consisted of healthy tissue. These parietal grafts provoked a parietal metastasis that was treated radically by ablation and the placing of an underskin prosthesis, which ended in healing.

The second case involved a patient who had already presented a positive peritoneal cytology during a laparotomy carried out immediately after lymph node extraction. Neoplastic cells may have been grafted directly during this procedure. As in the previous case, a coelio-extractor had not been used. As a result, the extraction path may have been contaminated by the direct means used.

A third case, involving a vaginal neoplasm with a voluminous interiliac adenopathy, has been observed more recently. The extraction was not easy and necessitated a widening of one of the lateral incisions. It is probable that the wall was contaminated by the adenopathic node. Surgery then became necessary.

Lymphocysts

Three asymptomatic lymphocysts were discovered during echography following a panoramic retroperitoneal pelviscopy carried out after an in-sano conization for T1a2 microinvasive cervical cancer, for which a complete ablation had been accomplished via the conization. Endoscopic clips might potentially prevent this type of incident, although their effectiveness remains in doubt for this purpose. Draining is not sufficient to avoid lymphocysts, as these were noted at a time when the authors systematically undertook this step as part of this procedure. Lymphocysts are not a severe complication.

Other complications observed by other authors

The following complications have also been noted during extra-peritoneal dissection of lymphatic nodes:

- An epigastric hemorrhage made laparotomy necessary. It was caused by the transfixing of an artery during the placement of the 5-mm trocar. This type of accident may be avoided by transparietal transillumination.
- An obturatory paresis with recuperation has been observed.
- A vesicle wound with secondary parietal abscess has been noted.
- Two ureteral lesions were observed during the first attempt by surgeons new to this operation.

To date, no anesthetic complications have been observed.

Limits of endoscopic exploration

Panoramic retroperitoneal pelviscopy is used to explore a limited and preferential area: the "interiliac area" (see Fig 39.2). Panoramic retroperitoneal pelviscopy should be used only in the case of cancers with progressive development but not with "skip" metastases. This limitation arises because of the strict anatomic boundaries related to the technique. It is only possible to explore the interiliac area; it is not possible to use this approach in cases of lesions that may have spread irregularly outside it. Therefore only small cervical cancers may be assessed using this technique.

Conclusion

We have recently made a survey of 400 panoramic retroperitoneal pelviscopies carried out by different authors in France for cervical cancer. The complication rate noted in these cases is extremely low, with most problems having occurred while the technique was being perfected. Consequently, these complications should eventually disappear. Overall, "incidents" should continue to outnumber "accidents," as long as rigorous care is taken to select the indications for this technique.

Panoramic pelviscopy may, therefore, be recommended. It provides surgical precision when exploring lymphatic nodes, which is valuable in the prognosis of small cervical cancers.

REFERENCE

A complete bibliography and videotape of the technique are available in Dargent D, Salvat J. Envahissement ganglionnaire pelvien. Paris: Medsi McGraw Hill, 1989.

Complications of Laparoscopic Pelvic and Para-aortic Lymphadenectomy | 40

M. Dwight Chen and Jeffrey M. Fowler

Introduction

An estimated 82,000 gynecological malignancies were newly diagnosed in the United States in 1995 (1). Of these cases, approximately 60% were surgically staged as recommended by the International Federation of Gynecologists and Obstetricians (FIGO). Among the routine procedures performed at surgical staging is a dissection of the pelvic and para-aortic lymph nodes, as lymph node metastases represent a strong prognosticator in a variety of gynecological malignancies.

With the development of more-sophisticated instrumentation and techniques, the use of the laparoscope has been recently expanded to include the field of gynecologic oncology (2, 3). Laparoscopic staging (and, in particular, pelvic and para-aortic lymphadenectomy) has been successfully performed in both animal models and humans and has been proposed as a feasible alternative to laparotomy (4–6). Before discussing the potential complications of laparoscopic pelvic and para-aortic lymphadenectomy, we will briefly review how the laparoscope—and especially its use in dissecting pelvic/para-aortic lymph nodes—can be incorporated in the management of patients with cancer of the cervix, endometrium, and ovary.

Cervical cancer

The most significant experience to date with laparoscopic lymphadenectomy involves women with cervical cancer. Although cervical cancer remains a clinically staged disease as prescribed by FIGO, the discrepancy between clinical and surgical staging can be as high as 48%, especially in patients with bulky tumors or an advanced clinical stage (7). Surgical staging in these patients remains controversial because a major surgical procedure is required and the information derived may benefit only as

many as 7% of all surgically staged patients (7, 8). The use of a minimally invasive technique to surgically stage these patients may decrease operative morbidity, however.

The benefit of pretreatment laparoscopic pelvic lymphadenectomy in cervical cancer may become evident in two separate settings. For patients with early clinically staged disease (FIGO Stage IB-IIA), as many as 10% will have positive common iliac and para-aortic lymph node metastases (9). A laparotomy may be avoided in those patients found to have unresectable disease, and definitive radiation therapy may be initiated sooner. On the other hand, in patients with advanced cervical cancer (FIGO Stage IIB-IVA) a pretreatment pelvic lymphadenectomy can be performed to tailor radiation therapy to reflect the extent of disease.

Current interest lies in combining the laparoscopic pelvic lymphadenectomy with newly developed techniques in performing radical hysterectomy—that is, with laparoscopy-assisted radical vaginal hysterectomy (modified Schauta procedure) or laparoscopic radical hysterectomy (10, 11).

Endometrial cancer

Pelvic and para-aortic lymph node status is also a powerful prognosticator in endometrial cancer. Thus, laparoscopy can also aid in the staging of patients with this disease. Childers *et al.* first reported the use of the laparoscope to perform a lymph node dissection, procurement of peritoneal cytology, and mobilization of the adnexae; this procedure was then combined with a vaginal hysterectomy to complete the surgical staging (12). In addition, this technique can be used to surgically assess those patients who were incompletely staged at their primary surgery (13). This strategy may assist the gynecologic oncologist in planning any adjuvant therapy.

Ovarian cancer

The use of laparoscopy in the management of ovarian cancer was first described in 1973 (14). As the instrumentation and techniques have been refined, two separate applications of the laparoscope in ovarian cancer have emerged. Patients are sometimes referred to the gynecologic oncologist after incomplete staging for presumed early-stage disease. Careful and systematic surgical staging is crucial, as patients can have occult metastases found only with random biopsies (15). In particular, lymph node involvement has been found in as many as 24% of patients with apparent Stage I disease (16).

Another group of patients with ovarian malignancies who may benefit from a laparoscopic procedure are women who present with disseminated peritoneal disease at initial surgery. With complete clinical response after induction chemotherapy, a second-look procedure may be performed to assess disease status. If it was not performed at the initial surgery, pelvic and para-aortic lymph node sampling is included because the retroperitoneum can act as a "sanctuary" for ovarian cancer cells. In one study, the laparoscopic approach was favorably compared with laparotomy in detecting persistent disease (17).

Patient selection

Laparoscopic pelvic/para-aortic lymphadenectomy is not indicated for all patients. Those patients with significant medical problems (especially if they are cardiac or pulmonary in nature) may not be able to tolerate prolonged intra-abdominal insufflation with carbon dioxide.

In addition, a relative contraindication for laparoscopic lymphadenectomy may be a history of multiple previous abdominal surgeries, any intra-abdominal inflammatory process, or extensive peritoneal adhesions. In such patients, it may be prudent to use an open technique to prevent injury to other vital organs.

Laparoscopic procedures in obese patients can prove problematic for several reasons: (1) the pneumoperitoneum may cause difficulties with mechanical ventilation; (2) technical limitations with the trocars and instruments may arise with an enlarged abdominal girth; and (3) it may be difficult to adequately retract the bowel out of the operative field because of the additional exposure required by para-aortic lymph node dissection. The use of steep Trendelenburg position in these patients may only exacerbate any potential ventilatory difficulties.

Procedure

After standard preoperative evaluation, all patients undergo a full mechanical and antibiotic bowel preparation as well as surgical antibiotic prophylaxis. General endotracheal anesthesia is administered with the patient in the supine position; the procedure is easier to perform if both arms are tucked to the sides. Central venous monitoring is used at the discretion of the anesthesiologist and the attending surgeon. Prior to beginning the laparoscopic procedure, a nasogastric tube is passed into the stomach.

All laparoscopic lymphadenectomies are performed by a team of two surgeons alternating as first assistant and operator. The laparoscopic equipment includes a camera attached to a 10-mm laparoscope with a light source, two video monitors, and a high-flow carbon dioxide gas insufflator. Irrigation solution, consisting of warm normal saline with 1000 international units of heparin per liter, is delivered by a high-pressure suction/irrigation apparatus. During the procedure, 5-mm laparoscopic scissors are used for sharp dissection and 5-mm laparoscopic graspers are employed for retraction and blunt dissection. When needed, monopolar cautery is provided by an electrosurgical generator and transmitted through the laparoscopic scissors.

Either four or five trocar sites can be used for laparoscopic surgery. For both techniques, a 10-mm trocar site is placed superior to the umbilicus in the midline and functions as the camera port. In the five-trocar approach, two 5-mm ports are placed directly lateral to the camera port, just lateral to the inferior epigastric vessels. Two 12-mm ports are inserted in each lower quadrant of the abdomen, 2 cm medial and 2 cm inferior to the anterior superior iliac spine. This method, though requiring a second assistant to direct the laparoscope, provides the surgeon with an additional port site from which to operate. Alternatively, for the four-port technique, a 12-mm port is placed in the midline 3 cm above the symphysis pubis, and two 5-mm ports are placed just lateral to the inferior epigastric vessels at approximately the midpoint between the two larger ports. The benefit of this approach is that it requires the services of only the surgeon and one assistant. All ports are secured to the skin with 2-0 suture.

After the ports are established, washings are obtained with the suction/irrigator apparatus. The patient is placed into steep Trendelenburg and all pelvic structures are inspected. Any adhesions to the anterior abdominal wall are sharply lysed, and the small bowel is displaced into the upper quadrants. Laparoscopic exploration of the abdomen and pelvis is then completed in a clockwise fashion.

The retroperitoneal spaces are accessed by incising the peritoneum lateral to the pelvic vessels after transecting the round ligaments with electrocautery; the pararectal and paravesical spaces are then developed. The pelvic lymph node dissection is performed by removing the nodal tissue surrounding the lower common iliac, external iliac, and hypogastric vessels, as well as within the obturator fossa above the obturator nerve.

Monopolar electrocautery is used to carry out hemostasis and sealing of lymphatics. Endoscopic clips are rarely necessary.

At the surgeon's discretion, a para-aortic lymphadenectomy can be performed with the same technique and instrumentation. The right para-aortic lymph nodes are accessed by incising the peritoneum over the upper portion of the right common iliac artery and extending this incision up along the aorta. The operator on the left side of the table then sharply dissects in the areolar plane between the lymph nodes and the peritoneum. Elevation of this peritoneal window permits lateral retraction of the ureter out of the operative field and visualization of the vena cava and aorta. Right-sided para-aortic lymphadenectomy is then performed.

The left-sided para-aortic lymphadenectomy is performed by incising the peritoneum over the left common iliac artery so that the sigmoid colon and inferior mesenteric artery can be lifted out of the field of dissection. The left ureter is also identified and retracted laterally.

Complications

Vascular injury

Vascular injuries from the insertion of insufflation needles or trocars are discussed elsewhere in this book. Important points reiterated here are that all instrument placements should be performed under direct visualization, that low insufflation pressures (less than 15 mm Hg) should be used when insufflating with the Veress needle to decrease the risk of an air embolism, and that the operator must use care to avoid perforation of the epigastric vessels.

The removal of the pelvic and para-aortic lymph nodes requires meticulous dissection of soft tissue adjacent to vessels in the lower abdomen and pelvis. Any undue traction on the lymphatic tissue during dissection can cause avulsion of perforating vessels and lead to significant hemorrhage. Major bleeding is more likely to be venous (versus arterial) in origin because it is easier to injure the thinner-walled veins. A frequent site of vessel injury involves the accessory vessels in the obturator fossa, which typically originate from the undersurface of the external iliac vessels. In performing the para-aortic lymphadenectomy, the precaval fat pad often contains perforating vessels that must be cauterized or clipped. Meticulous skeletonization of the lymph nodes is necessary to isolate these perforating vessels. In addition, after the ureter has been identified, the ovarian vessels can be ligated with a stapler or clips.

The use of the laparoscope in performing pelvic and para-aortic lymphadenectomy may actually assist the operator in identifying and controlling intraoperative bleeding. Because of the laparoscope's magnification capabilities, the development of the retroperitoneal spaces and removal of nodal tissues can be performed with greater precision. Any small vessel injury can be easily visualized and controlled, usually with electrocautery or surgical clips. In addition, the intra-abdominal pressures created with the pneumoperitoneum will help tamponade any minor bleeding encountered. Vascular pedicles can be secured with endoscopic bipolar electrocautery, stapler, or suture ligature.

If major bleeding does occur, direct pressure with a laparoscopic instrument can be an effective remedy. Alternatively, a sponge can be placed through one of the larger trocar sleeves to assist in blotting and direct tamponade. In all cases, the use of a high-pressure suction/irrigation apparatus is invaluable in improving visualization and evacuating any pooled blood or fresh clots.

Gastrointestinal injury

Injury to the gastrointestinal tract can occur several ways during a laparoscopic pelvic lymphadenectomy. An incidental bowel perforation will typically occur with the placement of the Veress needle or the first trocar. As mentioned earlier, a nasogastric tube should be placed immediately after intubation to decompress the patient's stomach. If the surgeon expects that the patient will have significant peritoneal adhesions, an open laparoscopy can be performed. Alternatively, the Veress needle can be inserted in either the left or right upper quadrant in an effort to avoid adhesions of bowel to the anterior abdominal wall (18). After all trocars are placed, the laparoscope should be used to evaluate the site of the first trocar, as any trocar can pass entirely through a loop of decompressed bowel. If a bowel perforation is suspected, the trocar should be left in place and an immediate laparotomy performed.

Bowel injury during surgery is either mechanical or thermal in nature. A preoperative mechanical bowel preparation may decrease active peristalsis and allow the small intestine to be easily swept out of the pelvis and lower abdomen. As a consequence, a small bowel loop may be less likely to inadvertently enter the operative field during the use of electrocautery. When using monopolar electrocautery, the field of dissection should be inspected and clearly defined to minimize thermal injury to the bowel. This step is especially important if a para-aortic lymphadenectomy is being contemplated.

Mechanical bowel injuries usually arise during lysis of adhesions. Concern for this complication is particularly relevant in patients who have undergone a previous surgery for advanced ovarian cancer, as they tend to form the most extensive and dense adhesions. Because the laparoscope provides only a two-dimensional view of the surgical procedure, any thick adhesion may contain loops of small bowel that are difficult to appreciate.

Standard surgical techniques to lyse adhesions (i.e., tension/countertension) should be used. If an injury to the intestine occurs, then immediate laparotomy is indicated; only those surgeons who are proficient in endoscopic suturing should attempt to repair any bowel injury via the laparoscope.

Genitourinary injury

Injury to the bladder is rare during this procedure, although perforation of this organ with an accessory trocar has been described. A urethral catheter should be placed preoperatively. In developing the paravesical spaces, care must be taken to avoid lacerating the lateral bladder wall; this injury can be avoided by first identifying the superior vesical artery and dissecting the paravesical space lateral to it.

The operator must always identify the ureter before performing a lymphadenectomy, especially where it crosses the bifurcation of the common iliac artery into the external iliac and hypogastric vessels. At this location, the ureter is most easily identified while developing the pararectal space. Medial displacement of the ureter will enable the operator to remove lymphatic tissue from these vessels. Similarly, if a para-aortic lymph node dissection is performed, lateral retraction of the ureter can prevent trauma or thermal injury.

Nerve injury

As is the case with an open laparotomy, the main risk for nerve injury during laparoscopic pelvic lymphadenectomy is transection of the obturator nerve. Before removing any lymphatic tissue from within the obturator fossa, the surgeon should identify the obturator nerve and any vessels in the fossa. Direct and constant visualization of the nerve during the node dissection should then largely prevent any injury. In addition, the dissection must be meticulous to avoid unnecessary bleeding, which might require excessive use of clips or electrocautery.

"Incomplete" lymphadenectomy

Most gynecologic oncologists would agree that a thorough lymph node dissection is required in the surgical treatment of women with cervical cancer. Therefore, it is important to confirm that an adequate lymphadenectomy can be performed laparoscopically. This critical issue was investigated at the University of Minnesota by first removing the lymph nodes via the laparoscope, and then evaluating the completeness of the procedure by laparotomy. The overall laparoscopic lymph node yield was as high as 90%. More importantly, no patient with negative nodes at laparoscopy demonstrated positive nodes at laparotomy. In addition, a significant improvement of lymph node yield was noted with time, indicating the existence of a "learning curve" for this procedure (19, 20).

Postoperative adhesions

One concern with the laparoscopic technique described here is that the lymphadenectomy is performed transperitoneally. Convincing evidence has shown that patients with cervical cancer who undergo transperitoneal staging laparotomies have a higher incidence of major postirradiation enteric complications when compared with those who have extraperitoneal staging laparotomies; this discrepancy is thought to reflect an increase in postoperative intraperitoneal adhesion formation with the transperitoneal approach (7, 21).

Evidence suggests that fewer adhesions are formed after transperitoneal laparoscopic surgery versus the same procedure performed by laparotomy (22). In addition, preliminary data in a porcine model indicated no difference in postoperative adhesions after pelvic lymphadenectomy by laparoscopy when compared with extraperitoneal laparotomy; however, the statistical power of this study was low and further research is needed (23). Laparoscopic techniques, including minimal peritoneal injury, vigilant hemostasis, minimal bowel manipulation, no irritation with dry sponges/pads, and reduced drying of tissues that results from an open laparotomy wound, may contribute to a decrease in adhesion formation after laparoscopic surgery. Even in light of these data, new instruments and techniques are currently being developed to perform extraperitoneal laparoscopic pelvic lymphadenectomy.

Conclusion

Laparoscopic pelvic lymphadenectomy is clearly a feasible alternative in a selected group of patients with gynecological malignancies. It is also clear that this complex technical procedure has a steep learning curve; only surgeons with adequate training and experience in both gynecologic oncology and operative laparoscopy should attempt this surgery. Although the potential complications from this procedure are many, they can usually be handled proficiently by an experienced operator. To date, very few data exist about the safety and efficacy of operative laparoscopy compared with more traditional approaches. Prospective clinical trials will be necessary to further define the role of laparoscopy in gynecologic oncology.

REFERENCES

1. Parker SL, Tong T, Bolden BA, Wingo PA. Cancer statistics, 1996. Ca Cancer J Clin 1996;46:5–27.
2. Grimes DA. Frontiers of operative laparoscopy: a review and critique of the evidence. Am J Obstet Gynecol 1992;166:1062–1071.
3. Diamond MP. Pelviscopy. Clin Obstet Gynecol 1991;34:371.
4. Schuessler WW, Vancaillie TG, Reich H, Griffith DP. Transperitoneal endosurgical lymphadenectomy in patients with localized prostate cancer. J Urol 1991;145:988–991.

5. Querleau D, LaBlanc E, Castelain B. Laparoscopic pelvic lymphadenectomy in the staging of early carcinoma of the cervix. Am J Obstet Gynecol 1991;164:579–581.

6. Herd J, Fowler JM, Shenson D, Lacy S, Montz FJ. Laparoscopic paraaortic lymph node sampling: development of a technique. Gynecol Oncol 1992;44:271–276.

7. LaPolla JP, Schlaerth JB, Gaddis O, Morrow CP. Influence of surgical staging on the evaluation and treatment of patients with cervical carcinoma. Gynecol Oncol 1986;24:194–206.

8. Potish RA, Twiggs LB, Okagaki T, Prem KA, Adcock LL. Therapeutic implications of the natural history of advanced cervical cancer as defined by pretreatment surgical staging. Cancer 1985;56:956–960.

9. Morrow CP, Curtin JP, Townsend DE. Synopsis of gynecologic oncology, 4th ed. New York: Churchill Livingstone, 1993: 111–152.

10. Querleu D. Laparoscopically assisted radical vaginal hysterectomy. Gynecol Oncol 1993;51:248–254.

11. Nezhat CR, Burrell MO, Nezhat FR, Benigno BB, Welander CE. Laparoscopic radical hysterectomy with paraaortic and pelvic node dissection. Am J Obstet Gynecol 1992;166:864–865.

12. Childers JM, Surwit EA. Combined laparoscopic and vaginal surgery for the management of two cases of stage I endometrial cancer. Gynecol Oncol 1992;45:46–51.

13. Childers JM, Spirtos NM, Brainerd P, Surwit EA. Laparoscopic staging of the patient with incompletely staged early adenocarcinoma of the endometrium. Obstet Gynecol 1994;83:597–600.

14. Bagley CM, Young RC, Scheine PS, Chabner BA, DeVita VT. Ovarian carcinoma metastatic to the diaphragm—frequently undiagnosed at laparotomy. Am J Obstet Gynecol 173;116: 397–400.

15. Buchsbaum HJ, Brady MF, Delgado G, et al. Surgical staging of ovarian carcinoma: stage I, II, and III (optimal): a Gynecologic Oncology Group study. Surg Gynecol Obstet 1989;169:226–232.

16. Burghardt E, Girardi F, Lahousen M, Tamussino K, Stettner H. Patterns of pelvic and para-aortic lymph node involvement in ovarian carcinoma. Gynecol Oncol 1991;40:103–106.

17. Childers JM, Lang J, Surwit EA, Hatch KD. Laparoscopic surgical staging of ovarian cancer. Gynecol Oncol 1995;59:25–33.

18. Childers JM, Brzechffa PR, Surwit EA. Laparoscopy using the left upper quadrant as the primary trocar site. Gynecol Oncol 1993;50:221–225.

19. Fowler JM, Carter JR, Carlson JW, et al. Lymph node yield from laparoscopic lymphadenectomy in cervical cancer: a comparative study. Gynecol Oncol 1993;51:187–192.

20. Fowler JM, Twiggs LB. Lymph node yield from laparoscopic lymphadenectomy in cervical cancer: accuracy of laparoscopic assessment of lymph nodes. In: Querleu D, Childers J, Dargent D, eds. Laparoscopic surgery in gynecologic oncology. Oxford, UK: Blackwell Science, 1995.

21. Weiser EB, Bundy BN, Hoskins WJ, et al. Extraperitoneal versus transperitoneal selective paraaortic lymphadenectomy in the pretreatment surgical staging of advanced cervical cancer: a Gynecologic Oncology Group study. Gynecol Oncol 1989;33:283–289.

22. Luciano AA, Maier DB, Koch EI, Nulsen JC, Whitman GF. A comparative study perspective of postoperative adhesions following laser surgery by laparoscopy versus laparotomy in the rabbit model. Obstet Gynecol 1989;74:220–224.

23. Fowler JM, Hartenbach EM, Reynolds HT, et al. Pelvic adhesion formation after pelvic lymphadenectomy: comparison between transperitoneal laparoscopy and extraperitoneal laparotomy in the porcine model. Gynecol Oncol 1994;55:25–28.

41 | Difficulties with Microlaparoscopy

Stefan Rimbach, Diethelm Wallwiener, and Gunther Bastert

Introduction

Laparoscopy has replaced open surgery in many fields of gynecological therapy with great benefits to patients. The endoscopic approach has dramatically reduced the invasiveness of both diagnostic and operative interventions. For example, trocar access has replaced incisional laparotomy in most instances in the laparoscopic diagnosis and management of pelvic adhesions, endometriosis, tubal pregnancy, distal tubal disease, and ovarian cysts.

Recently, *micro*laparoscopy using small-diameter fiber-optics and specially designed microtrocars has been introduced to further minimize patient trauma by reducing the access size even more (1–3). The equipment marketed to date has been developed and designed not only for direct optical control of the placement of the Veress needle (4, 5), but also for performing diagnostic and minor operative laparoscopic interventions with or without general anesthesia (1, 6).

Both the technically delicate instrumentation and the intended surgical indications imply specific difficulties that will be described in this chapter. As microlaparoscopy represents a rather new technique, experience with its use is naturally limited. Most of the issues discussed below will likely appear in a different perspective with further technological development and more widespread clinical use of this method. The objective of this chapter therefore is to draw attention to some currently critical aspects of microlaparoscopy to aid in optimizing its application in clinical routine.

Concept of the "optical Veress needle" and the microlap-microtrocar systems

Gynecological laparoscopy usually begins with two blind steps: puncture of the peritoneal cavity with the Veress needle for pneumoperitoneum insufflation, followed by the insertion of a (10-mm) trocar that gives the laparoscope optical access to the intraperitoneal space. Only

then does true "endoscopy" start, with the surgeon obtaining the first sight into the cavity.

Whereas the overall complication rate of laparoscopy has proved low—approximately 2–3 per 1000 cases—and has not varied much over the past years (7–10), the initial blind steps continue to carry a significant risk of relevant complications. In fact, serious and potentially fatal complications such as large-vessel and bowel lacerations typically occur during this phase of the procedure (11–13).

Patients with suspected intra-abdominal adhesions after previous (multiple) laparotomy incur an even markedly higher risk for visceral injury (14). Although rare in number (9, 15), such complications must not be neglected because of their severe consequences (16–18).

None of the various published reports on equipment and techniques—from the Veress insufflation needle itself (19) to open laparoscopy (20, 21), sonographic localization of abdominal wall adhesions (14), and indirect testing of the insufflation needle position (22)—has so far been able to eliminate this danger. Only direct optical control of the access puncture would prevent injury to intraperitoneal organs or structures.

The concept of an "optical" Veress needle tries to combine this requirement with the idea of blunt needle insertion. Two systems are currently available with these characteristics. The first consists of a 1.2-mm micro-fiber-optic component integrated into a modified Veress needle (Storz, Germany). The optical component replaces the inner blunt part of the needle, whereas the outer sharp part remains essentially unchanged. Gas insufflation works via a side port. The second option is a microlap system (Imagyn, United States) that uses a regular but long Veress needle that is charged with a microtrocar slid over the needle. The needle and trocar are inserted together; the needle is then withdrawn and the microtrocar remains in place, giving access for a micro-fiber-optic of 1.95-mm diameter.

Insufflation needle placement control and "pathfinding" in high-risk patients

In our experience with a pilot series of 78 cases, both systems allowed mostly successful optical control of the tip localization when used to check on correct intraperitoneal positioning *before insufflation*. Once the access to the peritoneal cavity is assured, the CO_2 can be insufflated and a 10-mm trocar safely inserted—if necessary under microlaparoscopic visual control. In high-risk patients with suspected anterior abdominal wall adhesions, the micro-optic/trocar or needle system can also be inserted at sites different from the umbilical area, as determined by the individual situation. It will then serve as a "pathfinder" for regular laparoscopic access.

Impaired vision—technical aspects and consequences

Only the optical Veress needle (not the microlap-microtrocar system) allows *insertion under vision*. This advantage is relative, however. Once the optic tip touches subcutaneous fatty tissue or meets blood or secretion, the vision becomes impaired by filmy lens contamination. In such cases, continuous irrigation of small amounts of fluid during insertion using a syringe on the needle side port may support or restore clear vision.

A second difficulty that frequently impairs optical information during insertion is the "white-out phenomenon," in which light is reflected because of close tissue contact. Using low light intensity and a fast automatic-

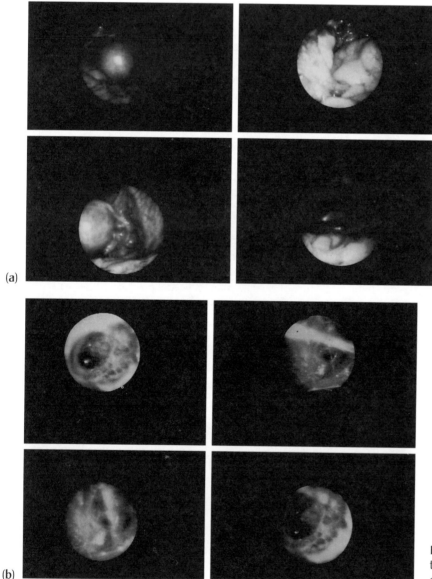

(a)

(b)

Fig. 41.1 (a) Correct intraperitoneal position of the Veress needle. (b) Preperitoneal position as detected by the optical Veress needle.

shutter camera may improve the image quality in such instances.

As a result of such problems, in clinical routine the modified Veress needle is usually inserted first and only then loaded with the optic. This technique, however, negates the original idea of preventing injury by continuous visual control.

The unquestionable advantage in this strategy lies in its ability to make an early diagnosis of misplacement of the access device, especially prior to CO_2 insufflation. Preperitoneal position can be detected immediately by direct optic assessment (Fig. 41.1), which is obviously much more reliable than indirect tests.

Preperitoneal needle or microtrocar position

At the same time, the use of either system may facilitate preperitoneal positioning, especially in obese patients. Careful previewing and handling are required to prevent this complication. Once the optical Veress needle is inserted and intraperitoneal position confirmed, it may be necessary to remove the micro-optic to permit gas flow sufficient for building up the pneumoperitoneum. When the optic is detached, care should be given so as not to withdraw the needle with it, which would probably result in preperitoneal insufflation. This potential difficulty can be avoided by using variable-length optical Veress needles.

The risk for obese patients also exists with the microlap system. The microtrocar is necessarily shorter than the puncturing insufflation needle, and the correct intraperitoneal position can be controlled only when the needle is already withdrawn. In some cases, the needle tip has been intraperitoneal prior to being removed even though the microtrocar tip was just preperitoneal—a situation not possible to recognize or prevent.

Bowel perforation

A much more severe complication than preperitoneal insufflation, bowel perforation can occur in case of anterior abdominal wall adhesion. The use of a microlaparoscopic system for puncture control can hardly prevent this complication if the insertion process is not monitored continuously. As discussed earlier, a number of technical difficulties only rarely allow such perfect monitoring with the optical Veress needle, and not at all with the microlap system. Nevertheless, those minimal access methods still provide an unquestionable advantage (3, 23).

The only alternative to endoscopy would be the much more invasive procedures of open laparoscopy or primary laparotomy. Neither of these techniques completely eliminates the risk of bowel injury, however. If the endoscopic approach is attempted, the risk of relevant visceral laceration is undoubtedly reduced by microendoscopic access.

Even if an intestinal perforation cannot be prevented by this strategy, it will be small and will be *known*. With microendoscopic control, the complication will be diagnosed before insufflation and before insertion of the 10-mm trocar. Thus a much larger injury and the dangerous situation of unknown visceral injury (9, 17, 18) are avoided. The patient can be adequately monitored and treated postoperatively.

In our experience with microlaparoscopy in high-risk patients, three such perforations occurred. All of these punctures were successfully diagnosed by the micro-optic (Fig. 41.2), with two of the lesions being undetectable in

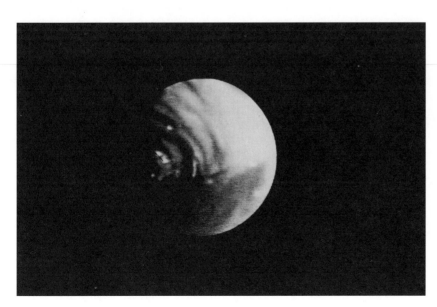

Fig. 41.2 Bowel perforation as detected by the optical Veress needle.

subsequent 10-mm laparoscopy. None required interventional consequences such as laparoscopic or open repair. No postoperative complications occurred.

Diagnostic and minor operative microlaparoscopy—indications and controversies

In addition to its use for safer access to the peritoneal cavity, microlaparoscopy has been applied to a number of indications. The spectrum of reported uses ranges from diagnostic to minor operative laparoscopic procedures. For example, diagnostic microlaparoscopy has been successfully performed for pelvic pain and inflammatory disease, chromopertubation, endometriosis, adhesions, uterine malformations, sterilization reversal potential, surgical feasibility on ovarian cysts, fibroids, ectopic pregnancy, and second-look procedures after cancer therapy (2, 3, 6, 23–25). It proved especially useful for simultaneous control during operative hysteroscopy or during falloposcopy (23, 24). Even interventional laparoscopy for indications such as tubal ligation, laser treatment of endometriosis, laser and conventional adhesiolysis, biopsy in case of endometriosis or cancer recurrence, and ZIFT procedures has proved successful (1, 2, 6, 24).

This broad spectrum of indications reported from pilot series proves feasibility but does not indicate optimal results. The image quality of small-diameter-fiber-optics as used for microlaparoscopy cannot compare to the image produced by a 10-mm lens-optic. Neither the light intensity nor the optical resolution nor the field of vision matches the quality available with macrolaparoscopy. As a result, controversies exist in estimating the role of microlaparoscopy in routine clinical use. Whereas some feel that this technology can compete with 10-mm laparoscopy for selected indications (1, 2, 6), others point out its obvious reduction of picture size and compromised clarity (24).

The critical question, however, is not primarily the surgeon's comfort in image interpretation but microlaparoscopy's diagnostic accuracy, which should not be compromised by the lower image quality. Whereas our experience indicates difficulties in exactly diagnosing the extent of subtle lesions (e.g., in endometriosis or ovarian cancer recurrences), a prospective study proved correct diagnoses in 13 of 14 infertility patients (6). Nevertheless, we currently recommend employing 10-mm laparoscopy in case of negative results to exclude false-negative diagnosis. This approach obviously implies some remaining risk of missing the diagnosis, as in the one case of peritoneal carcinosis diagnosed by neither microlaparoscopy nor 10-mm laparoscopy (6).

To achieve optimal technical conditions for successful microlaparoscopic diagnosis, the equipment should include a light source and camera unit with measurement technology adapted to the small picture size of the micro-fiber-optic. Choosing a different access site (e.g., in the lower abdomen rather than the umbilicus) will also bring the optic closer to the pelvis and therefore produce better image quality. A possible positive side effect of this approach is a reduction in the risk for large-vessel injury (6).

In addition, microlaparoscopy is associated with a certain learning curve (24), which is defined by the understanding and adequate handling of those fragile fiber-optics and microtrocars. It is especially complicated by the fact that the endoscopic surgeon "looks with different eyes" than in traditional procedures.

After the learning curve is completed and the operating room is well equipped, minor operative procedures should become possible in clinical routine; major laparoscopic interventions, on the other hand, will require the development of additional macrotechniques (25).

Office microlaparoscopy

The methodological limitations of microlaparoscopy are well matched to the clinical needs of patients for whom it is appropriate. In case of extensive laparoscopic surgery, the access certainly is not responsible for the overall invasiveness of the procedure and for operative patient trauma.

Selected patients would definitely profit from moving some minor procedures from the operating room to the physician's office. Microlaparoscopy could be an important tool that facilitates the adoption of a number of outpatient office interventions (2, 6, 24, 25).

The procedures reported to be carried out in this setting (2, 6, 24, 25) were performed under intravenous sedation and local anesthesia. In contrast to laparoscopy under general anesthesia, the pneumoperitoneum should not exceed 0.5–3 l in such cases, with individual levels of tolerance determining not only the CO_2 volume and pressure but also the duration of the procedure (2, 6, 24).

Conclusion

Microlaparoscopy represents a promising new technique that will certainly enlarge diagnostic and therapeutic possibilities in gynecological endoscopy. It will also contribute to the safety of laparoscopy in high-risk patients. Both technological and methodological improvements will be necessary to overcome specific limitations and difficulties, however.

In the future, more clinical experience will define the role of microlaparoscopy in comparison with 10-mm laparoscopy and select indications in which the unquestionable further reduction of invasiveness justifies the inherent operative-technical compromises.

By facilitating the spread of certain outpatient and office procedures carried out under local anesthesia, microlaparoscopy will most probably bring advantages for many patients and reduce health care costs. Nevertheless, an uncritical overuse of the method could result in the most relevant difficulty with this technology.

REFERENCES

1. Dorsey JM, Tabb CR. Mini-laparoscopy and fiber optic lasers. Obstet Gynecol Clin N Am 1991;18:613–617.
2. Risquez F, Pennehouat G, Fernandez R, Confino E, Rodriguez O. Microlaparoscopy: a preliminary report. Human Reproduction 1993;8:1701–1702.
3. Rimbach S, Wallwiener D, Bastert G. Minimal access endoscopy. Gynaecol Endoscopy 1994;3(suppl1):30.
4. Rimbach S, Wallwiener D, Bastert G. Die optische Veress-nadel—entwicklung und erste anwendung im experimentellen modell. Minim Invas Med 1994;5:166–168.
5. Schaller G, Kuenkel M, Manegold BC. The optical "Veress-needle"—initial puncture with a minioptic. Endosc Surg Allied Technol 1995;3:55–57.
6. Bauer O, Gerling W, Husstedt W, Felberbaum R, Diedrich K. Diagnostische mikrolaparoskopien mit 2-mm-optiken. Geburtsh u Frauenheilk 1995;55:473–476.
7. Chamberlain G, Brown JC, eds. Gynaecological laparoscopy: report on the confidential enquiry into gynaecological laparoscopy. London: Royal College of Obstetricians and Gynaecologists, 1978.
8. Peterson HB, Hulka JF, Phillips JM. American Association of Gynecological Laparoscopists' 1988 membership survey on operative laparoscopy. J Reprod Med 1990;35:587–589.
9. Chapron C, Querleu D, Mage G, Madelenat P, Dubuisson JB, Audebert A, Erny R, Bruhat MA. Complications de la coeliochirurgie gynécologique. J Gynecol Obstet Biol Reprod 1992;21:207–213.
10. Lehmann-Willenbrock E, Riedel HH, Mecke H, Semm K. Pelviscopy/laparoscopy and its complications in Germany. J Reprod Med 1992;37:671–677.
11. Erkrath KD, Weiler G, Adebahr G. Zur aortaverletzung bei laparoskopie in der gynäkologie. Geburtsh u Frauenheilk 1979;39:687–689.
12. Lignitz E, Püschel K, Saukko P, Mattig W. Iatrogene blutungskomplikationen bei gynäkologischen laparoskopien—bericht über zwei fälle mit tödlichem verlauf. Z Rechtsmed 1985;95:295–306.
13. Baadsgaard SE, Bille S, Egelblad K. Major vascular injury during gynecologic laparoscopy. Acta Obstet Gynecol Scand 1989;68:283–285.
14. Caprini JA, Arcelus JA, Swanson J, Coats R, Hoffman K, Brosnan JJ, Blattner S. The ultrasonic localization of abdominal wall adhesions. Surg Endoscopy 1995;9:283–285.
15. Mintz M. Risks and prophylaxis in laparoscopy. A survey of 100,000 cases. J Reprod Med 1977;18:269–272.
16. Borten M. Laparoscopic complications. Toronto: BC Decker, 1986:285–295.
17. Krebs HB. Intestinal injury in gynecologic surgery. A ten-year experience. Am J Obstet Gynecol 1986;155:509–514.
18. Ravina JH, Madelenat P. Plaies viscerales et vasculaires au cours de la coelioscopie d'exploration: causes–responsabilites–prevention. Contr Fertil Sex 1984;12:929–930.
19. Veress J. Neues Instrument zur ausführung von brust—oder bauchpunktionen. Dt Med Wschr 1938;41:1480–1481.
20. Hasson HM. Open laparoscopy versus closed laparoscopy. A comparison of complication rates. Adv Planned Parenthood 1978;13:41–43.
21. Chi IC, Feldblum PJ, Balogh SA. Previous abdominal surgery as a risk factor in interval laparoscopic sterilization. Am J Obstet Gynecol 1983;145:841–846.
22. Semm K. Pelviscopy—operative guidelines. Kiel, Germany, 1992.
23. Rimbach S, Wallwiener D, Bastert G. Microendoscopy (abstract). Contracept Fertil Sex 1995;9:39.
24. Van der Wat IJ. Micro endoscopy: a new approach in gynecological endoscopy (abstract). Contracept Fertil Sex 1995;9:69.
25. Déchaud H, Hédon B. What is the importance of microlaparoscopy in gynaecology? (abstract). Contracept Fertil Sex 1995;9:69.

Cervical and Uterine Complications During Insertion of the Hysteroscope

42

Rafael F. Valle

Endoscopy is the visualization of body cavities, either through natural or artificially made openings, utilizing endoscopes to avoid major disruption or surgery. Hysteroscopy permits observation of the endocervical canal and uterine cavity with an endoscope introduced into the cervical canal and advanced under vision until the uterine cavity is reached. Fiberoptically transmitted light provides illumination; the endocervical canal and uterine cavity are slightly distended with an appropriate medium to obtain a panoramic view of the uterine cavity. Hysteroscopy properly performed under proper indications and absence of contraindications has practically no complications. However, because some blind manipulations may be required in sounding the uterine cavity or dilating the endocervical canal, uterine perforation may occur, particularly if less than optimal attention is given to details (1–3).

Traumatic complications

Traumatic complications during a hysteroscopic procedure include cervical laceration, uterine perforation, hemorrhage, and infection.

Laceration of the cervix can occur while placing a tenaculum at the anterior or posterior lip of the cervix, particularly if excessive traction is exerted, especially during hysteroscopic surgery. This complication is seldom reported, and can be avoided by gentle manipulation of the cervix. Laceration of the cervix caused by the endoscope has not been reported and is unlikely, as the endoscope is introduced into the cervical canal under vision and follows a straight line until the junction with the uterine corpus. Bleeding can occur following the insertion of the endoscope, if abrasion of a friable ectocervix occurs and if the endoscope is not advanced under direct vision and abrades the epithelium of the endocervical canal or the uterine lining. Bleeding, following diagnostic hysteroscopy, is unusual; when it occurs, partial or total uterine perforation should be suspected. Also, early pregnancy could cause bleeding as well as abrasion or injury to a submucous myoma.

Infection is unusual, particularly if care is taken to screen those patients harboring vaginal, cervical, or uterine infection, or those with silent signs of early pelvic inflammatory disease. Although infection can be introduced through the endocervical canal into the uterine cavity by an improperly sterilized endoscope, this problem seldom occurs. Care should be taken to screen out patients with infections and to perform the procedures with meticulous attention to maintaining sterile conditions. Salat-Baroux *et al.* (4) reported four minor contaminations in over 7000 hysteroscopic procedures, detected by culturing the tip of the endoscope before and after the procedure. The organisms found were the same as those found at the cervix; therefore, these organisms could be introduced into the uterine cavity by the hysteroscopic procedure.

Uterine perforation

The frequency of uterine perforation is unknown, but is estimated at 1–2 per 100. Lindemann (5, 6) reported six fundal perforations among 5220 hysteroscopic examinations and two uterine perforations among 450 patients who underwent tubal sterilization by cornual coagulation. Neuwirth (7) reported one perforation during dissection of intrauterine adhesions and a partial perforation with myometrial penetration in a second patient. Valle and Sciarra (8) reported five uterine perforations among 187 patients treated for intrauterine adhesions, all recognized at the time of intrauterine dissection; three of the five occurred during the division of severe connective tissue adhesions, and two occurred at the time of insertion of an intrauterine contraceptive device following lysis of severe intrauterine adhesions. None of the perforations required specific treatment. A survey on operative hysteroscopy by the American Association of Gynecologic Laparoscopists showed that among 7293 operative hysteroscopies, a uterine perforation not requiring transfusion occurred in 91 patients, for a rate of 13.0 per 1000. A follow-up report on 17,298 operative hysteroscopic procedures demonstrated that a uterine perforation occurred in 296 patients, for a rate of 11.0 per 1000. Whether the perforations occurred during insertion of the endoscope or during operative procedures was not discussed (9, 10).

Uterine perforation during insertion of the hysteroscope can best be estimated from the occurrence of uterine perforation during dilatation and curettage, which has a rate of 6–13 per 1000, or the introduction of plastic cannulas of Vabra type or similar aspiration devices, which carries a risk of perforation of about 4 per 1000 (11).

Thus, uterine perforation may occur during sounding of the uterine cavity or during cervical dilatation, when the endoscope is forcibly advanced without panoramic vision, or when the lens becomes obstructed by blood, mucus, or debris, and the hysteroscope comes in direct contact with the uterine wall. In these situations, the endoscope should be withdrawn, cleansed, and reinserted again under direct vision (Figs. 42.1–42.3).

Insertion of the hysteroscope

Before attempting hysteroscopy, two important areas related to the technique should be well understood: direction of view of the hysteroscope, and the anatomy of the cervix and uterus.

Direction of view of the hysteroscope

Most hysteroscopes have a foreoblique view (150° angle or 30° angle), revealing the lateral aspects of the uterus and uterotubal junctions upon slight rotation of the

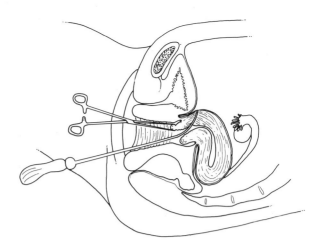

Fig. 42.2 Anterior uterine perforation by uterine sound in retroverted uterus.

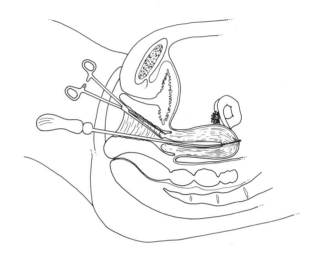

Fig. 42.3 Fundal perforation by uterine sound in midpositioned uterus.

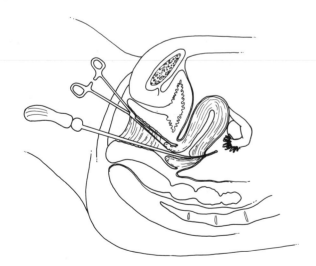

Fig. 42.1 Posterior uterine perforation by uterine sound in anteflexed uterus.

endoscope. Unlike in laparoscopy, where a 0° or 180° view is adequate, in hysteroscopy a relatively small cavity is inspected, and a foreoblique view is advantageous. Therefore, when the hysteroscope is placed at the ectocervix, the view is somewhat upward, not parallel to the endocervical canal, and this occurs when the light cord connection is down, which marks the orientation of most endoscopes. Therefore, the endoscope should be advanced by driving it slowly through the preformed tunnel without pressing the instrument against the cervical or uterine wall. This foreoblique view is most advantageous once the endocervical canal is bypassed, during examination of an anteverted or retroverted uterus. The "black spot," or fundal area of the uterus, should be pursued without moving the instrument laterally or against the uterine wall (12, 13) (Figs. 42.4 and 42.5).

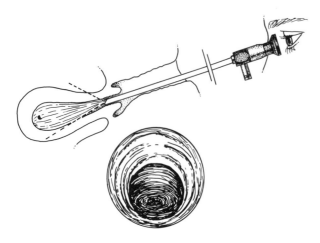

Fig. 42.4 Foreoblique (30°) hysteroscope in cervical canal, producing slight anterior deviation of view.

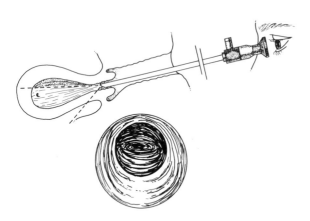

Fig. 42.5 Foreoblique (30°) hysteroscope rotated 180°, producing slight posterior deviation of view.

The resectoscope is usually oriented, at the time of initial insertion into the cervical canal, with the light-transmitting cable connection upward, so as to visualize the chosen electrode directed down. Therefore, when using telescopes that deviate the vision from the straight line, 0° or 180°, the vision provided will be slightly deviated posteriorly, as when the hysteroscope is introduced with the light cord connection directed upward.

Anatomy of the cervix and uterus

The uterus has two major portions, the cervix and, immediately contiguous, the corpus. The cervix is cylindrical, 2.5–3 cm in length, and has an external opening that communicates with the vagina; in general, it has an opening 2–3 mm or larger in multiparous women, and a small portion of the endocervix can easily be seen, except in postmenopausal women. The endocervical canal has

distinct longitudinal crests of endocervical mucosa called the plicae palmatae. At the junction with the corpus, the isthmus—a flattened, narrow, short canal between the upper portion of the cervix and uterine corpus—is the entrance to the uterine body. At this junction, the uterus bends forward or backward; the bend may be markedly pronounced in acutely anteverted or retroverted uteri. At this junction, perforations can most easily occur. Therefore, the endoscope should be gently introduced at the level of the internal os, and advanced under direct vision. The uterine cavity measures about 4–5 cm longitudinally and both uterine walls, anterior and posterior, are in apposition, forming a potential cavity that must be distended to achieve a panoramic view during hysteroscopy. The uterine walls are about 2 cm thick, but at the cornual regions they may become only 0.5 cm thick (14). Anteriorly, the close proximity of the uterine corpus to the urinary bladder may predispose injury to that organ, should perforation of the anterior uterine wall occur. Because vascularization comes from the lateral aspects of the uterus, from the isthmus to the uterine corpus, perforation in this area must be evaluated to rule out a possible vessel injury with a hematoma extending into the broad ligament.

Dilatation of the cervical canal will be necessary to admit an endoscope, 5 mm outside diameter (OD) or larger.

Conditions predisposing to uterine perforation

Benign conditions

Benign conditions predisposing to uterine perforation are severe cervical stenosis, acutely anteverted or retroverted uterus, and the postmenopausal uterus. Cervical stenosis may be encountered in patients who have had cryosurgery or any type of surgery to the cervix, and occasionally in patients without this history. These patients may require probing and dilatation under general anesthesia; if difficulty is encountered, probing could be performed under sonographic guidance, and a small-caliber endoscope (4 mm OD) inserted under direct view. The acutely anteverted or retroverted uterus usually can be easily examined utilizing a small-caliber endoscope inserted under direct view. Dilatation of the endocervical canal should be done gently, with tapered Praat-type dilators, until the cervix can be bypassed and a small-caliber endoscope inserted. Further uterine dilatation can be easily accomplished once the angle of the uterocervical junction is observed. The same procedure is performed for the acutely retroverted uterus.

Postmenopausal patients may develop atrophic cervical stenosis and may also require sounding or gentle dilatation, if the diagnostic hysteroscope cannot be introduced under direct vision. Examination should be performed with gentleness in an atraumatic, unhurried way.

Pathologic conditions

These conditions comprise distortion of the uterus secondary to myomas; occlusion of the uterine cavity secondary to adhesions; uterine anomalies with hypoplastic cornua; hypoplastic uterus (?); unsuspected endometrial carcinoma; exposure to diethylstilbestrol (DES). They are detailed below.

Distortion of the uterus

When there is marked distortion of the uterus, particularly by uterine leiomyomas at the lower portion of the uterus and at the cervix, introduction of the hysteroscope may be difficult and should be done cautiously, under complete panoramic visualization. The endoscope usually can be driven slowly around the myoma; the amount of cavity that can be observed will depend on the size of the leiomyoma. Should the leiomyoma completely occlude the entrance of the uterine cavity, observation should be made at the level of the endocervix and internal os. A diagnostic flexible hysteroscope, 3–4 mm in outer diameter, is useful in these situations.

Occlusion by intrauterine adhesions

Adhesions occluding the uterine cavity and obstructing the passage of the hysteroscope should be divided and uterine cavity symmetry reestablished. Extensive intrauterine adhesions require concomitant laparoscopy to monitor their dissection. When the uterine cavity is totally occluded, visualization should begin at the endocervix and the adhesions should be divided before advancing the hysteroscope.

Uterine anomalies with hypoplastic cornua or cavities

Avoiding abrasion of the uterine walls, the operator should observe first one horn and then the other, without blind sounding or manipulation of the uterine horns with probes or dilators, to avoid perforation, particularly at the cornual regions. If cervical dilatation is necessary, the dilators should not be advanced beyond the internal cervical os.

Hypoplastic uterus (?)

Although unusual, a hypoplastic uterus can occur, and should be evaluated with diagnostic hysteroscopes introduced only under direct vision.

Endometrial carcinoma

Pathologic conditions of the endometrium, particularly endometrial carcinoma with myometrial invasion, may alter the normal consistency of the uterine wall into a softer and more friable tissue, predisposing the uterus to perforation by trauma or injury to these areas. When endometrial carcinoma is suspected, before or during hysteroscopy, the procedure must be performed with utmost care, gentleness, and attention to details.

DES uterus

The T-shaped uterus usually resulting from exposure to DES has thick cervical and uterine walls and the cavity may be somewhat smaller than a normal uterus. It is vulnerable to uterine perforation if the instrument is not introduced smoothly or if there is marked distortion of uterine cavity symmetry. Knowledge of DES exposure is important to avoid unnecessary intrauterine manipulation.

Diagnostic hysteroscopy

The possibility of uterine perforation varies according to whether diagnostic or operative hysteroscopy is being performed and with the size of the hysteroscope used.

Because diagnostic hysteroscopy is performed with a small-caliber endoscope, less than 4 mm OD, cervical dilatation is not required and the endoscope is introduced under direct vision into the cervical canal. With small-caliber endoscopes, the best medium to distend the uterine cavity is carbon dioxide gas, and the insertion begins at the ectocervix while the gas is flowing. The endoscope is advanced, and once the internal cervical os is bypassed, the gas distends the uterine cavity and panoramic view of this area begins. When bubbles, debris, or blood clots obstruct the view, the endoscope should immediately be withdrawn. Because the endocervical canal and uterine cavity are relatively small areas, the endoscope is advanced slowly and cautiously, without pressure, considering the angle of view of the endoscope, to avoid trauma of the lateral uterine walls, and to observe in detail the anatomy of the endocervical canal. Should bubbles preform in the uterine cavity, the endoscope should be withdrawn slightly to allow bubbles to disappear before again advancing the endoscope (Figs. 42.6–42.10). A continuous-flow diagnostic hysteroscope, 5–6 mm in outer diameter, utilizing low-viscosity fluids for uterine distention, is a good option in these situations.

Because the endoscope does not permit insertion of instruments through an operating channel, due to its small caliber, no attempt at surgery with the tip of the endoscope should be made, to avoid possible false passages in the uterine wall and even perforation. Should filmy adhesions be disrupted in this manner, this

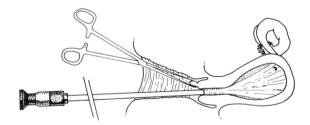

Fig. 42.6 Diagnostic hysteroscope introduced under direct view from ectocervix.

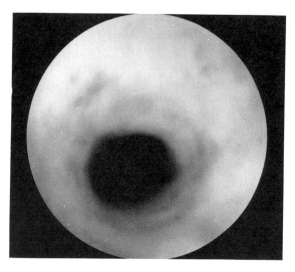

Fig. 42.7 Initial portion of endocervical canal seen as hysteroscope is inserted.

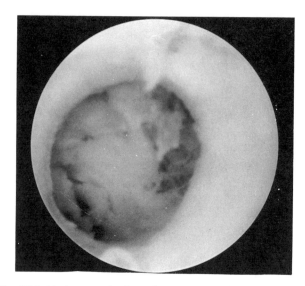

Fig. 42.9 Hysteroscopic view of uterine cavity from internal cervical os.

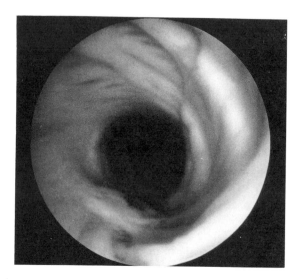

Fig. 42.8 With gas flowing throughout endocervical canal, hysteroscope is advanced and plicae palmatae observed.

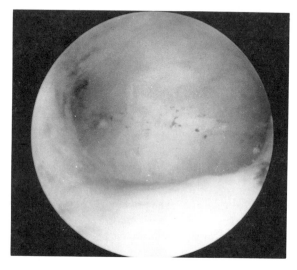

Fig. 42.10 Panoramic hysteroscopic view of normal uterine cavity. Right tubal opening can be seen.

maneuver should be performed with utmost care and gentleness.

Operative hysteroscopy

When operative hysteroscopy is performed, the hysteroscope usually has a 7–8 mm OD, and in most patients, requires cervical dilatation. The addition of this procedure to hysteroscopy, therefore, predisposes the patient to problems associated with dilatation and curettage, such as laceration of the cervix from the tenaculum, sounding of the uterine cavity, and cervical dilatation causing uterine perforation or reopening of false passages previously created by dilators. Before undertaking

a blind approach, the endoscopist should observe under direct vision the passage through which the hysteroscope is to be introduced. Furthermore, blind introduction of the hysteroscope should be undertaken only until the level of internal cervical os; if visual insertion from the ectocervix cannot be accomplished when using operative hysteroscopes, panoramic visualization of the uterine cavity should also begin at the internal os (Fig. 42.11).

While insertion of laminaria tents prior to hysteroscopic or resectoscopic operative procedures may be beneficial in selected patients with severe cervical stenosis, the possibility of infection should be kept in mind. It

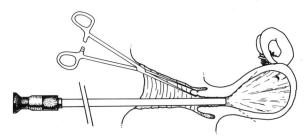

Fig. 42.11 Operative hysteroscope at level of internal os with uterine cavity distended.

may be necessary to prophylactically treat these patients with broad-spectrum antibiotics.

To summarize, uterine perforation may be avoided by:

1. Appropriate technique with gentle insertion;
2. No forceful entry;
3. Introduction and advancement of the hysteroscope under direct vision from the ectocervix to the level of the internal os;
4. Advancement of the hysteroscope only under an unobstructed panoramic view when the uterine cavity is reached;
5. Use of continuous-flow hysteroscopes in the presence of bleeding;
6. Removal of mucus, blood clots, and debris with a polyethylene catheter;
7. Selective use of laminaria tents in patients with marked cervical stenosis.

Operative procedures predisposing to perforation

Hysteroscopic operative procedures that may predispose to perforation, particularly when the uterine cavity is distorted, are the division of uterine septa; severe intrauterine adhesions; some myomectomies for broad-based, sessile, and large leiomyomas endometrial–myometrial resections; and tubal cannulation. These procedures benefit from concomitant laparoscopy and/or sonography in selected patients (15–19).

When operative hysteroscopy is performed, excessive manipulation with a hysteroscope should be avoided while forceps or instruments are in place. Particularly when laser fibers are being used, the operation should be performed with an unobstructed panoramic view and with complete control of the instruments or fibers and complete view of the distal tip.

When using optical, fixed, operative instruments, the chances of perforation increase because the panoramic view of the uterine cavity may be impaired; therefore, these instruments should be used with utmost care, and only when visualization of the uterine cavity permits their manipulation.

The resectoscope provides excellent visualization due to its continuous-flow system. Nonetheless, when introducing the instrument, uterine perforation can occur, particularly if large-caliber resectoscopes (more than 9 mm OD) are used. Furthermore, when using the resecting loop in an attempt to remove a submucous myoma that invades the uterine wall, uterine perforations can occur. Similarly, if endometrial–myometrial deep resections are attempted, particularly at the uterine cornual regions, perforations may occur. The activated loop that perforates the uterus may also damage adjacent organs such as bowel and/or large vessels. It is therefore important to evaluate carefully those patients in whom these perforations occur. These patients will benefit from laparoscopy; should laparoscopy fail to reveal damage to adjacent organs and tissue, attentive observation following the procedure is important to detect early signs of infection or bowel damage.

Management of perforations

When perforation of the uterus occurs, it is important to stop the procedure immediately and withdraw the instrument, assessing where and how the perforation happened. If it occurred during diagnostic hysteroscopy, the location should be assessed, along with the size of the perforation, the condition of the patient, and the presence of bleeding or unusual pain. If the perforation occurred during sounding or dilatation of the endocervical canal, in the absence of any symptoms, observation after discontinuation of the procedure is best.

If the perforation occurred during operative hysteroscopy with a large-caliber endoscope, and the patient is under local anesthesia but does not develop heavy

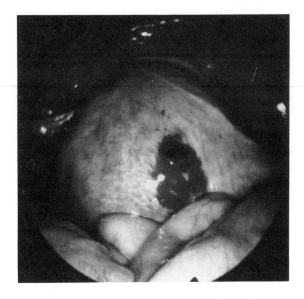

Fig. 42.12 Laparoscopy showing slight bleeding following fundal uterine perforation with uterine sound.

active bleeding, observation may be sufficient. However, if the perforation happened during operative hysteroscopy and there is active bleeding, or if the perforation is lateral or anterior, laparoscopy should be performed to assess damage. When a perforation is encountered during operative hysteroscopy and manipulations with biopsy forceps or scissors have been performed without awareness of the previous perforation, laparoscopy should also be performed.

Most uterine perforations do not require active treatment, unless bleeding persists, and that is unusual. Nonetheless, special alertness to perforations is important during surgery, particularly when utilizing laser fibers and/or electrocoagulation (Figs. 42.12–42.16).

Follow-up of patients with uterine perforations

Depending on the type and site of the perforation, the important feature is immediate follow-up for signs of pain or bleeding. When large perforations occur, and/or energy modalities such as laser or electrocoagulation are used, longer monitoring is important for early signs of infection, such as fever and pain.

The patient should be aware that a perforation occurred if she becomes pregnant later and a vaginal delivery is contemplated.

In large uterine perforations, a hysterosalpingogram three months after the perforation may be helpful to establish complete healing of the uterine wall. Future obstetric surveillance will depend on the size and type of the perforation.

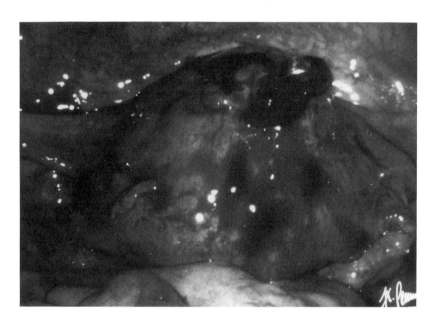

Fig. 42.13 Laparoscopic view of distal end of curette at the time of fundal uterine perforation. (Reproduced courtesy of Dr. K. Semm.)

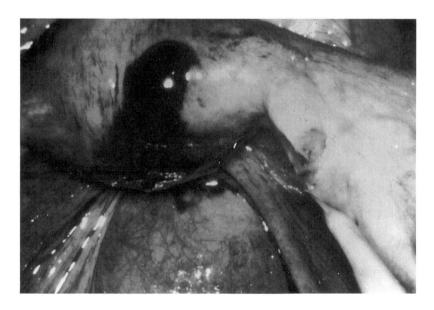

Fig. 42.14 Active bleeding from fundal perforation. (Reproduced courtesy of Dr. K. Semm.)

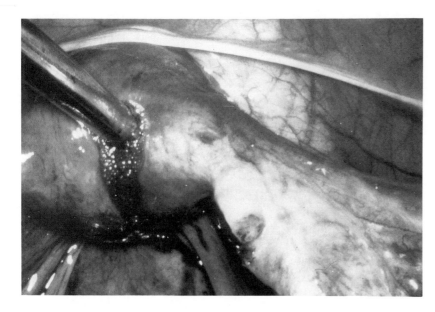

Fig. 42.15 Endocoagulation used for homostasis of fundal perforation. (Reproduced courtesy of Dr. K. Semm.)

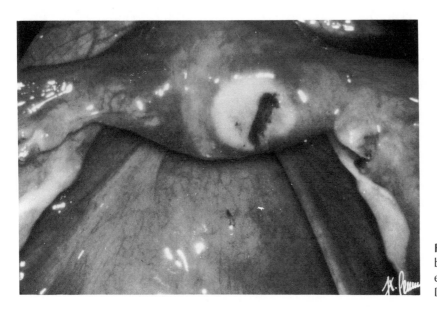

Fig. 42.16 Bleeding controlled and blanching of tissue following application of endocoagulation. (Reproduced courtesy of Dr. K. Semm.)

Summary and conclusions

Most hysteroscopic complications, particularly uterine perforations, are avoidable. Attention to detail and technique, and strict adherence to all stages of the hysteroscopic examination and operations, established indications, and absence of contraindications should result in a technique free of complications. Prevention is the best treatment, with attention being paid to individual patients, particularly when predisposing factors are present. When complications, especially perforations of the uterus, occur, they must be recognized, verified, and treated appropriately. Immediate and long-term follow-up of patients sustaining these complications should also be ensured.

REFERENCES

1. Siegler AM. Adverse effects. In: Siegler AM, Lindemann HJ, eds. Hysteroscopy. Principles and practice. Philadelphia: Lippincott, 1984:108–111.
2. Valle RF. Hysteroscopy. In: Wynn R, ed. Obstetrics and gynecology annual, vol 7. New York: Appleton-Century-Crofts, 1978: 245–283.
3. Valle RF, Sciarra JJ. Current status of hysteroscopy in gynecologic practice. Fertil Steril 1979;32:619.
4. Salat-Baroux J, Hamou JE, Maillard G, Chouraqui A, Verges P. Complications from microhysteroscopy. In: Siegler AM, Linde-

mann HJ, eds. Hysteroscopy. Principles and practice. Philadelphia: Lippincott, 1984:112–117.

5. Lindemann HJ. Komplicationen bei der CO_2-hysteroskopie. Arch Gynakol 1975;219:257.

6. Lindemann HJ, Mohr J. CO_2-hysteroscopy: diagnosis and treatment. Am J Obstet Gynecol 1976;124:129.

7. Neuwirth RS. Hysteroscopy. In: Friedman EA, ed. Major problems in obstetrics and gynecology, vol 8. Philadelphia: WB Saunders.

8. Valle RF, Sciarra JJ. Intrauterine adhesions: hysteroscopic diagnosis, classification, treatment, and reproductive outcome. Am J Obstet Gynecol 1988;158:1459.

9. Peterson HB, Hulka JF, Phillips JM. American Association of Gynecologic Laparoscopists' 1988 membership survey on operative hysteroscopy. J Reprod Med 1990:35:590.

10. Hulka JF, Peterson HB, Phillips JM, *et al*. Operative hysteroscopy. American Association of Gynecologic Laparoscopists' 1991 membership survey. J Reprod Med 1993;38:572–573.

11. Grimes DA. Diagnostic dilatation and curettage. A reappraisal. Am J Obstet Gynecol 1982;142:1.

12. Valle RF. Hysteroscopy for gynecologic diagnosis. In: Gynecologic endoscopy and instrumentation. Baggish MS, ed. Clin Obstet Gynecol 1983;26:253. Harper and Row Publishers.

13. Valle RF. Technique of panoramic hysteroscopy. In: Baggish MS, Barbot J, Valle RF, eds. Diagnostic and operative hysteroscopy. A text and atlas. Chicago: Mosby Year Book Medical Publishers, 1989:94–101.

14. Baggish MS. Anatomy of the uterus. In: Baggish MS, Barbot J, Valle RF, eds. Diagnostic and operative hysteroscopy. A text and atlas. Chicago: Mosby Year Book Medical Publishers, 1989: 18–25.

15. McCausland M, Fields GA, McCausland AM, *et al*. Tuboovarian abscesses after operative hysteroscopy. J Reprod Med 1993; 38:198–200.

16. Siegler AM. Risks and complications of hysteroscopy. In: van der Pas H, van Herendael B, van Lith D, Keith L, eds. Hysteroscopy. Proceedings of the First European Symposium on Hysteroscopy. A.Z. Jan Palfijn, O.C.M.W. Antwerp, Belgium. Sept. 2–3. Boston: MTP, 1982:75–80.

17. Gentile GP, Siegler AM. Inadvertent intestinal biopsy during laparoscopy and hysteroscopy: a report of two cases. Fertil Steril 1981;38:402.

18. MacDonald R, Phipps J, Singer A. Endometrial ablation: a safe procedure. Gynaecol Endosc 1992;1:7–9.

19. Sullivan B, Kenny P, Seibel M. Hysteroscopic resection of fibroid with thermal injury to sigmoid. Obstet Gynecol 1992;80:546–547.

43 | Complications from Uterine Distention During Hysteroscopy

Franklin D. Loffer

Relatively few complications are associated with hysteroscopy. Many large series, in fact, have reported no serious problems. Complications usually are related to the specific surgical procedure being performed rather than to some aspect of the hysteroscopic technique, with the exception of problems related to uterine distention (1). All panoramic hysteroscopic cases require uterine distention and therefore the potential of complications related to this step exists for all hysteroscopic procedures. These problems usually relate to excessive absorption of the media, an idiosyncratic reaction to the media, or a combination of the two. While complications related to uterine distention are not common, the hysteroscopist must be familiar with their avoidance and their management.

Types of distending media and their methods of insufflation

Three types of distending media are used in hysteroscopy: carbon dioxide, low-molecular-weight 32% dextran-70 (Hyskon; Pharmacia Laboratories, New Jersey), and low-viscosity fluids. Carbon dioxide is more commonly used for diagnostic work, while Hyskon and low-viscosity fluids are typically employed for operative procedures. They can, however, be used interchangeably.

Carbon dioxide is usually preferred for diagnostic office hysteroscopy because it requires no clean-up and provides an excellent view as its index of refraction is essentially the same as that of air. The low viscosity of CO_2 is both an advantage and disadvantage, however. On the one hand, it allows a higher flow rate to be carried through the small-diameter sheath of the diagnostic hysteroscope than do the liquid media. On the other hand, uterine distention may prove difficult if any leakage from the uterus occurs. Other disadvantages of CO_2 include the expense of the insufflating machine and bubbles that may obscure visualization. Carbon dioxide

insufflation must be attempted only with insufflators that deliver low flow and low pressures. Several models specifically designed for hysteroscopy can be used in either an office or a surgical suite. The hysteroscopist should have the ability to vary pressures, which is the most critical factor in uterine distention, with the assurance that the flow rate will not be excessive. It is seldom necessary to exceed 100 mm Hg pressure or 100 mL/minute flow rate.

Thirty-two percent dextran (Hyskon) is a crystal clear, highly viscous branched polysaccharide with a molecular weight of 70,000. Its major advantage as a uterine-distending medium is the fact that it is immiscible with blood, which facilitates visualization. Although its high viscosity makes administration difficult, leakage is rarely a problem once distension has been achieved. Hyskon can be administered through an IV tubing using a large syringe or by means of commercially available pumps. Control of intrauterine pressure is difficult, however, because its high viscosity results in a lag in transmission of the infusion pressure.

The low-viscosity fluids include those solutions prepared for intravenous administration or for urological endoscopic use (2). Continuous-flow hysteroscopes are designed to use these fluids. The intravenous solutions include 5% or 10% dextrose and water, Ringer's lactate, saline, or a combination of these preparations. The solutions developed for urological use but suitable for uterine distention are 1.5% or 2.2% glycine and 3% or 5% sorbitol. Although sorbitol is also combined with mannitol to promote diuresis of intravasated fluid, hyponatremia can occur with this solution (3). A 5% mannitol solution has been suggested as a better distention media for use in hysteroscopy (4); it has been used in urology as well (5). Water is not an appropriate uterine-distending medium because intravasation can produce hemolysis of the red blood cells (6).

Saline and Ringer's lactate both contain electrolytes and avoid the risk of hyponatremia. They are the distension media of choice, except when a unipolar resectoscope is being used. In such cases, the electrical current will become dissipated throughout the uterine cavity and will not create the desired effect at the resectoscope electrode.

The urological fluids are supplied in 3000 cc bags, which decrease the frequency with which the bag must be changed. While glycine is an amino acid solution, sorbitol and mannitol are sugars. As a result, these two fluids are tacky when they dry on the gloves and the surgical field. The low-viscosity media have the advantage of being readily available and require no special instrumentation for infusion (other than appropriate tubing). They can be administered by an inflated pressure cuff around the bag, by commercially available mechanical pumps, or by gravity.

Pressure cuff systems that cannot provide constant pressure are difficult to use since the pressure will decrease as the bag empties (7). Mechanical pumps should be designed to provide continuous pressure and a flow rate that varies with pressure. Mechanical pumps that provide only continuous flow usually create excessive pressures and should not be used. Commercially available, pressure-dependent hysteroscopic pumps that allow the hysteroscopist to set the exact amount of pressure desired are advantageous only in that they avoid the inconvenience of elevating the bag high enough to provide adequate gravity pressure. This convenience must be balanced against the cost of the disposables required by these systems and the fact that pumps are *not* inherently safer than gravity. Some, for example, can be set to use excessive pressure.

The author prefers to create distention pressure by gravity. A low-viscosity bag 1 m (100 cm) above the patient uses gravity to create a pressure of 73 mm Hg (100 cm H_2O), which provides adequate uterine distention. An elevation of 1.5 m (150 mm H_2O) will result in 110 mm Hg of pressure.

All low-viscosity systems should use a large-bore, urological-type tubing for inflow because smaller, IV-type tubing may limit the flow and hence the volume of fluid available to replace the outflow from cervical leakage or from the discharge through a continuous-flow hysteroscope. When outflow exceeds the inflow, pressure may prove inadequate to distend the uterine cavity.

Low-viscosity fluids are generally not used for office-based procedures because a large volume often leaks and must then be collected. Several commercial systems have been introduced to help avoid this problem.

Pressures required for uterine distention and good visualization

The uterine cavity can be adequately distended by pressure in the range of 60 to 75 mm Hg. Little intravasation or tubal passage will occur at this level. Pressures exceeding 100 mm Hg are virtually never needed and will only increase the transtubal passage and intravasation.

High infusion pressures are not necessary to clean the uterine cavity of blood and debris to provide good visualization. Clear visualization may be achieved in three ways (8): overdilation of the cervix; a continuous-flow hysteroscope; and an outflow catheter.

Overdilation cannot be used with CO_2. When applied with Hyskon or low-viscosity media, this technique results in variable distention and intrauterine pressures and uses large volumes that are hard to measure accurately. This technique should be employed only with those hysteroscopes that rule out the use of continuous flow or an outflow catheter.

Continuous-flow hysteroscopes are designed for use with the low-viscosity fluids. To have a continuous flow, the hysteroscope must include both an inner sheath to provide a channel for introducing clean distending media into the uterine cavity and an outer sheath, preferably with holes at the distal end to remove the soiled distending media from the cavity. The tubing to these channels must not be reversed. Note, however, that many hysteroscopes are not designed with a double sheath. Adapters are available to convert hysteroscopes to continuous flow (Zimmer Company, Dover, Ohio). Outflow may be obtained by gravity, a mechanical pump system, or wall suction. The author prefers to use wall suction on low and leave the outflow stopcock of the hysteroscope only slightly opened. When necessary, this stopcock can be opened completely. If left continuously open, an unnecessarily large amount of fluid is used, which complicates measuring intake and output.

When a continuous-flow hysteroscope is not available, an outflow catheter may be used if the hysteroscope includes an operative channel. The catheter, a 7 French wide-bore tubing (10468B7 Karl Storz Endoscopy America, Los Angeles, California), is passed into the uterine cavity through the operating channel. When CO_2 is used to distend the uterus, a syringe containing a small amount of saline is attached to the tubing. This fluid is then injected through the catheter into the uterine cavity to clear away blood and debris. The syringe controls the removal of the saline and prevents the loss of the CO_2 distention. Because Hyskon is so viscous, active aspiration with a syringe is required to clear the cavity. When low-viscosity fluids are used, the intrauterine pressure passively forces the soiled media out of the outflow catheter. Occasionally aspiration is needed to remove mucus or larger pieces of debris.

Factors affecting uterine distention

To distend the uterus for panoramic hysteroscopy, the intrauterine pressure of the distending medium must be great enough to overcome the resistance of the uterus.

Distention of the uterus alone does not guarantee good visualization. Instead, the intrauterine pressure must also be high enough to prevent bleeding into the uterine cavity.

Intrauterine pressure is usually 10 to 15 mm Hg less than the infusion pressure (9). It will be the same *only* when no inflow or outflow from the uterus occurs—it can *never* be greater. This pressure will be less during filling and replacing outflow from the uterus. Outflow of the medium occurs from four sources: (1) leakage around the cervix or from the equipment; (2) intentional outflow through a catheter or a continuous flows system to clear the cavity; (3) passage through the fallopian tubes; and (4) intravasation into the vascular system. A combination of these factors usually produces total outflow.

In addition to infusion pressure of the medium, the flow rate must be sufficient to keep the uterus distended. Inflow rate is limited by the smallest diameter found in the tubing and hysteroscope channels. The length of the inflow tubing and the viscosity of the medium will also affect resistance to flow. Compensating for excessive outflow by increasing inflow pressure is not safe because it may lead to intravasation. If appropriate pressure is used and adequate uterine distention is not achieved, the hysteroscopist should verify the absence of leakage from the cervix or any part of the equipment; he or she should also ensure that the outflow stopcock used to clear the cavity is not fully open and that no obstruction appears in the system, such as a closed stopcock or bent tubing. If no obstruction or apparent excessive outflow is found, then a uterine rupture or significant intravasation may exist.

Carbon dioxide has the lowest viscosity of all distending media. Thus the size or length of the inflow channel is not a limiting factor for this medium, but outflow can occur readily and result in a loss of intrauterine distention. In contrast, the high viscosity of Hyskon requires that considerable pressure be applied to drive this fluid through the tubing and hysteroscope. It is difficult to titrate the inflow of Hyskon against its outflow because of the slowness which with it flows into the uterine cavity. Maintenance of the pressure initially needed for infusion, once uterine distention has been achieved, may create excessive intrauterine pressure and intravasation. The low-viscosity fluids provide a distension system much easier to control. With this medium, infusion pressure is readily transmitted to the uterine cavity as long as inflow tubing with an adequate diameter is used.

Types of problems with uterine distention

It is an artificial conceit to divide problems of uterine distention into specific causes as a relationship frequently exists between these causes and the problems they create.

Nevertheless, the roles of excessive absorption, idiosyncratic reactions, rupture of viscous, hypothermia, concomitant laparoscopy, and misuse of equipment will be reviewed as though they were independent of other factors.

Excessive absorption

Excessive absorption, apparently the most common problem related to uterine-distending media, is frequently associated with excessive pressure. This relationship appears to be overlooked by many hysteroscopists as reports of excessive absorption often do not make reference to the distending pressures used. A critical threshold at which significant intravasation will occur has been suggested to be the mean arterial pressure (10). The uterus is more than adequately distended with 60 to 75 mm Hg or less of pressure. Higher pressures will not provide better visualization and will only increase the amount and rapidity of intravasation and transtubal passage.

Significant excessive absorption usually occurs when large vascular channels are opened. This complication primarily arises when cervical–lower uterine segment lacerations are caused during dilation or in operative procedures where disruption of the endometrial surface has opened vascular channels in the myometrium (11). When large channels are opened, excessive intravasation can occur even when appropriate distension pressures are used (12, 13). In such circumstances, however, excessive pressure will compound the problem. Most uterine bleeding that interferes with visualization is venous and not arterial. Since the intrauterine pressure should remain higher than the venous pressure, some intravasation will always occur. Therefore, the amount of intravasation also increases in longer cases.

Gonadotropin-releasing hormone agonists (14, 15), oxytocin (12, 16), and vasopressin (17) may aid in decreasing the amount of intravasation. However, use of vasopressin may be associated with hypotension, hypertension, and cardiac abnormalities (18); this agent has also been severely criticized because of its antidiruetic effects (19).

Transtubal passage into the peritoneal cavity is seldom, if ever, a basis of excessive absorption if appropriate pressures are maintained.

The use of commercially available fluid pumps will not guarantee prevention of fluid overload, and these devices should not provide a false sense of security. None measures true intrauterine pressure—indeed, the need to do so has been questioned (20).

The combination of excessive pressure and an open vascular tree most readily leads to excessive absorption. If large vascular channels are opened, clinically significant intravasation can nevertheless occur in diagnostic and intrauterine surgical procedures even though appropriate pressures are used.

Idiosyncratic reactions

Another common type of complication is an adverse reaction to normally tolerated amounts of the distending medium. While such reactions are usually dose-related, they may occur from only a small amount of medium.

Rupture of viscous

Although generally listed as a complication, this problem is more a theoretical concern than a practical one. Rupture of either the uterus or the fallopian tubes would require excessive pressure in combination with an obstruction to a ready outflow of the distending medium. It has only been reported once (21).

Hypothermia

The possibility of hypothermia exists only when large volumes of low-viscosity fluids are used. Low-molecular-weight dextran is not used in sufficient volumes and CO_2 does not carry with it sufficient ability to absorb heat to make hypothermia a concern.

Concomitant laparoscopy problems

Diagnostic and operative laparoscopy is frequently used in conjunction with diagnostic or operative hysteroscopy. Under these circumstances the patient may be exposed to additive effects. For example, excessive amounts of CO_2, Hyskon, or low-viscosity fluids could be absorbed if they were used in both intrauterine and intraperitoneal procedures. Hypothermia could result if a large amount of intra-abdominal irrigating fluid was combined with a low-viscosity distending medium.

Misuse of equipment

Although this problem may not technically belong in a discussion of uterine distention media, it warrants mentioning. The use of a laparoscope insufflator or any instrumentation not specifically designed to provide pressure and flow rates appropriate for the hysteroscopic use of CO_2 carries excessive risks; consequently, its use should be avoided. In addition, sapphire tips used in conjunction with the Nd:Yag laser may require cooling. When employed during intrauterine surgery, the junction of the fiber and the tips should not be cooled with any gas because the flow required for cooling varies from several hundred to several thousand milliliters per minute. These flows are excessive for intrauterine distention and can result in high intrauterine pressure and excessive absorption. During the intra-abdominal use of the Nd:Yag sapphire tip, the same risks of abdominal overdistention should also be avoided.

Problems associated with carbon dioxide

The extent of complications associated with CO_2 is not known. Considering the thousands of hysteroscopies that have been performed with this medium, it is apparent that it is very safe when used at pressures of 100 mm Hg or less and flow rates of less than 100 mL/min. Complications are more prone to occur with excessive pressure or flow rates (22–25).

In addition to the published reports, the author is aware of three unpublished cases related to this problem. One patient died when the hysteroscope was hooked directly to the CO_2 tank without the use of a proper insufflator (26). In a second case, the patient suffered extensive brain damage when a prototype insufflator delivered an excessive flow rate of carbon dioxide. The third occurred in the author's own practice and dealt with a patient undergoing lysis of intrauterine adhesions. A commercially available hysteroscope insufflator set to deliver a maximum of 100 mL of CO_2 per minute was used; the pressure was set at 100 mm Hg. Laparoscopic monitoring of the dissection was being carried out at the same time. The laparoscope insufflator was set to deliver intra-abdominally a maximum of a 1 liter of CO_2 per minute at 25 cm of H_2O pressure (18.4 mm Hg). Approximately 30 minutes after the start of the procedure, the patient suddenly developed cardiac irregularity and had a cardiac arrest. During the resuscitative period gas was heard in the ventricle. The patient was resuscitated successfully and had no residual damage. The hysteroscopic insufflator was checked and found to be delivering pressures and flow rates in excess of those indicated on the dial. Insufflators—like electrical generators—should be periodically checked for accuracy.

Embolization of CO_2 has been reported to occur in 52% of patients when the flow rate equals 100 cc per minute. This complication is observed more frequently with intrauterine manipulation and at pressures of 60 to 120 mm Hg (57.7%) than at pressures less than 60 mm Hg (14.7%) (27). As a result, precordial stethoscope cardiac monitoring has been recommended (25). Other authors using lower flow rates (40–60 mL/min) have not identified embolization (28).

Excessive absorption of CO_2 results from either excessive flow rate or excessive pressure. The CO_2 must enter the vascular system through uterine vessels opened by excessive pressure or surgery. Peritoneal absorption is not a significant factor. The risk increases in prolonged procedures, cases involving disruption of the endometrial surface, or hysteroscopy with concomitant laparoscopy. When excessive absorption occurs, pCO_2 increases and pO_2 decreases, which results in a metabolic acidosis and resultant cardiac irregularity (29, 30).

Avoidance of this problem involves the use of appropriate pressures and flow rates as well as adequate ventilation (CO_2 is readily dissociated from the hemoglobin molecule in patients with normal respiratory function). To treat significant embolization, the patient is turned on her left side.

Idiosyncratic reactions do not occur with carbon dioxide. In addition to metabolic imbalance related to excessive absorption, problems might potentially arise in patients with sickle-cell disease trait or pulmonary insufficiency. The possibility of these latter two problems is considered theoretical given that no cases have been reported. Avoidance would rely on the use of a distending medium other than CO_2 in these patients. Treatment would be symptomatic and supportive.

Hypothermia is a potential risk with the high flows used in laparoscopy (31). It probably does not represent a significant risk with the low flows used in hysteroscopy.

Problems related to concomitant laparoscopy are associated with peritoneal absorption and/or inadequate ventilation and hypothermia. They have been discussed previously.

Misuse of equipment could occur if an inappropriate gaseous distending medium, such as nitrous oxide (32) or air, was used. Excess absorption and death have resulted when a laparoscope insufflator was used or a gas (33) to cool Nd:Yag sapphire tips. These problems may be avoided through appropriate use of equipment. Cooling of the sapphire tips can be done with the same medium used to distend the uterus (34). Saline, Ringer's lactate, or a combination of dextrose and water is appropriate.

The occurrence of a gas embolism during hysteroscopy may not necessarily be related to CO_2 uterine distention (35, 36). One reported case (24) may have involved a room-air embolism, as cardiovascular collapse occurred four minutes after cessation of uterine distention.

In summary, the risks of carbon dioxide are minimal. Excessive absorption of CO_2 is difficult to achieve because this gas is highly soluble in blood and readily escapes the body with adequate ventilation. When excessive absorption does occur, metabolic changes result and are manifested by cardiac irregularity and ultimately arrest. Avoidance involves the use of appropriate flow rates and pressures. In operative cases, the author prefers to perform only the most minor surgical procedures with carbon dioxide. Adequate respiration can help avoid problems related to CO_2. Should a problem occur, the administration of oxygen and hyperventilation are required.

Problems associated with Hyskon

The many reports of problems associated with Hyskon as a uterine-distending medium probably reflect the fact that it is commonly used rather than that it carries an increased risk relative to other media. The frequency of problems appears to be low during hysteroscopy (37) and in obstetrical cases where large amounts were given for thromboembolism prophylaxis (38).

Hyskon is a plasma expander, with the osmotic properties of 100 mL of dextran-70 being able to expand plasma volume by 860 mL (39). Excessive absorption may result in high left ventricular output failure. Only a few authors have attributed the pulmonary problems of Hyskon as being related to its plasma expansion properties, however (40, 41). A review of those cases that attribute a direct toxic effect of Hyskon on the lungs (described later in this section) shows that they do not always address other important factors, such as the amount of Hyskon actually introduced into the vascular system; the contribution to plasma expansion by IV fluids; the shifting of fluids from the third space; and the slow clearance of Hyskon (42). We believe that most cases of coagulopathies and adult respiratory syndrome may actually be related to excessive absorption.

Hyskon's manufacturer states that patients are at an increased risk of pulmonary edema if: (1) the procedures last more than 45 minutes, (2) large areas of endometrium are traumatized, and (3) more than 500 cc of Hyskon is infused. In addition, it recommends an infusion pressure between 100 and 150 mm Hg. These warnings do not fully reflect the issues that put patients at risk, however. The amount retained by the patient is important—not the amount infused into the uterus. Fluid that spills from the cervix cannot have an effect on the patient. In addition, the arbitrary limitation of time is questionable as the number of vascular channels open actually dictates the amount of Hyskon that can be intravasated. Opened vascular spaces during disruption of the endometrium surface are also a significant factor (11). Peritoneal absorption that occurs when Hyskon passes through the fallopian tubes appears to carry little risk (43).

Pulmonary problems can be avoided by use of appropriate pressures during operative procedures to avoid intravasation. Hyskon is not readily cleared from the vascular system, which makes management difficult. Treatment is symptomatic and includes diuretics, oxygen, and supportive measures.

Because idiosyncratic reactions are more common with dextran-40 than dextran-70 (Hyskon), only the higher-molecular-weight product should be used for hysteroscopy. The idiosyncratic reactions that have been attributed to Hyskon 70 include noncardiogenic pulmonary edema, intravascular coagulopathies, allergic reactions, and anaphylaxis.

The interpretation that noncardiogenic pulmonary edema arises from a direct effect on the lungs by Hyskon (44–47) has been disputed (39, 48–51). The pulmonary problems and coagulopathies probably have another basis. Many reports of these complications do not state the actual volume of the Hyskon retained by the patient and therefore ignore the possible role played by introduction of excessive amounts of Hyskon into the vascular system followed by resultant fluid overload. Furthermore, these reports do not account for fluid brought into the intravascular space and contributing to pulmonary edema that may come from surrounding tissues (not just surgical IV fluids). Likewise, they do not address the prolonged retention and therefore prolonged effects of the intravascular dextran.

Intravascular coagulopathy has been suggested to be an idiosyncratic reaction like pulmonary edema (46, 47). It more likely relates to the volume of intravasated Hyskon as the anticlotting properties of dextran are affected by the amount used (49).

Treatment of pulmonary edema and coagulopathies is symptomatic but is complicated by the slowness with which Hyskon is cleared from the vascular system. Such problems can be prevented by use of appropriate pressure and monitoring of the amount of Hyskon retained by the patient.

Allergic reactions are idiosyncratic reactions. Anaphylaxis has been reported (52–55), and minor allergic reactions can also occur. In the author's series of 244 tubal plug sterilization procedures using Hyskon, one patient developed allergic reactions manifested by skin changes (56). Treatment is symptomatic. Although prevention of these idiosyncratic problems is theoretically possible by hapten inhibition (57), this approach has not found widespread acceptance.

Hypothermia should not be a concern because of the small volumes used. The only specific problem that might arise with concomitant laparoscopy is excessive absorption if Hyskon were left in the peritoneal cavity. Misuse of equipment is, to the author's knowledge, not likely, although a pump has been incriminated in a massive air embolism resulting in death (58).

In summary, complications related to Hyskon are rare, but they may prove difficult to manage when they occur because of the medium's slow clearance from the body. Excessive absorption occurs most commonly during surgical procedures and with excessive infusion pressure. Pulmonary edema, coagulopathies, and allergic reactions can develop. Prevention is difficult except for avoiding excessive absorption.

Problems associated with low-viscosity fluids

The risks of low-viscosity fluids have been emphasized by clinicians because they frequently are associated with life-threatening problems. Complications of these fluids include generalized edema, pulmonary edema, hyponatremia, hyperglycemia, and combinations of these problems. An incidence of fluid overload of 0.4% has been reported in one large series (59). A survey of general gynecologists found a complication rate that varied between 1.4% and 3.4% (60–62).

Excessive absorption can result from or be worsened by excessive pressures of uterine distention (10, 63). This problem occurs more frequently in surgical procedures where myometrial vessels are opened (3). Fluid overload may cause generalized edema. In these cases, development of pulmonary edema may depend on the patient's

cardiac reserve (59, 64–71). Hyperglycemia may result when the intravasated fluid contains glucose (72). Hyponatremia is a major life-threatening risk if non-isotonic electrolyte solutions, such as dextrose in water, glycine, or sorbitol, are used (64, 65, 72–77). Metabolic alterations may occur in addition to hyponatremia hemodilution and the expansion of intravascular volume. Sorbitol—an isomer of mannitol—can produce hyperlactatemia in metabolically compromised patients. Postoperative nausea and vomiting are noted more frequently in patients with a lower serum sodium (78).

Fluid overload may occur even when appropriate infusion pressures are used. Therefore, strict monitoring of intake and output is essential in all cases. This goal is difficult to accomplish if calculations are based on the visual reading of bags used and collection canisters. All bags are overfilled by as much as 10%, and canister labels can prove difficult to read. Addition and subtraction errors are also common. Intake and output machines based on the weight of fluid used can simplify the problems of intake and output (79, 80). The author has used a commercially available system (Aquintel, Inc., Mountain View, California) for this purpose and found it very helpful.

Should a significant deficit between intake and output develop, either lower pressures or discontinuation of the procedure should be considered. In the author's experience, pressures of 75 mm Hg or less rarely lead to excessive intravasation and fluid deficits, even in prolonged cases, usually remain less than 1000 cc. Once a deficit of 1000 cc has developed, however, opening of large vessels must be suspected as further rapid fluid intravasation then occurs (81). This observation has been confirmed by at least one other author (12). Risks from fluid absorption do not appear to be a problem with deficits of less than 1500 cc (82).

Fluid overload and hyponatremia in hysteroscopy represent acute problems and should be treated aggressively. Therapy consists of a loop-acting diuretic such as furosemide, electrolyte replacement, and oxygen (83). The diuretic will facilitate the excretion of the water overload, and sodium bicarbonate or hypertonic saline (3%) will treat the nondilutional hyponatremia. Hypernatremia levels should be avoided. Central pontine myelinolysis from rapid elevation of sodium does not appear to be a problem in acute hyponatremia.

The goals of treatment in acute hyponatremia are to reduce excessive cellular water and to increase plasma sodium concentration only to the degree necessary that the patient returns to normal respiration and remains seizure-free and alert (84). Failure to recognize and treat hyponatremia may have fatal consequences (85–89). Prevention is achieved by avoiding excessive absorption. This process includes avoiding high pressures, recognizing potential high-risk patients (90), and monitoring fluid intake and output to determine when a problem is developing.

Idiosyncratic reactions are associated only with the combination of excessive free ammonia and glycine (6, 91). Glycine is a nonessential amino acid. Diminution in the liver and kidneys results in the formation of glyoxylic acid and ammonia. Reports conflict as to glycine's role in increasing free ammonia levels in the blood. This increase may be responsible for encephalopathy in patients manifesting a water intoxication syndrome after excessive glycine absorption. No evidence suggests that existing liver disease increases this risk. Oral 1-arginine may be useful as a protective and/or therapeutic agent (92).

Hypothermia has not been reported. Hysteroscopists should consider this complication to be a distinct risk with low-viscosity fluids, however, as large volumes of these media are frequently used. It is advisable to have fluids at least at room temperature and preferably warmed. The practice of some hysteroscopists of cooling the distending medium to decrease bleeding and improve endometrial ablation results by vasoconstricting the uterus seems ill advised. It is unlikely that such a vascular organ can be significantly vasoconstricted.

Problems associated with laparoscopy would relate to hypothermia if large amounts of abdominal irrigating fluid were used and to fluid overload and electrolyte imbalance if they were not suctioned out. Misuse of equipment with low-viscosity fluids occurs when excessive pressures are used for insufflation. This problem can arise even with commercial pumps.

In summary, risks related to the low-viscosity fluids are primarily the result of excessive intravasation and can result in life-threatening hyponatremia as well as pulmonary edema. These risks are easily monitored by tracking fluid intake and output and are treated with diuretics and electrolyte replacement.

Is there a most appropriate uterine distention medium?

No uterine distending media is best suited for all cases. Each option has its own advantages and drawbacks. As a result, the hysteroscopist should be aware of the advantages and potential problems of each distending medium and be comfortable with each as a method for uterine distention in panoramic hysteroscopy. Excessive pressure for distention is the single greatest risk that the physician can control. Patients in whom myometrial vessels have been opened are at greatest risk.

REFERENCES

1. Loffer FD. Complications of hysteroscopy—their cause, prevention, and correction. J Am Assoc Gynecol Laparosc 1995;3:11–26.
2. Shirk GJ, Kaigh J. The use of low-viscosity fluids for hysteroscopy. J Am Assoc Laparosc 1994;2:11–21.
3. Kim AH, Keltz MD, Arici A, et al. Dilutional hyponatremia during hysteroscopic myomectomy with sorbitol-mannitol distension medium. J Am Assoc Gynecol Laparosc 1995;2:237–243.
4. Indman PD. Editorial. J Am Assoc Gynecol Laparosc 1995;3:1–2.
5. Allgen LG, Norlen H, Kolmert, et al. Absorption and elimination of mannitol solution when used as an isotonic irrigating agent in connection with transurethral resection of the prostate. Scand J Urol Nephrol 1987;21:177–184.
6. Madsen PO, Madsen RE. Clinical and experimental evaluation of different irrigating fluids for transurethral surgery. Invest Urol 1965;3:122–129.
7. Loffer FD. Laser ablation of the endometrium. In: DeCherney AH, ed. Hysteroscopy. Philadelphia: WB Saunders, 1988:77–89 (Obstet Gynecol Clinic of N Am, vol 15.)
8. Loffer FD. Hysteroscopy. In: Stangel JJ, ed. Infertility surgery. A multimethod approach to female reproductive surgery. Norwalk: Appleton and Lange, 1990:80–81.
9. Shirk GJ, Gimpelson RJ. Control of intrauterine fluid pressure during operative hysteroscopy. J Am Assoc Gynecol Laparosc 1994;1:229–233.
10. Garry R, Hasham F, Kokri MS, Mooney P. The effects of pressure on fluid absorption during endometrial ablation. J Gynecol Surg 1992;8:1–10.
11. Baggish MS, Davauluri C, Rodriquez F, et al. Vascular uptake of Hyskon (dextran 70) during operative and diagnostic hysteroscopy. J Gynecol Surg 1992;8:211–217.
12. Garry R, Mooney P, Hasham F, et al. A uterine distension system to prevent fluid absorption during Nd:Yag laser endometrial ablation. Gynaecol Endosc 1992;1:23–27.
13. Vulgaropulos SP, Haley LC, Hulka JF. Intrauterine pressure and fluid absorption during continuous flow hysteroscopy. Am J Obstet Gynecol 1992;167:386–391.
14. Vercellini P, Ragni G, Colombo A, et al. Gonadotropin releasing hormone agonist treatment before hysteroscopic metroplasty. Gynaecol Endosc 1993;2:153–157.
15. Vercellini P, Trespidi L, Bramante T, Panayma S, Mauro F, Crosignani PG. Gonadotropin releasing hormone agonist treatment before hysteroscopic endometrial resection. Int J Gynecol Obstet 1994;45:235–239.
16. Shelley-Jojnes DC, Garry R, Mooney P, Kumar CM, Kokri M. The use of syntocinon in the management of excessive fluid absorption during endometrial ablation. Aust NZ J Obstet Gynaecol 1994;34:205–207.
17. Corson SL, Brooks FP, Serden SP, et al. Effects of vasopressin administration during hysteroscopic surgery. J Reprod Med 1994;39:419–423.
18. Nezhat F, Admon D, Nezhat CH, et al. Life-threatening hypotension after vasopressin injection during operative laparoscopy, followed by uneventful repeat laparoscopy. J Am Assoc Gynecol Laparosc 1994;2:83–86.
19. Arieff AI, Ayus JC. Hyponatremic encephalopathy after endometrial ablation. JAMA 1994;271:345.
20. Loffer FD. The need to measure intrauterine pressure—myth or necessity? J Am Assoc Gynecol Laparosc 1994;2:1–2.
21. Seigler AM, Valle RF, Lindemann JH, Mencaglia L. Therapeutic hysteroscopy. Indications and techniques. St. Louis: CV Mosby, 1990.
22. Porto R. Hysteroscopie. In: Encyclopedie. Paris: Medico-Chirurgie, 1974. Cited in: Seigler AM, Valle RF, Lindemann HJ, Mencaglia L. Therapeutic hysteroscopy. Indications and techniques. St. Louis: CV Mosby, 1990.
23. Mahmoud F, Fraser IS. CO_2 hysteroscopy and embolism, Gynaecol Endosc 1994;3:91–95.
24. Brink DM, DeJong P, Fawcus S, et al. Carbon dioxide embolism following diagnostic hysteroscopy. J Obstet Gynaecol 1994; 101:717–718.
25. Brundin J, Thomasson K. Cardiac gas embolism during carbon dioxide hysteroscopy: risk and management. European J Obstet Gynecol and Reprod Biology 1989;33:241–255.
26. Obstetrician connected in sterilization death is placed on probation. Obstet Gynecol News 1974;9:4.
27. Rythen-Alder E, Brundin J, Notini-Gudmarsson A, Melcher A, Thomasson K. Detection of carbon dioxide embolism during hysteroscopy. Gynaecol Endosc 1992;1:207–210.

28. Siegler AM. A comparison of gas and liquid for hysteroscopy. J Reprod Med 1975;15:73–75.
29. Gallinat A. Carbon dioxide hysteroscopy: principles and physiology. In: Seigler AM, Lindemann HJ, eds. Hysteroscopy: principles and practice. Philadelphia: Lippincott, 1984:45–48.
30. Corson SL, Hoffman JJ, Jackowski J, Chapman GA. Cardiopulmonary effects of direct venous CO_2 inflation in ewes. A model for CO_2 hysteroscopy. J Reprod Med 1988;33:440–444.
31. Ott DE. Laparoscopic hypothermia. J Laparoendoscopy 1991;1:127–131.
32. Hulf JA, Corall JM, Strunin L, Knights K, Newton J. Possible hazards of nitrous oxide for hysteroscopy. Brit Med J 1975;1:511.
33. Baggish MS, Daniell JF. Death caused by air embolism associated with neodynium; yttrium aluminum-garnet laser surgery and artificial sapphire tips. Am J Obstet Gynecol 1989;161:877–888.
34. Loffer FD. Fluid cooling of artificial sapphire tips of laser. Am J Obstet Gynecol 1990;163:681.
35. Weissman A, Kol S, Peretz BA. Gas embolism in obstetrics and gynecology—a review. J Reprod Med 1996;41:103–111.
36. Corson SL, Brooks PG, Soderstrom RM. Gynecologic endoscopic gas embolism. Fertil Steril 1996;65:529–533.
37. Ruiz JM, Neuwirth RS. The incidence of complications associated with the use of Hyskon during hysteroscopy: experience in 1783 consecutive patients, J Gynecol Surg 1992;8:219.
38. Ankum WM, Vonk J. The spring balance: a simple monitoring system for fluid overload during hysteroscopic surgery. Lancet 1994;343:836–837.
39. Lukascko P. Noncardiogenic pulmonary edema secondary to intrauterine instillation of 32% dextran-70. Fertil Steril 1985;44:560–561.
40. Golan A, Sieder M, Buhar M, Ron-El R, Herman A, Caspi E. High output left ventricular failure after dextran used in an operative hysteroscopy. Fertil Steril 1990;54:939–941.
41. McLucus B. Hyskon complications in hysteroscopic surgery. Obstet Gynecol Survey 1991;46:196–200.
42. Arturson G, Wallenius G. The renal clearance of dextran of different molecular size in normal humans. Scand J Clin Lab Invest 1964;1:81–86.
43. Tulandi T, Hilton J. Effects of intraperitoneal 32% dextran-70 or blood coagulation and serum electrolytes. J Reprod Med 1985;30:431–434.
44. Zebella EA, Moise J, Carson SA. Noncardiogenic pulmonary edema secondary to intrauterine installation of 32% dextran-70. Fertil Steril 1985;43:479–480.
45. Leake JF, Murphy AA, Zacur HA. Noncardiogenic pulmonary edema: a complication of operative hysteroscopy. Fertil Steril 1987;48:497–499.
46. Mangar D, Gerson JI, Constantine RM, Lenzi V. Pulmonary edema and coagulopathy due to Hyskon (32% dextran-70) administration. Anesth Analg 1989;68:686–687.
47. Jedeikin R, Olsfanger D, Kessler I. Disseminated intravascular coagulopathy and adult respiratory distress syndrome: life threatening complications of hysteroscopy. Am J Obstet Gyecol 1990;162:44–45.
48. Loffer FD. Explanation of mechanism of Hyskon solution reaction needed. Am J Obstet Gynecol 1990;163:2029.
49. Ljunstrom K. Safety of 32% dextran 70 for hysteroscopy. Am J Obstet Gynecol 1990;163:2029.
50. Schinagl EF. Hyskon (32% dextran 70), hysteroscopic surgery and pulmonary edema. Anesth Analg 1990;70:223–224.
51. Witz CA, Schenken RS, Silverberg KM, et al. Complications associated with the absorption of hysteroscopic fluid media. Fertil Steril 1993;60:745–756.
52. Users reminded about adverse reactions to Dextran. FDA Drug Bulletin 1983;13:23–24.
53. Taylor PJ, Cummings DC. Hysteroscopy in 100 patients. Fertil Steril 1979;31:301–308.
54. Trimbos-Kemper TCM, Veering BT. Anaphylactic shock from intracavitary 32% dextran-70 during hysteroscopy. Fertil Steril 1989;51:1053–1054.
55. Ahmed N, Falcone T, Tulandi T, et al. Anaphylactic reaction because of intrauterine 32% dextran 70 instillation. Fertil Steril 1991;55:1014–1016.
56. Loffer FD. Hysteroscopic sterilization with the use of the formed, in-place silicone plugs. Am J Obstet Gynecol 1984;194:261–270.
57. Heinonen PK. For heavy users of dextran who don't read Acta Chirurgica Scandinavica. Fertil Steril 1990;53:1109.
58. Nachum Z, Kol S, Adir Y, Melamed Y. Massive air embolism—a possible cause of death after operative hysteroscopy using a 32% dextran-70 pump. Fertil Steril 1992;58:836–838.
59. Garry R, Erian J, Grochmal S. A multicare collaborative study into the treatment of menorrhagia by Nd:Yag laser ablation of the endometrium. Brit J Obstet Gynecol 1991;98:357–362.
60. Peterson HB, Hulka JF, Phillips JM. American Association of Gynecologic Laparoscopists' 1988 membership survey of operative hysteroscopy. J Reprod Med 1990;35:590–591.
61. Hulka JA, Peterson HB, Phillips JM, et al. Operative hysteroscopy: American Association of Gynecologic Laparoscopists' 1991 membership survey. J Reprod Med 1993;38:572–573.
62. Hulka JA, Peterson HA, Phillips JM, et al. Operative hysteroscopy: American Association of Gynecologic Laparoscopists' 1993 membership survey. J Am Assoc Gynecol Laparosc 1995;2:131–132.
63. Garry R. Safety of hysteroscopic laser surgery. Lancet 1990;336:1013–1014.
64. Goldrath MH, Fuller TA, Segal S. Laser photovaporization of endometrium for the treatment of menorrhagia. Am J Obstet Gynecol 1981;140:14–19.
65. Goldrath MH. Intrauterine laser surgery. In: Keye WR, ed. Laser surgery in gynecology and obstetrics, 2nd ed. Chicago: Yearbook Medical Publishers, 1989:151–165.
66. Lomano JM. Photocoagulation of the endometrium with Nd:Yag laser for the treatment of menorrhagia. J Reprod Med 1986;31:148–150.
67. Lomono JM, Feste JR, Loffer FD, Goldrath MH. Ablation of the endometrium with the neodymium yag laser: a multicenter study. Colposcopy Gynecol Laser Surg 1987;2:203–207.
68. Goldfarb HA. A review of 35 endometrial ablations using the Nd:Yag laser for recurrent menometrorrhagia. Obstet Gynecol 1990;76:833–835.
69. Feinberg RI, Gimpelson RJ, Golder DE. Pulmonary edema after photocoagulation of the endometrium with the Nd:Yag laser—a case report. J Reprod Med 1989;34:431–434.
70. Morrison LMM, Davis J, Sumner D. Absorption of irrigating fluid during laser photocoagulation of the endometrium in the treatment of menorrhagia. Brit J Obstet Gynecol 1989;96:346–352.
71. Davis JA. Hysteroscopic endometrial ablation with the neodymium-Yag laser. Br J Obstet Gynaecol 1989;96:928–932.
72. Carson SA, Hubert GD, Schriock ED, Buster JE. Hyperglycemia and hyponatremia during operative hysteroscopy with 5% dextrose in water distension. Fertil Steril 1989;51:341–343.
73. Van Boven MJ, Singelyn F, Donnez J, Gribomont BF. Dilutional hyponatraemia associated with intrauterine endoscopic laser surgery. Anesthesiology 1989;71:449–500.
74. Complications and precautions in operative hysteroscopic surgery. In: Donnez J, ed. Laser operative laparoscopy and hysteroscopy. Leuven, Belgium: Nauwelaerts Printing, 1989;299–306.
75. Magos AL, Baumann R, Turnbull AC. Safety of transcervical endometrial resection. Lancet 1990;336:44.
76. Baumann R, Magos AL, Kay JDS, Turnbull AC. Absorption of glycine irrigating solution during transcervical resection of the endometrium. Br Med J 1990;300:304–305.
77. Boto TCA, Fowler CG, Cockroft S, Djahanbakch O. Absorption of irrigating fluid during transcervical resection of the endometrium. Br Med J 1990;330:748.
78. Istre O, Skajaa J, Schjoensby AP, et al. Changes in serum electrolytes of the transcervical resection of endometrium and submucous fibroids with the use of glycine 1.5% for uterine irrigation. Obstet Gynecol 1992;80:218–222.
79. Ankum WM, Vonk J. The spring balance: a simple monitoring system for fluid overload during hysteroscopic surgery. Lancet 1994;343:8.
80. Chandler CJ, Ford PM. Monitoring of fluid overload during hysteroscopic surgery. Lancet 1994;343:1368.
81. Loffer FD. Removal of large symptomatic intrauterine growths by the hysteroscopic resectoscope. Obstet Gynecol 1990;76:836–840.

82. Byers GF, Pinion S, Parkin DE, Chambers WA. Fluid absorption during transcervical resection of the endometrium. Gynaecol Endosc 1993;2:21–23.

83. Arieff AI, Ayus JC. Treatment of symptomatic hyponatremia: neither haste or waste. Critical Care Med 1991;19:748–751.

84. Berl T. Treating hyponatremia: what is all the controversy about? Ann Intern Med 1990;113:417–419.

85. Arieff AI. Hyponatremia, convulsions, respiratory arrest and permanent brain damage after elective surgery in healthy women. N Eng J Med 1986;314:1529–1539.

86. Fraser CL, Arieff AI. Fatal central diabetes mellitis and insipidus resulting from untreated hyponatremia: a new syndrome. Am Int Med 1990;112:113–119.

87. Ayus JC, Wheeler JM, Arieff AI. Postoperative hyponatremic encephalopathy in menstruant women. Ann Intern Med 1992;117:891–897.

88. Baggish MS, Brill AI, Rosenswieg B, *et al.* Fatal acute glycine and sorbitol toxicity during operative hysteroscopy, J Gynecol Surg 1993;9:137–143.

89. Arieff AI, Ayus JC. Endometrial ablation complicated by fatal hyponatremic encephalopathy. JAMA 1993;270:1230–1232.

90. Molnar BG, Broadbent JAM, Magos AL. Fluid overload risk score for endometrial resection. Gynaecol Endosc 1992;1:133–138.

91. Roesch RP, Stoelting RK, Lingeman JE, Kahnoski JR, Bacakes DJ, Gephardt SA. Ammonia toxicity resulting from glycine absorption during a transurethral resection of the prostate. Anesth 1983;58:577–579.

92. Kirwan PH, Ludlow J, Makepeace P, Layward E. Hyperammonaemia after transcervical resection of the endometrium. Brit J Obstet Gynaecol 1993;100:603–604.

Venous Air Embolism During Operative Hysteroscopy | 44

Philip G. Brooks

Introduction

A rare, but devastating complication of operative hysteroscopy is venous air entrapment and subsequent room-air embolization. While this phenomenon has been reported to occur during neurosurgical (1) and urological (2) surgery and at caesarean section (3), its occurrence during operative hysteroscopy has been cited only in obscure instances except as a complication of the inappropriate use of a dextran pump (4). Two cases were reported in letters to the editor of an anesthesia journal (5, 6), and one case was described in a letter to a British medical journal (7). Corson, in a recent publication on endoscopic air embolism in general (8), included several cases of hysteroscopic air embolism complications, some of which are included in this chapter. The author has been asked to review seven additional cases of this complication, either as a consultant for a hospital peer-review process or as an expert in a litigation. This chapter will describe these cases and the pathogenesis of this problem, with recommendations for its prevention and management when it occurs. Because some cases are still pending, they will be presented anonymously and with intentional minor changes.

Pathogenesis

In neurosurgery, when procedures are performed with the patient in the sitting position in order to gain access to posterior lesions, it is well recognized that, unless the brain is bathed in saline solution, opening venous sinuses in the calvarium or dura will permit venous air aspiration. This situation arises due to the fact that, because the heart is below the level of the brain, a negative intravenous pressure occurs with each diastolic relaxation of the heart (1). Such an event occurs in 25% to 50% of such neurosurgical operations, depending on the detection method. Once the air enters the venous circulation, foaming appears in the right side of the heart and blood outflow becomes obstructed, increasing the pulmonary arterial pressure. Early in the development of the problem, end-tidal CO_2 declines; ultimately, circulatory collapse and cardiac arrest occur. Because the pressure increases in the right side of the heart to levels higher than those in the left heart, the previously closed foramen ovale may open in more than 15% of adult patients, resulting in paradoxical embolism to the brain and other organs (1).

In gynecological procedures, the identical mechanism exists. Instead of the patient in the sitting position, however, his or her head is tipped down, putting the heart below the level of the uterus. If the surgeon opens some of the large sinuses deep in the myometrial wall and leaves an open passage to the outside, room air is aspirated into the venous circulation.

Review of cases

In addition to the three cases cited earlier from letters to the editors, seven cases of venous air embolism personally reviewed by the author are summarized in Table 44.1. Five of the patients were undergoing hysteroscopy for the management of abnormal uterine bleeding, one of which was following a spontaneous abortion. The other two were undergoing repair of intrauterine defects for fertility reasons, one a congenital defect (septum) and one an acquired defect (uterine synechiae). Five of these patients were stated to be in a Trendelenburg position, one was reported not to be tipped, and the other had no statement as to the degree of tip. Difficulty with dilating the cervix was reported in three of the seven procedures, two indicated no such difficulty, and no information was available on the other two. No correlation was found between the development of air embolism and the distention medium used, with three procedures employing carbon dioxide at appropriate flow and pressure, and three using different low-viscosity liquids; the remaining case had not yet started the hysteroscopy, as the first sign

Table 44.1. Summary of cases of venous air embolism occurring at operative hysteroscopy.

Case No.	Reason for Surgery	Trendel. Position?	Difficult Dilation?	Distention Medium	Time to Sign of Trouble	Clinical Signs	Result
1.	Uterine septum	Yes	n/s	CO_2	35 s	↓ E-T CO_2 ↓ PO_2	D.I.C., death
2.	Abnormal bleeding	n/s	yes	CO_2	9 min	Bradycardia; Doppler = bubbles, both sides of heart; septal defect	Coma, death
3.	Abnormal bleeding	yes	no	CO_2	10 min	Mill-wheel murmur; ↓ E-T CO_2 ↓ PO_2; Doppler = bubbles, both sides of heart	Hyperbaric chamber, survived
4.	Menorrhage	yes	yes	none	"after D&C only"	Bradycardia; ↓ E-T CO_2; CVP line withdrew bubbles	Death
5.	Menorrhage	no	yes	glycine	15 min	↓ E-T CO_2 ↓ PO_2; mill-wheel murmur.	Resuscitated, recovered
6.	Incomplete abortion	yes	no	Ringer's lactate	15 min	↓ PO_2 ↓ E-T CO_2; CVP line withdrew >50 cc bubbles	Death
7.	Synechiae	yes	n/s	saline	<10 min	↓ PO_2; bradycardia; inguinal crepitance; gas recovered from femoral vein and cardiac taps	Death

n/s = not stated.
E-T = end-tidal.

of trouble occurred at the end of a preceding dilation and curettage.

All of the complications emerged within 15 minutes after beginning the actual operative procedure. In each case the earliest signs of problems were dramatic changes noted by the anesthesiologist. These signs included either a sudden fall in end-tidal CO_2 measurements, bradycardia, a fall in oxygen saturation, or the presence of the classic sign of air in the heart, a mill-wheel type of murmur auscultated over the precordium. Confirmation of the presence of gas in the circulation was achieved in two cases with the use of emergency echocardiography and by needle or central venous pressure catheter aspiration in three others.

Five of the seven patients died from the complication, with the other two recovering. One recovery was attributed to the brilliance of the anesthesiologist in turning the patient onto her right side, rapidly infusing physiologic saline solution intravenously, confirming the condition with a transesophageal echocardiogram, and ordering the transfer of the patient to a hyperbaric chamber.

Discussion

Drawing from the understanding of the development of venous air embolism during other surgical procedures, a fairly clear pattern emerges as to how this complication happens during operative hysteroscopy. Very often—if not for every procedure—the patient's position on an operating table places the level of the heart and vena cava below the level of the uterus; this differential is often accentuated by requesting that the head of patient be tipped even more downward (Fig. 44.1), mainly so that weighted specula stay in place better. With the current use of video cameras for hysteroscopic procedures, almost no other reason exists to tip the patient.

When operative instruments are to be used, their larger caliber requires that the cervix be dilated more than with diagnostic instruments. This process can result in either occult lacerations and false passages at the level of the internal cervical os, or in partial penetrations into the

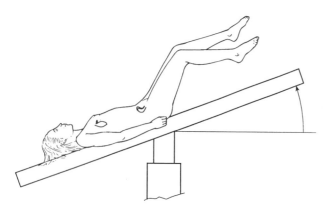

Fig. 44.1 Hysteroscopy in the Trendelenburg position.

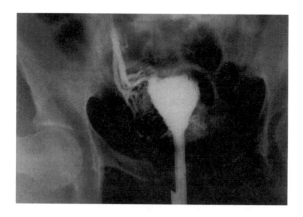

Fig. 44.2 Hysterogram showing a fistulous communication between the uterine cavity and a major uterine blood vessel, created by a deep biopsy. (Photo courtesy of Ray Garry, M.D.)

myometrial wall at the top of the fundus from a partly blunt dilator "popping" through the cervix after considerable force is applied to dilate the canal. At that point, while the surgeon is assembling and readying the operative instruments, the cervix and vagina are left open to room air and the negative pressure in the vascular tree literally sucks the air in.

Evidence for large sinus communication with the venous circulation has been shown brilliantly by Garry (9). In this research, following a biopsy deep into the myometrial wall, dye instilled at intrauterine pressure higher than venous pressure was seen radiographically to flow into the venous system at flow rates sufficient to give a clear venogram (Fig. 44.2). That cardiorespiratory function is altered so soon after the beginning of the procedure attests to the fact that the bubbles noted must be room air, as carbon dioxide (used in three of the cases) has a wide margin of safety at the flow rates and pressures used in hysteroscopy, even if insufflated directly into the venous circulation (10). Because of its high solubility in plasma, it would take much more time or much higher flow rates to create this condition using carbon dioxide.

Detection and management

Figure 44.3 shows the sensitivity of methods used to detect the presence of gas in the heart and great vessels and to monitor the subsequent physiological changes (8). Echocardiography, either by transesophageal probe or by precordial Doppler, may be the most sensitive technique to detect as little as 0.5 mL of gas bubbles in the heart (1). Neither method is widely used by anesthesiologists, especially for "low-risk" gynecological procedures, because of the high false-positive readings obtained. As noted in the case summaries, however, both techniques were used to define and document the event.

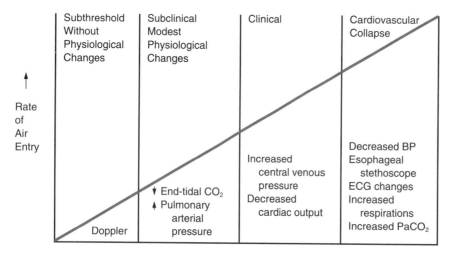

Fig. 44.3 Venous air embolism monitoring, showing the development of abnormal cardiorespiratory parameters as more air enters the vascular system. [Courtesy of Stephen L. Corson, M.D. (8).]

As more air enters the bloodstream, the fall in end-tidal CO_2 is highly sensitive and specific for embolism. Most patients undergoing general anesthesia today are monitored by capnography, making this one of the most important early signs. If a central venous pressure catheter is placed, either prior to the procedure (for high-risk patients) or during the procedure (as difficulties arise), elevation of intracardiac and pulmonary arterial pressures can be detected and monitored. Aspiration of the bubbles, when detected, can assist in the correction of the problem. As more gas is entrapped, the increasing resistance to blood flow results in hypoxia, decreased cardiac output, hypotension, tachypnea, and cardiac arrest. Resuscitative efforts at this point might be aided by stopping the source of the air inflow, turning the patient onto her right side, attempting to aspirate the bubbles as much as possible and flushing the circulation with a large saline bolus.

Prevention

The events in venous air embolism are so sudden and so severe as to make their management extremely difficult. Consequently, this complication often results in death or severe disability. It is obvious that prevention is the most important lesson from the review of this problem.

To begin with, avoid putting the patient in the Trendelenburg position. As noted earlier, the use of video cameras essentially eliminates the need to tip the patient head-down. Dilate the cervical canal with care, attempting to avoid lacerations and partial penetrations into the myometrial wall. After the dilation, do not leave the cervix and vagina open to room air for any length of time. If the instruments were not prepared before the dilation is performed, allow the vagina to close or place a wet gauze sponge or packing against the cervix while they are assembled. Another suggestion would be to leave the last dilator in the cervical canal until the surgeon is ready to insert the hysteroscope and start the distention gas or liquid flowing. The best protection against a complication due to venous air embolism is understanding how it develops.

REFERENCES

1. Shapiro HM, Drummond JC. Neurosurgical anesthesia and intracranial hypertension. In: Miller RD, ed. Anesthesia, 3rd ed. New York: Churchill Livingstone, 1990:1737–1789.
2. Albin MS, Ritter RR, Reinhart R, Erickson D, Rockwood A. Venous air embolism during radical retropubic prostatectomy. Anesth Analg 1992;74:151–153.
3. Lowenwirt IP, et al. Nonfatal venous air embolism during caesarean section: a case report and review of the literature. Obstet Gynecol Surv 1994;49:72.
4. Nachum Z, Kol S, Adir Y, Melamed Y. Massive air embolism—a possible cause of death after operative hysteroscopy using a 32% dextran-70 pump. Fertil Steril 1992;58:836–838.
5. Michael A. Endometrial ablation and air embolism (letter). Anaes Intens Care 1993;21:475.
6. Eugster D. Cardiac arrest during endometrial ablation (letter). Anaes Intens Care 1993;21:891–892.
7. Wood SM, Roberts FL. Air embolism during transcervical resection of endometrium (letter). Br Med J 1990;300:945.
8. Corson SL, Brooks PG, Soderstrom RM. Gynecologic endoscopic gas embolism. Fertil Steril 1996;65:529–533.
9. Garry R. Endometrial laser ablation. References Gynecol Obstet 1994;2:188–195.
10. Corson SL, Hoffman JJ, et al. Cardiopulmonary effects of direct venous CO_2 insufflation. J Reprod Med 1988;33:440–445.

Suboptimal Visualization at Hysteroscopy

45

Philip G. Brooks

Introduction

The single most important factor in performing either diagnostic or operative hysteroscopy is the need for a clear view. No accurate assessment of the uterine cavity or performance of precise and safe operative procedures is possible when the view is obscured by poor distention, poor light transmission, the presence of bubbles or particulate debris, or, especially, the presence of even small amounts of blood. This chapter will describe the techniques used to avoid these problems and their management when encountered.

Basic principles for good visualization

Whenever possible, hysteroscopy should be performed in the first half of the menstrual cycle and when no menstrual bleeding or abnormal uterine bleeding is present. Endometrium in the latter half of the cycle becomes thicker, more irregular, more vascular, and more friable. In addition to being mistaken for polypoid or hyperplastic tissue, secretory endometrium is likely to break apart and produce fragments that obscure the view. When employing a liquid distending medium, such fragments could also plug the small outflow ports or cause clouding of the medium.

While it is preferable to perform hysteroscopy in the absence of bleeding, waiting is not always feasible. In those instances, selection of the proper distention medium is essential, with high-viscosity liquids (such as dextran-70) being nonmiscible with blood, or with low-viscosity liquids (e.g., dextrose, saline, sorbital, glycine) and a continuous-flow system used to dilute and rinse away the blood.

When neither high-viscosity liquids nor continuous-flow instrumentation is immediately available, blood can be aspirated or rinsed from the uterine cavity with a syringe and a 3- or 4-mm soft Silastic catheter, such as that used by anesthesiologists for aspirating secretions within endotracheal tubes.

Occasionally, such as in preparation of the endometrium prior to ablation or suppression of blood loss to allow the treatment of anemia prior to any surgical intervention, drugs that inhibit the thickness and vascularity of the endometrium can prove very effective in reducing the chance of a poor image at hysteroscopy. In a study comparing endometrial histology after the administration of progestins (oral and injectable), danocrine, and a GnRH analog (leuprolide acetate-depot), we found that the GnRH analog provided the best suppression of all elements (thickness, glands, and vascularity); progestins were the least successful, with much abnormal vascularity resulting after their administration (1).

It is impossible to discuss adequacy of the view during hysteroscopy without mentioning the role of the light source and optics. Most hysteroscopy is performed with rigid 4-mm telescopes, although flexible hysteroscopes, with their promise of increased safety, have recently captured the interest of many hysteroscopists. The miniaturization of telescopes, however, has resulted in a reduced transmission of light into the uterus and back to the viewer. In most cases of rigid hysteroscopy with direct viewing through the eyepiece, a simple 150-W light source will provide an adequate image. When beam-splitting types of teaching attachments or video cameras are used, the additional reduction of light may require light sources of higher intensity, such as that provided by xenon bulbs. In addition, flexible hysteroscopes must utilize bundles of many tiny fibers that result in a necessary loss of light transmission through the spaces between the fibers. The Olympus Company (Olympus Corporation, Lake Success, New York) enhances light transmission via focusing lenses at the ends of its light cables that decrease divergence of the light rays.

Although beam-splitters and video cameras reduce the amount of light in and out of the uterus, they offer a significant advantage in minimizing the risks of a suboptimal view. Without them, trying to teach hysteroscopy or to show a visitor what the surgeon sees can prolong the procedure, increasing the likelihood of blood or bubbles obscuring the view. For the patient's sake, the rule should always be "complete the inspection first, then do the demonstrating to others."

In addition to using the most appropriate telescopes and light sources possible, several tips about technique will help to provide optimal visualization at hysteroscopy.

Whenever possible, the first instrument into a cervical canal should be the hysteroscope. Uterine sounds and cervical dilators are rarely necessary, provide very little useful information, and may fracture the small endocervical vessels, causing blood and mucus to be pushed up ahead of the telescope and greatly obscuring the view. Although the hysteroscope also fractures blood vessels, the bleeding it produces will remain behind the tip of the telescope and will be of little significance. This consideration is particularly important with CO_2 hysteroscopy where blood and bubbles, once developed, are hard to overcome.

When beginning a CO_2 hysteroscopy, always start with a low flow rate and a low pressure, and increase them once inside the endometrial cavity, if needed, An initially high flow rate may cause more bleeding and produce bubbles from the mucus present in the uterus or cervix. Our recommendation is to start with flow rates of 30 to $50\,cm^3$ per minute at most.

Once inside the uterine cavity, advance the hysteroscope directly to the top of the fundus, where most of the pathology and important anatomy are found. Inspect the rest of the lower segment and cervical canal on the way out. With this strategy, if bleeding begins during the procedure, the important viewing will be finished by the time it obscures the view.

As mentioned earlier, large amounts of blood can be aspirated with suction through a small cannula or rinsed out with some liquid, such as saline or a combination or dextrose and water. When using a hysteroscope with an operating channel, a small catheter can be inserted under direct visualization to aspirate blood and debris from the area of interest.

If only small amounts of blood or mucus on the lens of the hysteroscope clouds the view, gently touching the tip of the telescope to the top of the fundus usually cleans the lens. There is no need to remove the instrument and thus lose the uterine distention.

An experienced hysteroscopist should anticipate the possibility of encountering bleeding during diagnostic or operative procedures. When difficulties are encountered it is essential to be familiar with the availability and uses of other instrumentation and distention media. Changing from carbon dioxide or low-viscosity liquids to high-molecular-weight dextran (which is not miscible with blood) allows the distention medium to push the blood aside to allow visualization of the area immediately ahead of the hysteroscope. Switching to a continuous-flow system and a low-viscosity liquid allows continuous rinsing of blood out of the uterine cavity. In addition, when using liquid media delivered by gravity or infusion pump, surface bleeding vessels often can be compressed by slightly increasing the intrauterine pressure, thereby temporarily reducing the bleeding in order to complete the procedure.

The use of dilute pitressin to constrict small vessels and reduce bleeding is very beneficial. Injection of four to six units directly into cervical stroma produces transient ischemia, reducing the interference by bleeding (2). Because the cervix is dense, a large volume of liquid is difficult to inject. Therefore, a moderately concentrated solution of 10 units of pitressin in $10\,cm^3$ of saline (one unit per cm^3) is used, with approximately two units injected into each of three separate areas of the cervix.

False passages and uterine perforation

Perforation of the uterus is a rare complication of hysteroscopy. It can occur when the cervix is dilated to move the hysteroscope into the endometrial cavity (most often needed with the use of operative sheaths and accessory instruments) or when mechanical incision or use of laser or electrical energy results in penetration through the uterine wall. Often, the first hint that perforation has occurred is an obstruction of the view. In most cases of uterine perforation, immediate laparoscopy should be performed to ensure that the perforation has not lacerated parametrial vessels or damaged adjacent or adherent organs, and to verify that excessive bleeding at the perforation site does not exist.

When perforation occurs, the operator usually has no choice except termination of the procedure. Occasionally, if the perforation is small and not bleeding as viewed laparoscopically, it may be occluded with a blunt instrument inserted through an accessory laparoscopic cannula or squeezed closed with a grasping forceps sufficiently to provide adequate distention to complete the operation.

A note about false passages: Especially when larger diameter sheaths are employed to introduce operating instruments (e.g., resectoscopes, scissors), forceful dilation of the cervical canal can produce troughs or tunnels into the myometrium. Obviously, inserting the hysteroscope into a false passage produces a very poor view of the endometrial cavity. The tip-off that the telescope has entered a false passage is the appearance of the myometrial fibers, a criss-crossing network with spaces between the fibers. When this view is encountered, the first step is to stop the advancement of the telescope. Next, slowly retract the telescope until the correct passage is found and then try to advance it into the correct space. The pressure of the telescope and the distention medium will usually compress the false passage to reduce the bleeding and the loss of distention liquid into the myometrial vascular or lymphatic spaces.

Problems specific to distention

General

It is imperative to have good uterine distention to obtain an adequate panoramic view of the cavity. When a poor view is believed to reflect a lack of distention of the cavity, the surgeon should check that all tubing is connected correctly and that inflow stopcocks are open and outflow ones are closed (unless a continuous-flow system is employed). Next, verify whether the sheath or sheaths have accidentally come apart from the telescope due to inadvertent unlocking of the connecting catch or lock.

Finally, check for leakage around the sheath through an overly dilated cervix or one that is lacerated or patulous from childbirth or other causes. The use of laminaria tents has been recommended to assist in dilating the cervix for operative hysteroscopy (3). Occasionally, their use results in overdilation. When leakage of gas or liquid medium occurs through such a dilated cervix, the canal can be constricted using an additional tenaculum placed anteroposteriorly across the cervix at one side of the canal or with one of several instruments especially designed for this problem. A four-toothed tenaculum designed by Dr. Richard Gimpelson (Richard Wolf Medical Instruments Company, Rosemont, Illinois) (Fig. 45.1) and a conical canal-reducing device designed by Dr. Steven L. Corson (Karl Storz Endoscopy America, Inc., Culver City, California) (Fig. 45.2) are very handy to have available when this problem occurs.

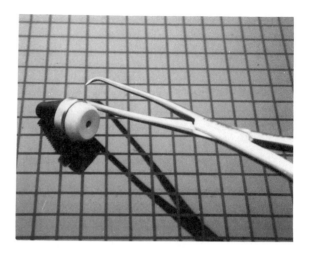

Fig. 45.2 The Corson cervical adapter reduces the size of the cervical canal, affording a tight seal and improving uterine distention.

Carbon dioxide distention

When used as a distention medium, carbon dioxide should be administered initially at very low flow rates to minimize the production of bubbles from the cervical mucus or the blood. In addition, a gas medium is inappropriate when electrosurgery is being used intrauterine, as the production of smoke or steam will cloud the view.

Distention with low-viscosity liquids

Suboptimal views may be produced when using these liquids by the immediate discoloring of the fluid by blood, as these media are highly miscible with blood. To correct this problem, the circulation or turnover of the liquid through the endometrial cavity should be increased. This step can be done by increasing the height of the inflow source (bags or bottles, if using gravity as inflow force) or by increasing the flow rate of the low-viscosity mechanical pump. Unfortunately, this process also increases the pressure driving the liquid, which heightens the risks of intravascular intravasation or regurgitation through the oviducts. The author prefers to increase the turnover of liquid inside the uterus by increasing the outflow via greater suction (negative) pressure attached to the outflow ports. This technique produces increased circulation without higher intrauterine pressure.

Occasionally, at the end of a procedure using low-viscosity liquid (as with resectoscopic ablations), excessive bleeding is observed when the inflow is halted. Usually this condition signifies that the inflow pressure was higher than the intravascular pressure, compressing the surface vessels and closing them during the procedure. To find the precise location of the bleeding points, the author prefers to open the inflow and outflow ports

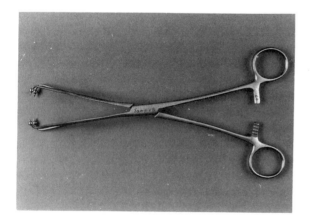

Fig. 45.1 The Gimpelson hysteroscopy tenaculum compresses the patulous cervical canal around the hysteroscope, affording a tight seal and improving uterine distention.

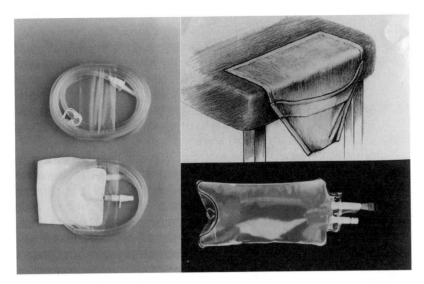

Fig. 45.3 Disposable fluid system for office liquid hysteroscopy (Disten–U–Flo, Circon ACMI, Stamford, Connecticut): tubing set (left), fluid pouch (top right), bag of fluid (bottom right). (Photos courtesy of Circon Corporation.)

and rinse the blood away. The outflow port is then closed, followed by the inflow port. If no leakage occurs, the pressure stays high and no bleeding is encountered. Next, the outflow port is opened slowly. The endometrial cavity should collapse gradually, and the reduction of intrauterine pressure results in bleeding from the open vessels that can be coagulated with electrosurgery or another method. This procedure can be repeated until all bleeding points are precisely delineated and stopped.

Until recently, continuous-flow equipment capable of rinsing debris and blood from the uterine cavity while maintaining optimal uterine distention was available only for operative procedures, such as that using the gynecological resectoscope. Diagnostic procedures using narrow-caliber instruments, especially for office hysteroscopy, could not be performed easily or with continuously rinsing low-viscosity liquids as no continuous-flow instrumentation of the caliber desired for painless and relatively atraumatic diagnostic hysteroscopy was available.

In recent years, several instrument companies have developed dual-channeled, continuous-flow sheaths for use with standard or miniaturized hysteroscopes and with physiologic low-viscosity fluids (e.g., saline, Ringer's lactate). In addition, in conjunction with Circon ACMI (Stamford, Connecticut), a very cost-effective fluid system has been designed. It consists of sterile, disposable inflow and outflow tubing, 250 or 500 cm³ bags of Ringer's lactate or normal saline solution, an under-buttocks fluid pouch to collect any fluid leaking from the vagina, and a collection bag at the end of the outflow tubing (Figs. 45.3 and 45.4).

Another problem occurring with low-viscosity liquids that obscures the view is the formation of bubbles, either from air in the inflow tubing or from carbon dioxide when cells are desiccated with laser or electrical energy. These bubbles always rise to the anterior part of the cavity. They can be removed by pushing the part of the

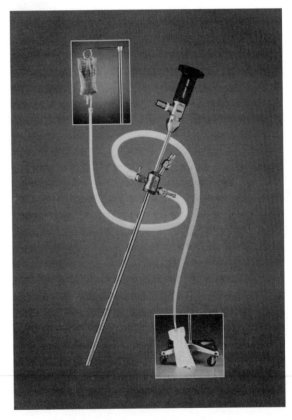

Fig. 45.4 Office hysteroscopy fluid system, assembled and attached to 5.5-mm continuous-flow sheath and telescope. (Photo courtesy of Circon Corporation.)

hysteroscope with the outflow ports into the bubbles and sucking them out the outflow system or by inserting a small cannula through the operating channel and aspirating the bubbles.

High-viscosity liquids

Because this medium is nonmiscible with blood, the view becomes obscured only when too little liquid is being infused, such as when the surgeon changes syringes during manual administration, or if particulate debris floats directly in front of the telescope. These problems are corrected by increasing the inflow, removing the debris with a suction catheter inserted into a separate channel, or removing the telescope and sheath and extracting the debris with a grasping or ovum forceps. Particulate debris often represents a greater problem with high-viscosity liquids because, with low-viscosity liquids, the debris falls to the bottom (posterior) part of the uterus and obscures the view only when it reaches a large volume, as when resecting a large myoma or polyp.

In conclusion, suboptimal visualization during hysteroscopy renders the procedure useless, but can be avoided or managed by understanding the use of accessory instruments or by switching to a distention medium and/or instrumentation system that can readily correct the problem. Rarely is it necessary to abandon the procedure for lack of a good view.

REFERENCES

1. Brooks PG, Serden SP, Davos I. Hormonal inhibition of the endometrium for resectoscopic endometrial ablation. Am J Obstet Gynecol 1991;164:1601–1609.
2. Corson SL, Brooks PG, Serden SP, Batzer FR, Gocial B. The effect of vasopressin administration during hysteroscopic surgery. J Reprod Med 1994;39:419–423.
3. Townsend DE, Richart RM, Paskowitz RA, Woolfork RE. "Roller-ball" coagulation of the endometrium. Obstet Gynecol 1990;76:310–314.

46 | Uterine Perforation: Endoscopic Complications and Treatment

Gerald J. Shirk

Introduction

Any invasive technique involving the uterine cavity carries with it the risk of uterine perforation. The current trend of treating and diagnosing many gynecological conditions by endoscopic visualization has increased both the risk and the incidence of this surgical complication. The procedures that may lead to perforation include uterine sounding, D&C, endometrial biopsy, insertion of an intrauterine device (IUD), therapeutic or elective abortion, hysteroscopy (both diagnostic and operative), and laparoscopy. Although this event has the potential to become a catastrophic complication, perforation does not always need to end with disastrous results if approached appropriately. The immediate concerns are intra-abdominal hemorrhage, trauma to intra-abdominal anatomical structures, the introduction of infection, the loss of a mechanical device intra-abdominally (in the case of an IUD), and thermal damage and/or fluid overload during operative hysteroscopy. Immediate recognition, evaluation, and treatment should significantly reduce immediate postoperative complications, diminish the development of long-term sequelae, and avoid disturbances in reproduction.

Anatomical and clinical correlates

When discussing uterine perforation and the appropriate clinical response, the significant issues are its incidence, the anatomical location in the uterine cavity, the patient's age, the type of procedure, the type of equipment used, the clinical setting, and the frequency with which this complication goes unrecognized and unreported by either ignorance or design.

Incidence

The incidence of uterine perforation reflects the type of procedure and the clinical experience of the surgeon. The inexperienced operator is associated with a greater occurrence of this problem, so teaching facilities generally have higher risk factors. In addition, each procedure may have differences in incidence due to technical or difficulty factors. The standard D&C in a reproductive female, for example, carries a perforation risk ranging from 0.6% to 1.3%. This risk increases to 2.6% in the postmenopausal female and to 5.1% for postpartum bleeding. The reported incidence of IUD-related perforation varies from 0.0% to 8.7%. Elective first-trimester abortions have an incidence of uterine perforation varying from 0.02% to 1.5% (1). Diagnostic hysteroscopy is associated with an incidence of 0.1% (2). The incidence of perforation during operative hysteroscopy has been reported to range from 1% to 3% (3). The difficulty of the operative procedure and problems with visualization influence the occurrence rates as well (4, 5). Operative hysteroscopy may involve both mechanical perforation and perforation by thermal energy without mechanical disruption of the uterine wall (6).

Documenting the perforation incidence for each procedure is important, but it is more important to know the type of serious injury that can occur during any given procedure.

Type of equipment used

Each instrument used in these procedures is associated with a unique set of risks and mechanism of causing injury. Diagnostic D&C, for example, remains the most common gynecological surgical procedure. The most frequent cause of perforation during this procedure is cervical dilation. Dilators are generally rigid, smooth metal rods that pose little risk to intra-abdominal structures (1). The main risk focuses on the introduction of infection, although the potential for blunt vascular injury must be considered.

The other tools used during a D&C are sharp rigid curettes, grasping forceps, and large aspiration curettes. The use of a sharp, rigid curette has been responsible for more serious injuries than any other instrument used to traumatize the uterine cavity. This tool has the potential to produce blunt and sharp injury. Its use is also indirectly responsible for most dilator injuries, as the need to create enough cervical dilation for introduction of the sharp curette causes the operator to increase the mechanical force and thereby increase the risk of fracturing the cervix or perforating the fundus. The blunt injuries are similar to the dilator injuries. The major risk from a sharp curette derives from its cutting action during the withdrawal process, which can lead to its introduction into the peritoneal cavity or broad ligament and subsequent damage to vital structures. Perforation with a sharp curette should be assumed to have created a major injury until proved otherwise (1).

The use of a small-bore suction curette (<7 mm) is less likely to create a major injury. Conversely, the use of a large-bore suction curette can cause serious problems. Intra-abdominal activation of the curette may produce significant trauma to the colon, small intestine, adnexa, vascular structures, and urinary tract structures (7). The traction forces from the suction curette can potentially pull bowel or other tissues into the wound, trapping these structures in the uterine wall defect (8).

Grasping forceps can cause two types of injury. First, they may perforate the uterine wall during forward manipulation and cause injuries similar to a sharp curette. Second, they may cause perforation by avulsion of the uterine wall. This type of injury has generally occurred in association with the mechanical transcervical removal of large submucosal leiomyoma (1).

Insertion of an intrauterine device carries the obvious risk of placing a foreign object in an unintended anatomical area. In particular, the IUD may perforate the fundus and enter the abdominal cavity. There it may introduce infection or cause an adhesive response (9). It may also perforate laterally and cause vascular injury. In the acutely retroflexed or anteflexed uterus, perforation may occur in the cervix.

Perforation during diagnostic hysteroscopy is unlikely because the introduction of the hysteroscope is performed under direct visualization. However, a number of these injuries do occur because of forceful advancement of the hysteroscope without visualization of the endocervical canal or the uterine cavity. This injury is a blunt type of injury (2).

The advent of advanced operative hysteroscopic surgical procedures using mechanical or thermal devices to remove or ablate tissue in the uterine cavity has resulted in different types of injury. These mechanical injuries resemble those produced by other mechanical instruments. The unique complications are the thermal injuries, which may or may not involve the mechanical penetration of the myometrium. The earliest reports of these problems surfaced during studies of transcervical sterilization by the use of electrocautery (10). The use of the Nd:YAG laser for endometrial ablation has resulted in several reported and unreported thermal bowel injuries (6). These complications were assumed to result from mechanical perforation of the uterine wall by the fiber with direct laser injury. A recent study indicated, however, that thermal damage to the bowel occurred in one procedure using a very-high-power (110-W), noncontact technique without perforation of the uterine wall by the fiber (6). The perforation of the uterine wall was linked to the thermal energy. Use of the resectoscope has a similar potential to cause thermal injuries either directly or indirectly. Recent reports have described resection damage to vascular structures, bowel, urinary bladder, and ureter (11, 12). The increased use of these modalities by inexperienced operators has significantly increased these injuries. The operative hysteroscopic procedures with complete or partial perforation have been associated with fluid distention media complications that have resulted in several deaths (13, 14).

Anatomical site

The most important factor related to uterine perforation may be the anatomical site affected (15). The fundus is the most frequent area of perforation in the nongravid uterus. The anterior and posterior walls and the fundus possess no major vascular structures. In contrast, the cornual areas are linked to a significant risk of vascular injury as well as a risk of damaging future child-bearing ability. Perforations in these areas caused by either sharp or suction curettage are also associated with a significant risk of injury to other intraperitoneal structures. The structures most frequently damaged are the bowel, omentum, adnexa, and occasionally urinary tract structures. Perforation sites in the cervix, lower uterine segment, or lateral uterine walls are less common, but can involve significant vascular injury to the uterine artery, perforation of the rectosigmoid, or urinary tract injury (15).

Type of procedure

Elective abortions represent the majority of D&C procedures. The lower uterine segment and cervix in the gravid uterus are the most frequent sites of perforation in such cases. The sites most commonly exposed to trauma in the gravid uterus are all associated with a significant risk of major vascular injury (15). The use of a large-bore suction curette is associated with a large number of intraperitoneal injuries caused by perforation in the fundus. Activation of the curette while intra-abdominal may produce significant trauma. Perforation of the gravid uterus is always significant because of the high risk of anatomical injury, hemorrhage, or complications due to inadequate removal of the remaining products of conception.

Operative hysteroscopic procedures carry not only risks of perforation from mechanical and thermal factors (as previously discussed), but also risks associated with the distention media being used (13, 14). Low-viscosity fluids are the media most frequently employed for these procedures. A complete defect in the uterine wall can lead to the loss of large volumes of these fluids into the peritoneal cavity or other pelvic spaces. In contrast, a partial perforation increases the risk of intravascular intravasation by opening larger peripheral vascular structures in the myometrium (16). If isotonic saline is used, the fluid overload is similar to cardiac failure. This fluid complication can be treated with diuresis and aggressive supportive therapy.

The use of nonelectrolytic solutions for procedures involving electrosurgical devices can create a significant electrolyte imbalance called the transurethral prostatectomy (TURP) syndrome. The result of severe hyponatremia, the TURP syndrome includes both severe cardiac and neurologic sequelae if not aggressively and immediately treated (17). In operative hysteroscopic procedures, severe hyponatremia has been determined to be the cause of brainstem herniation with death (18). This unique catastrophic sequelae has been reported only in menstrual-age females. If 32% dextran-70 solution (Hyskon) is used in the electrosurgical procedure, complications may include electrolyte imbalance, anaphylactic reaction, or adult respiratory distress syndrome (19).

Patient's age

The differences in incidence and cause of uterine perforation in the reproductive female reflect the surgical difficulties of these endoscopic operations. In an invasive intrauterine procedure on a menopausal female, atrophic changes can lead to cervical stenosis, loss of tissue elasticity, decreased myometrial thickness, and variable uterine depth. The chance of involvement of the myometrium with a malignant process increases dramatically. In the menstruating female, aggressive minimally invasive surgical procedures come with increased risks of accidental or inadvertent perforation as already described. Any increase in the technical difficulty of an invasive procedure increases the risk of uterine perforation.

Clinical setting

The clinical setting may play two roles in determining uterine perforation risks. First, it may change the incidence for a procedure. Second, it will probably determine—at least in part—how aggressively the problem is managed.

The hospital setting usually dictates that the patient is either under anesthesia or significantly sedated. The sedation may or may not decrease the technical difficulties of the surgery. In general, the types of procedures carried out in this setting will be more aggressive and operative in nature. Such an environment will probably encourage aggressive management if uterine perforation occurs.

The office setting is, in general, associated with minimal sedation. The increased patient discomfort may increase the technical challenges. The setting is typically used for only minimally traumatic procedures, however, with technically difficult procedures being avoided. If a uterine perforation does occur, management is likely to be minimized. The lower use of large or sharp objects that might cause a perforation reduces the risk of bleeding or intra-abdominal trauma. Nevertheless, minimizing the clinical evaluation still could have dire consequences. Transferring the patient to a care facility that has resources to adequately observe or surgically evaluate the patient should be considered.

Unrecognized and unreported complications

An unrecognized perforation can lead to delayed recognition of collateral damage. When bleeding, damage to visceral structures, or infection is induced but goes untreated, the sequelae are generally far more significant. The surgeon who recognizes the perforation, but fails to follow through with appropriate evaluation and treatment of collateral damage for whatever reasons may create unnecessary problems for the patient and surgeon. The incidence of this problem is unknown, but fortunately the biological system can usually tolerate iatrogenic injury without dire consequences.

Evaluation of uterine perforation

The aggressiveness with which a patient with uterine perforation is evaluated depends on the factors already discussed. Recognition is necessary to start this process. Informing the patient, if she is lucid, or her responsible guardian, if she is anesthetized or sedated, represents an important second step. All procedures should be terminated when such a problem is recognized to prevent further injury and, in hysteroscopic procedures, complications from distention media and the thermal unit. The clinical assessment of the type of injury dictates the decision whether to observe or to surgically evaluate the extent of visceral injuries.

All patients require immediate prophylactic antibiotic treatment. The regimen used should cover the anaerobic and aerobic bacteria encountered in the vaginal flora and should be administered by the intravenous or intramuscular route.

Operative hysteroscopic procedures that result in excessive loss of distention media present a more complex problem. Massive, rapid fluid loss at the beginning of a procedure is generally due to uterine wall perforation by the cervical dilators. If this type of loss occurs later in the procedure, it reflects a complication other than perforation. The only safety mechanism for recognizing this potential catastrophic occurrence is frequent careful monitoring of fluid deficits during the procedure. Observation is an appropriate strategy only when the perforation is caused by a blunt instrument (i.e., uterine sound, dilators, or diagnostic hysteroscope) and the location is in the midline of the fundus. Because the immediate risk from these injuries is hemorrhage, monitoring of blood pressure and pulse, measurement of serial hemoglobin and hematocrit, and continual assessment of acute abdominal signs are necessary. The length of the period of observation can be arbitrary, but must be adequate to rule out vascular injury. The hospital setting is the most controlled location in which to undertake this evaluation.

In all other instances, uterine perforation requires surgical evaluation (20, 21). This assessment can be best accomplished with multiple-puncture diagnostic laparoscopy (the least traumatic surgical means of evaluation) performed under general anesthesia. The site of perforation should be well defined. The significance of any injuries can be determined only by careful visualization, including a complete inspection of the length of the small bowel. The injuries for which the surgeon should investigate are determined by the clinical and anatomical correlates. If distention fluid from an operative hysteroscopic procedure is noted, it should be removed from the abdominal cavity to avoid the development of possible fluid complications.

Surgical treatment

Surgical evaluation and recognition can prevent surgical injuries from evolving into catastrophic medical problems in most instances (20, 21). The increased general use of laparoscopy has provided a minimally traumatic means of surgical assessment of uterine perforation. In most situations the injury can be repaired by operative laparoscopic techniques. If a vascular injury occurs, the vessel can be dissected under laparoscopic visualization. Hemostasis can be achieved by thermal means, hemoclips, or ligation. Defects in the uterine wall that are bleeding may be sutured. Injection of a 1:50 dilute solution of vasopressin in the uterine wall may facilitate this procedure.

Damage to the adnexal structures should be treated by operative laparoscopic technique. Partially avulsed structures must be treated for hemostasis and reconstructed when possible. The same procedures used in treating adnexal pathology can be applied to treating traumatic injuries.

Injuries to the bowel, urinary tract, and some vascular structures require surgical or urological consults. These injuries should be treated in a fashion similar to other traumatic injuries to these structures. Operative laparoscopic procedures can replace most laparotomies in repairing these injuries. Indeed, the rapid advance of general surgical use of operative laparoscopy has made available the expertise and equipment necessary.

Reich has reported on the laparoscopic repair of urinary bladder injuries and bowel injuries (22). Urinary bladder injuries must be inspected for possible ureteral compromise before closure with the standard two-layer repair. Perforating injuries to the rectosigmoid can be closed if the defect is small; the patient without a prepared colon who has a significant laceration is not a candidate for primary laparoscopic repair, however. Small bowel lacerations can be sutured by advanced operative laparoscopic techniques. Animal studies have shown that small bowel anastomosis is possible with a laparoscopic stapling device. Such surgery does not require a prepped bowel and is much less likely to be associated with further complications.

Vascular injuries, except those involving the great vessels, can be treated with either mechanical or thermal hemostasis. Bipolar cautery can desiccate all pelvic vessels to achieve rapid hemostasis. In addition, hemoclips can provide a means of achieving hemostasis in a rapid fashion. Before treating any vascular injury, a copious saline wash of the area and identification of all anatomical structures should be undertaken. Isolation of the damaged vessel is ideal.

Conclusion

Uterine perforation is a common gynecological surgical complication. This chapter has reviewed the causes and risks of this surgical complication. When discussing uterine perforation and the appropriate clinical response, the significant issues are its incidence, the anatomical location in the uterine cavity, the patient's age, the type of procedure, the type of equipment used, and the clinical setting.

Uterine perforation is a common complication of procedures that require instrumentation of the uterine cavity. Generally the consequences of this event can be minimal with appropriate care, including early recognition and appropriate diagnostic evaluation of the patient. Most patients can be clinically observed, although surgical exploration is indicated for any patient who has a risk of significant bleeding or injury to the abdominal contents. Laparoscopy is the best diagnostic procedure available under most circumstances. By use of this technique, patients can be adequately evaluated and treated with minimal cosmetic damage and long-term disability.

Operative laparoscopic treatment should not be undertaken if it is associated with risks significantly greater than those noted for laparotomy treatment. The treatment with the least risks is always the best procedure, as complications of complications automatically become medical-legal problems. This approach will lessen the possibility of further patient harm.

REFERENCES

1. Ben-Baruch G, Menczer J, Shalev J, Romem Y, Serr DM. Uterine perforation rates and postperforation management. Isr J Med Sci 1980;16:821–824.
2. Lindeman HJ. CO_2 hysteroscopies today. Endoscopy 1979; 11:94.
3. Hulka JA, Peterson HB, Phillips JM, et al. Operative hysteroscopy: American Association of Gynecologic Laparoscopists' 1993 membership survey. J Reprod Med 1993;38:572–573.
4. Loffer FD. Complications of hysteroscopy—their cause, prevention, and correction. JAAGL 1995;3:11–26.
5. March CM, Israel R, March AD. Hysteroscopic management of uterine adhesions. Am J Obstet Gynecol 1978;130:653–657.
6. Perry CP, Daniell JF, Gimpelson RJ. Bowel injury from Nd:YAG endometrial ablation. J Gyn Surg 1990;6:199–203.
7. Freiman SM, Wulff GJL. Management of uterine perforation following elective abortion. Ob Gyn 1977;50:647–650.
8. McArdle CR, Goldberg RP, Rachlin WS. Intrauterine small bowel entrapment and obstruction complicating suction abortion. Gastrointest Radiol 1984;9:239–240.
9. Connell EB. Intrauterine devices. In: Kase NG, Weingold AB, eds. Principles and practice of clinical gynecology. New York: John Wiley & Sons, 1983:1033–1057.
10. Guerror RQ, Ramos RA, Duran AA. Tubal electrocoagulation under hysteroscopic control. Contraception 1973;7:195–201.
11. Sullivan B, Kenney P, Seibel M. Hysteroscopic resection of fibroids with thermal injury to the sigmoid. Obstet Gynecol 1992;80:546–547.
12. Kivnick S, Kanter M. Bowel injury from rollerball ablation of the endometrium. Obstet Gynecol 1992;79:833–834.
13. Shirk G, Kaigh J. The use of low-viscosity fluids for hysteroscopy. JAAGL 1994;2:11–21.
14. Witz CA, Schenken RS, Silverberg KM, et al. Complications associated with the absorption of hysteroscopic fluid media. Fertil Steril 1993;60:745–756.
15. Berek JS, Stubblefield PG. Anatomical and clinical correlates of uterine perforation. Am J Ob Gyn 1979;135:181–184.
16. Vulgaropulos SP, Haley LC, Hulka JF. Intrauterine pressure and fluid absorption during continuous flow hysteroscopy. Am J Obstet Gynecol 1992;167:386–391.
17. Bernstein GT, Loughlin KR, Grittes RF. The physiological basis of the TURP syndrome. J Surg Res 1989;46:135–141.
18. Arieff AI, Ayus JC. Endometrial ablation complicated by fatal hyponatremic encephalopathy. JAMA 1993;270:1230–1232.
19. Mangar D, Gerson JI, Constantine RM, Lenzi V. Pulmonary edema and coagulopathy due to Hyskon (32% dextran-70) administration. Anesth Anal 1989;68:686–687.
20. Ben-Baruch G, Menczer J, Frenkel Y, Serr DM. Laparoscopy in the management of uterine perforation. J Reprod Med 1982;27:73–76.
21. Lauersen NH, Birnbaum S. Laparoscopy as a diagnostic and therapeutic technique in uterine perforations during first-trimester abortions. Am J Ob Gyn 1973;117:522–526.
22. Reich H, McGlynn F. Laparoscopic repair of bladder injury. Ob Gyn 1990;76:909–910.

Complications of Hysteroscopic Myomectomy | 47

Robin L. Molsberry and Robert S. Neuwirth

Introduction

Hysteroscopy has proved to be of great value in the management of symptomatic submucous myomas as well as in the management of dysfunctional uterine bleeding not responsive to medical therapy (1–6). Hysteroscopic myomectomy is performed by morcellation and removal of the tumor or tumors through the cervix. The techniques are electrosurgical using the resectoscope, laser using fiberoptically conducted laser through the hysteroscope, or mechanical with hysteroscopic visualization. The limits of the surgery are dependent on the size of the uterus and the extent of the submucous myomas. The use of gonadotropin-releasing hormone agonists preoperatively has made a larger number of cases operable (7–9). A larger variety of myomatous lesions can be treated hysteroscopically by laser or electrosurgical techniques, which morcellate in combination with mechanical removal. It is important to be aware, however, of contraindications for hysteroscopic myomectomy: size of the uterine cavity greater than 10 cm, adnexal pathology, acute or recent pelvic inflammatory diseases, pregnancy, and cervical cancer.

These hysteroscopic methods have proved to be cost-effective in that they shorten hospital stay, reduce recovery time and disability, and have a decreased incidence of postoperative morbidity relative to that for transabdominal myomectomy. Morbidity is lessened both immediately and in the long term. Indeed a vaginal delivery is to be anticipated rather than a scheduled cesarean section. Longer experience has shown that the approach offers continued or restored fertility as well as control of menorrhagia for the preponderance of patients for at least 5–10 years (4, 10–12). The attractiveness of the hysteroscopic myomectomy must be tempered by the complications that can occur. This chapter will review potential as well as observed complications. Specifically reviewed will be those complications associated with electrosurgical hysteroscopic myomectomy.

Types of complications

As in any surgical technique, the array of problems to be encountered is numerous, potentially involving endoscopic equipment, the surgical anatomy, and the operator's surgical skill. Also potential sources for misadventure are electrosurgical equipment, reactions to biomaterials, infection, hemorrhage, and anesthesia.

The endoscopy system

The equipment for electrosurgical hysteroscopic myomectomy consists of several systems. These include the illumination system and the visual monitoring system, the hysteroscopic cannula itself, the distention system, and the electrosurgical system.

Illumination

Illumination system complications are rare. A potential complication may arise from the fiber-optic bundle being left detached against the surgical drapes or the patient's skin. Although the bundle tip conveys "cold light," the radiant energy—particularly with high-intensity light for television and photography—can cause severe burns and fire. Attention to the intensity of light and bundle tip must be constant. Over- or underillumination may cause hysteroscopic errors of interpretation, particularly when using video monitor systems with endoscopy. In addition, changes in uterine color due to lighting or filters may create inaccurate endoscopic interpretation. Obviously, there should always be a back-up lighting system, as light failure during an operative procedure can lead to an unforeseen emergency.

Optical monitoring

The optical monitoring system includes the endoscopic system (rigid lens or flexible) and video or visual reading of the ocular lens. The major problems arising from the optical system are clarity of vision and orientation. As hysteroscopy is conducted in a small, possibly incompletely distended, and bloody chamber, adequate vision is critical. Part of the vision problem may be related to the distention system, but complications due to poor vision may also stem from the small distances from the objective lens to the object. Magnification produces problems of orientation in terms of diameter of field as well as depth of field. For example, in resection of a myoma, particularly near the base, the procedure nearing completion can be hazardous as the resectoscope may appear to be resecting myoma while in reality be excavating the uterine wall, leaving a perforation or a weakened myometrium. This situation has occurred in our experience, particularly when the operating surgeon is earlier on the learning curve with this equipment. A solution is to withdraw the endoscope to the internal cervical os repeatedly, thus regaining orientation to the uterine cavity, and to employ simultaneous laparoscopy for identification of perforation or near perforation (13, 14). Video surgery demands constant awareness of orientation. Understanding the orientation of the video camera to the ocular lens, and in turn the resectoscope's relation to the endometrial cavity, is essential.

Other visual problems can arise from tissue fragments in the field obstructing and/or positioned on the objective lens. These problems will be discussed under "Distention systems" below.

Surgical anatomy

Traumatic complications can occur that are unique to hysteroscopic procedures because of the surgical anatomy. These complications involve either perforation or laceration of the uterine wall or a burn through the thickness of the myometrium. A distorted uterine cavity is the challenge.

Cervical lacerations can occur secondary to excessively forceful use of the tenaculum or by forceful cervical dilation. Gentleness at this step is mandatory. The cannula used for hysteroscopy can be a problem at the level of the cervix. Noncontinuous flow systems are of smaller diameter and thus the small resectoscope, 18 French or less, more readily passes the cervix. However, the operating loops associated with the smaller resectoscope are small and may be unsatisfactory for large myomas. The larger instruments, 21–28 French, may be difficult to pass and cause cervical lacerations. A possible approach is to initiate dilatation with the smaller caliber instruments. Alternatively, slow dilatation of the cervix and careful use of Goodell dilators will often overcome the resistance. Laminaria tents have been used.

The curves of the cervical canal can be a potential site for perforation and must be negotiated under visual control. Uterine perforation may occur in the lower uterine segment and in the fundus as well, far beyond the internal os. Probes inserted into the tubal ostia can create false passage and perforate the uterotubal junctions (15). Neuwirth has reported one uterine perforation occurring during dissection of intrauterine adhesions, and a partial perforation with myometrial penetration in another patient (16). Gentile and Siegler report an inadvertent intestinal biopsy using hysteroscopic resection for Asherman's syndrome (17). In 733 cases of hysteroscopic sterilization, there were seven uterine perforations (0.95%), with three cases of bowel injury and secondary peritonitis (0.4%). There was one death from bowel perforation and peritonitis (18). Multiple lacerations of the cervix may force termination of the procedure. Perforations, however, must be recognized, the procedure immediately terminated and the patient observed.

One particular problem of surgical anatomy occurs when a large submucus myoma protrudes from the wall on a base not more than 3×4 cm and filling much of the cavity. In this circumstance, the beginning of the procedure must be semi-blind. Certainly laparoscopy is appropriate if the surgeon is not comfortable with the anatomical situation. To reduce the risk of damage in the blind area behind the myoma, two techniques can be used. In the first technique, a cutting loop progressively excises a groove in the center of the myoma to see behind it as the morcellation is completed. The other technique (19) is to utilize a high-energy grooved electrode to vaporize a groove in the myoma to provide a view of the far side of the myoma. The vaporizing electrode is convenient, as no tissue chips are produced, but requires great control because it employs power in the 200-W range. The loop technique has the disadvantage of producing tissue chips that may block the view at the objective lens of the hysteroscope and require removal.

Distention systems

The uterine distention aspects of resectoscopic surgery are most important and a critical factor in patient safety. Adequate uterine distention is mandatory. The necessary pressure and flow of distention demand constant awareness of both. A pressure of 50–80 mmHg is necessary for hysteroscopic viewing as well as intraoperative hemostasis by a tamponade effect. The pressure must be enough to distend the uterus but not cause rupture. Two hundred millimeters of mercury is the accepted pressure limit. Exceeding the pressure to enter uterine veins and lymphatics may lead to distention medium being absorbed into both intravascular and extravascular spaces. In excess this fluid may lead to several potentially serious complications. These complications have been reported with both low-viscosity and high-viscosity distending agents (5%, dextrose in water, 1.5% glycine, and 32% dextran-70, respectively).

Fluid overload with secondary congestive heart failure has been reported as well as noncardiogenic pulmonary edema (20–22). The latter effect, seen with dextran uniquely, has been postulated to occur secondary to a direct toxic effect on pulmonary capillaries. Hemodilutional complications reported include hyponatremia, and hyperglycemia along with dilutional disseminated intravascular coagulopathy (23–25). As these complications seem to be dose-related (with the exception of noncardiogenic pulmonary edema), prevention of cardiovascular overload or hemodilutional problems can only be accomplished by maintaining a continuous and accurate balance between inflow and outflow. It is important to be aware as well that in the case of 32% dextran-70, hypertonicity enables each cubic centimeter of this medium infused to hold approximately $8\,cm^3$ of body fluids (26). If the absorbed amount of distending medium exceeds 2 liters of low-viscosity liquid or $500\,cm^3$ of high-viscosity liquid, the procedure should be terminated as quickly as possible and special attention paid to the possibility of congestive failure and/or hemodilution. The management may consist of monitoring oxygen saturation, vital signs, urine output, and giving supplemental oxygen as well as diuretics.

The fluid flow must also be adequate to wash the objective lens and to keep the field relatively free of blood and debris to maintain visibility in the operative field. Although liquid medium used for uterine distention enters the cul-de-sac in those patients with patent tubes, this occurrence in and of itself does not seem to cause any adverse effects.

The electrosurgical system

Problems with electrosurgery can be categorized as those due to perforation, burn, or hemorrhage. Perforation can occur during insertion, manipulation, or activation of the instrument. The problems with perforations have been mentioned above. Remember, however, that during manipulation and extension of the electrode, perforation can occur. Alternatively, withdrawal of an activated electrode, where the loop is cutting deeply through the myometrium so as to excavate it, may lead to perforation into the peritoneal cavity or the broad ligament. Only under unusual circumstances is it acceptable to activate the electrode during an extension maneuver of the loop away from the operator.

Burns can occur in a variety of ways. The wiring may be exposed to the patient's skin and/or have damaged insulation. The external electrode may not be properly connected, and thus the current leaves the patient's body via an ECG lead or other grounding line causing an exit burn. The external electrode surface area may not be completely in contact with the patient's skin or the electrolyte paste not properly applied. In such instances, the exit of the electrosurgical current will cause heat generation at the exit locus that may reach a temperature and time of exposure sufficient to cause a second- or third-degree burn. Most modern electrosurgical generators will give warning or not function if the circuit is not complete between the generator and the patient. Nonetheless, the potential for burn must be understood by the surgeon.

Excessive burns in the operative field may also occur. This complication is more likely to occur with coagulation current that causes greater penetration of heat into the tissues. If the power is set too high, or the time of current application too long, a deeper and broader burn will occur and may penetrate through the myometrium. Bowel and bladder injuries are also possible. Ways to avoid these complications are detailed below.

First, become thoroughly familiar with the output of the generator and electrodes at various power settings, times of exposure, and with various electrode tips. Second, use simultaneous laparoscopy to observe the uterus (13, 14). Finally, inject an electrolyte solution into the pelvis to diffuse the electrosurgical current and thereby avoid adjacent bowel or bladder burns should the uterine serosa become burned.

The evolution of an unsuspected burn may occur over a period of up to seven days. The more serious burn will manifest earlier. If bowel is involved, the patient may experience abdominal discomfort, nausea, and pain secondary to ileus with or without peritonitis. A bladder fistula may cause symptoms of cystitis and ultimately uroperitoneum or external drainage. If one is concerned about the possibility of a penetrating burn, laparoscopy will usually clarify the question. The uterine surface will have a focal perforation or coagulated serosa. The bowel and bladder must be carefully inspected to determine if any thermal injury has developed. Laparotomy may be required to completely rule out bowel involvement. Observation with early diagnosis and immediate repair are the key.

Hemorrhage is less common than one might expect from hysteroscopic myomectomy. It can occur from a resection into the myometrium or perforation, particularly laterally into the broad ligament. It can also occur during mechanical removal of morcellated fragments of myoma that are not completely transected. Laceration into the surrounding tissues may occur by pulling on these incompletely resected fragments leading to hemorrhage. Another cause of bleeding is the coagulation current, which may cause the electrode to stick to the uterine wall and pull away tissue, again causing bleeding. Important in avoiding hemorrhage is gentleness in removing fragments from the uterus and verification of their complete resection. Management consists of cauterization of bleeding points or tamponade with a balloon at a pressure approaching systolic blood pressure. The balloon can be used prophylactically to avoid postoperative bleeding. About 50% of our patients are treated with the balloon tamponade for several hours postoperatively primarily for prophylaxis, although occasionally to control heavy bleeding at the end of the procedure (1, 27, 28). In severe cases laparotomy for uterine repair or hysterectomy may be required. In our series we have had two laparotomies for hemorrhage—one handled by repair alone, the other by hysterectomy.

Approximately 3% of our hysteroscopic myomectomy patients have been transfused during or shortly after the procedure (12).

Surgical complications

By surgical complications, we mean those not specific to hysteroscopic myomectomy itself. Those discussed here include infection, allergic reactions, and anesthetic-related complications.

Infection is a rare complication of hysteroscopy (16, 29). The frequency of infectious morbidity has ranged from 1 in 34 to 7 in 4000. In one series of 773 cases of hysteroscopic sterilization, 0.7% were complicated by postoperative endometritis (18). Hysteroscopy can exacerbate latent salpingitis, resulting in acute salpingitis with possible peritonitis, fever, adnexal swelling, and tenderness. These infections respond favorably to antibiotics and prophylactic antibiotics should be used. In general, however, there is a much lower rate of infectious morbidity compared with the abdominal approach for myomectomy. In our hysteroscopic myomectomy series, we have seen two cases of adnexitis requiring antibiotic therapy.

Although we have not seen allergic reactions to 32% dextran-70 in our operative series, others (30) have reported this phenomena, albeit rarely. Previous sensitization is required for allergic reaction, whether secondary to intraperitoneal instillation or secondary to oral sensitization by exposure to sugar beets and cross-reactivity with bacterial antigens from streptococci, pneumococci, and others (31). Taylor and Cumming report a patient who received $150\,cm^3$ of 32% dextran-70 for operative intrauterine device (IUD) removal and suffered intraoperative anaphylaxis (32). As well, anaphylactic reactions to dextran have been reported after intraperitoneal instillation (33). Local types of allergic reactions have also been reported (i.e., skin rash).

Anesthesia problems are also rare. One postoperative pneumonitis has occurred in our series secondary to general endotracheal tube anesthesia in a patient with a flu-like syndrome. On occasion epidural anesthesia has been used, but the majority of our patients have had general anesthesia.

Conclusion

In summary, operative hysteroscopy has many merits, especially for endometrial ablation and myomectomy. However, as with any surgical procedure, there are risks inherent in the specific procedure as well as those due to nonprocedure-related events.

In the modern-day market-oriented health systems, reduction in cost and/or hospitalization and/or recovery time to achieve a specific therapeutic goal is emphasized. The complications are understandably deemphasized. This chapter has attempted to explore the negative aspects of this surgery. As in all things the merits must outweigh the risks.

REFERENCES

1. Neuwirth RS. Hysteroscopic management of symptomatic submucous fibroids. Obstet Gynecol 1983;62:509–511.
2. Neuwirth RS. A new technique for and additional experience with hysteroscopic resection of submucous fibroids. Am J Obstet Gynecol 1978;131:91–94.
3. Neuwirth RS, Amin HK. Excision of submucous fibroids with hysteroscopic control. Am J Obstet Gynecol 1976;126:95–99.
4. DeCherney AH, Polan ML. Hysteroscopic management of intrauterine lesions and intractable uterine bleeding. Obstet Gynecol 1983;61:392–397.
5. Van Caillie TG. Electrocoagulation of the endometrium with the ball-end resectoscope. Obstet Gynecol 1989;74:425–427.
6. Baggish MS, Baltoyannis P. New techniques for laser ablation of the endometrium. Am J Obstet Gynecol 1988;159:287–292.
7. Coddington CC, Collins RL, Shawker TH, Anderson R, Loriaux DL, Winkle CA. Long acting gonadotrophin hormone-releasing hormone analog used to treat uteri. Fertil Steril 1986;45:624–629.
8. Friedman AJ, Rein MS, Atlas-Harrison D, Garfield JM, Doubilet PM. A randomized, placebo-controlled, doubled-blind study evaluating leuprolide acetate depot treatment before myomectomy. Fertil Steril 1989;52:728–733.
9. Donnez J, Gillerot S, Bourgonjon D, Clerckx F, Nisolle M. Neodymium:Yag laser hysteroscopy in large submucous fibroids. Fertil Steril 1990;54:999–1003.
10. Siegler AM, Valle RF. Therapeutic hysteroscopic procedures. Fertil Steril 1988;50:685–701.
11. March CM, Israel R. Gestational outcome following hysteroscopic lysis of adhesions. Fertil Steril 1981;36:455–459.
12. Neuwirth RS. Hysteroscopic therapy of fibroids. Clin Consult Obstet Gynecol 1990;2:43–46.
13. Levine RU, Neuwirth RS. Simultaneous laparoscopy and hysteroscopy for intrauterine adhesions. Obstet Gynecol 1973;42:441–445.
14. Cumming DC, Taylor PJ. Combined laparoscopy and hysteroscopy in the investigation of the infertile couple. Fertil Steril 1980;33:475–478.
15. Siegler AM, Kemmann E. Hysteroscopy. Obstet Gynecol Surv 1975;30:567.
16. Neuwirth RS. Endoscopic procedures. In: Gold JJ, Josimovich, eds. Gynecological endocrinology New York: Plenum, 1987:295–588.
17. Gentile GP, Siegler AM. Inadvertent intestinal biopsy during laparoscopy and hysteroscopy, a report of two cases. Fertil Steril 1981;36:402–404.
18. Darabi KF, Richart RM. Collaborative study on hysteroscopic sterilization procedures. Obstet Gynecol 1977;49:48–54.
19. Brooks PG. Resectocopic myoma vaporizer. J Reprod Med 1995;40:791–795.
20. Golan A, Siedner M, Bahar M, Ron-El R, Herman A, Caspi E. High-output left ventricular failure after dextran use in operative hysteroscopy. Fertil Steril 1990;51:939–941.
21. Zbella EA, Moise J, Carson SA. Noncardiogenic pulmonary edema secondary to intrauterine instillation of 32% dextran-70 Fertil Steril 1985;43:479–480.
22. Leake JF, Murphy AA, Zacur HA. Noncardiogenic pulmonary edema: a complication of operative hysteroscopy. Fertil Steril 1987;48:497–499.
23. Van Boven MJ, Singelyn F, Donnez J, Gribomont BF. Dilutional hyponatremia associated with intrauterine endoscopic laser surgery. Anesthesiology 1989;71:499.
24. Carson SA, Hubert GD, Schriock ED, Buster JE. Hyperglycemia and hyponatremia during operative hysteroscopy with 5% dextrose in water distention. Fertil Steril 1989;51:341–343.
25. Jedeikin R, Olsfanger D, Kessler I. Disseminated intravascular coagulopathy and adult respiratory distress syndrome: life-threatening complications of hysteroscopy. Am J Obstet Gynecol 1990;162:44.

26. Neuwirth RS, Richart RM. Hysteroscopic resection of submucous leiomyoma. Contemp Obstet Gynecol 1985;25:103–123.
27. Neuwirth RS, Amin HK, Schiffman BM. Hysteroscopic resection of intrauterine scars using a new technique. Obstet Gynecol 1982;60:111–114.
28. Neuwirth RS. A new way to manage submucous fibroids. Contemp Obstet Gynecol 1978;12:101–104.
29. Valle RF, Sciarra JJ. Current status of hysteroscopy in gynecologic practice. Fertil Steril 1979;32:619–632.
30. Trimbos-Kemper TCM, Veering BT. Anaphylactic shock from intracavitary 32% dextran-70 during hysteroscopy. Fertil Steril 1990;51:1053–1054.
31. Kohen M, Mattikow M, Middleton E Jr, Butsch DW. A study of three untoward reactions to dextran. J Allergy 1970;46:309.
32. Taylor PJ, Cumming DC. Hysteroscopy in 100 patients. Fertil Steril 1979;31:301–304.
33. Borten M, Siebert CP, Taymor KL. Recurrent anaphylactic reaction to intraperitoneal dextran 75 used for prevention of postsurgical adhesions. Obstet Gynecol 1982;61:755–757.

48 | Hysteroscopic Resection of Uterine Leiomyomata and Postoperative Hemorrhage

Alan B. Copperman and Alan H. DeCherney

Introduction

With the first report of a successful transvaginal resection of intrauterine myomata using a urological resectoscope, Neuwirth *et al.* introduced a new era of hysteroscopic surgery (1). Technological advances in fiber-optics and improved instrumentation and operator experience continue to make this procedure easier, improve its efficacy, and lower its associated morbidity. While various complications from operative hysteroscopy have been reported (and are discussed in other chapters), postoperative hemorrhage remains a relatively rare complication. With careful patient selection, proper preoperative evaluation and preparation, good surgical technique, and prompt recognition and treatment of complications, hysteroscopic myomectomy has become safer, and intraoperative and postoperative hemorrhage even more rare.

Preoperative evaluation of patients must include a thorough evaluation of the uterine cavity. This assessment can be performed using a variety of modalities, including ultrasonography, office hysteroscopy, formal hysterosalpingograhpy, and saline sonohysterography (Fig. 48.1) (2). If evaluation reveals large intracavitary pedunculated fibroids, totally insessile fibroids, or fibroids too large or too numerous to operate on primarily, the patient can be placed on a GnRH analog for a period of two to four months and reevaluated until surgery is considered safe.

Preoperative myoma treatment with GnRH analogs has been reported to reduce fibroid volume and mean intrauterine volume by as much as 40% (3). One study documented its efficacy as a short-term treatment (Fig. 48.2) (4). While shrinking the fibroids may facilitate surgery, the difference in mean operative blood loss may not be statistically significant. Unfortunately, the decreased myoma volume is temporary. Unless combined with definitive surgical treatment, the fibroids often grow back to their pretreatment size. While the literature continues to grow regarding the effects of GnRH on intramural fibroid volume, it is not clear whether these data can be extrapolated to submucosal fibroids. At present, it seems reasonable to pretreat patients with extremely large fibroids (greater than 4 cm) and patients requiring preoperative correction of anemia caused by menometrorrhagia. Finally, endometrial inhibition with GnRH analogs provides a favorable operative environment. Although concern has been expressed that GnRH-agonists may cause histopathologic changes secondary to estrogen deprivation, a large series of patients receiving prolonged treatment showed no evidence of GnRH-related deleterious effects on microscopic examination of the specimen (5).

When approaching myomas transabdominally, gynecologists have introduced a variety of techniques in an effort to prevent intraoperative and postoperative bleeding. The Bonney clamp has been used to grip the uterine arteries (6), rubber shod forceps have been employed to occlude uterine and ovarian vessels, and, on occasion, tourniquets have been placed through the broad ligament at the level of the uterocervical junction to occlude uterine vessels. The injection of vasopression or neosynephrine around the tumor intraoperatively has been advocated by some in an attempt to minimize blood loss, although others have not found this technique necessary or helpful (7). Despite use of these and other techniques, as many as 20% of patients experience bleeding significant enough to require transfusion (8, 9). In a randomized trial designed to compare these modalities, they all appeared to have similar efficacy; instead, operating time, total weight of fibroids removed, and preoperative uterine size remain the most important risk factors for intraoperative blood loss (10).

Before the modern resectoscope became available, the only alternative to an abdominal procedure was a rather primitive technique that involved grasping and ripping

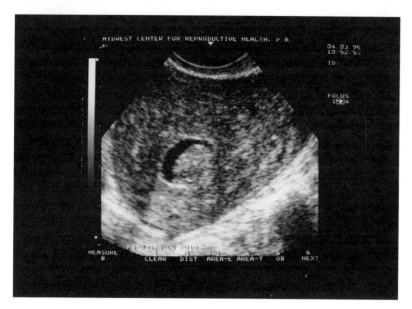

Fig. 48.1 Saline hystogram of a submucosal fibroid amenable to hysteroscopic resection.

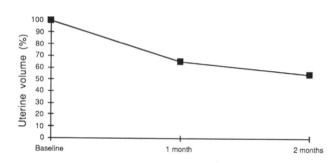

Fig. 48.2 Results of a short preoperative course of GnRH-agonist treatment on uterine volume in 27 patients with leiomyomas (4).

the fibroid from its uterine bed. Following cervical dilatation with laminaria tents, the myoma was grasped at its widest diameter and twisted to avulse it from its attachment. In one series, this procedure was performed successfully in 83 of 92 patients; in the remaining nine, all or part of the myoma could not be removed. Unfortunately, brisk hemorrhage followed removal of the myoma in five cases (11).

When the diagnostic hysteroscope was introduced, it became possible to visualize the uterine cavity before and after myomectomy. In an early case report, a 3 × 3 × 5 cm pedunculated fibroid was grasped with ovum forceps and twisted off its pedicle. Hysteroscopic examination of the uterine cavity revealed an intact cavity, although bleeding ensued. The operators were eventually able to control the bleeding by packing the uterus with 1-in. iodoform gauze. Packing was removed 12 hours later, and the patient's recovery was uneventful (1).

The hysteroscopic resection procedure

A thorough preoperative evaluation of the patient can often prevent episodes of intraoperative and postoperative hemorrhage. Certainly, attempting to elicit any history of abnormal bleeding and evaluating prothrombin time and activated partial thromboplastin time before operating on a patient with menometrorrhagia is prudent. Having the patient's blood typed and screened for atypical antibodies, assuring adequate anesthesia, and checking the adequacy of the surgical equipment are all steps that should be performed preoperatively as well.

Scattered reports exist in the literature of attempts to embolize large fibroids prior to myomectomy (12); it is unlikely, however, that this procedure will find widespread use prior to hysteroscopy. Hysterocopic resection of leiomyomata is then begun with the patient placed in the dorsal lithotomy position. The resectoscope is inserted, and flow of a distention medium is begun. Multiple fluids (and gases) have been evaluated for efficacy in this procedure. Many physicians prefer D5W or glycine over saline as physiological saline is too conductive for use with the resectoscope. Unfortunately, the low specific gravity of D5W makes visualization difficult if bleeding arises. Solutions of glycine (usually prepared in a concentration of 1.5 g/100 mL) have found wide use in transurethral prostatectomies and other urological procedures because they are nonviscous, clear, nonsticky, inexpensive, and well tolerated even if absorbed systemically. Because glycine mixes readily with blood, it rinses the blood rapidly out of the field of view (13). A combination of sorbitol and mannitol acts with similar efficacy.

The precise manipulation required for this procedure can also be facilitated by high-viscosity liquids, such as 32% dextran-70 (Hyskon, Pharmacia Labs, Piscataway, New Jersey). This medium minimizes transcervical loss of distending fluid. In addition, bleeding during manipulation occasionally becomes brisk and is more easily controlled via intermittent cauterization in this high-viscosity medium. The use of more than 300 cc of intravascular absorption of Hyskon has the potential to place the patient in cardiac arrest secondary to fluid overload. In addition, cases of anaphylaxis and coagulation disorders including disseminated intravascular coagulation have been associated with Hyskon (14, 15).

After distention is ensured, the gynecological resectoscope is inserted into the uterus under direct visualization. Use of a system that allows continuous flow of distending media is preferable. The distending fluid is brought to the resectoscope through large-bore urological tubing to ensure adequate flow, and standard operating-room wall suction or a gravity outflow is attached to the outflow channel. Initially, surgeons recommended a pure cutting current of 40 to 50 W, but it now appears that better results are achieved by beginning with 90 W. Small arterial bleeders are controlled with 50 W of pure coagulation current. To obtain the proper cutting effect, the generator should be activated immediately before the resection loop makes contact with the tissue. Care should be taken to coagulate sites of bleeding while performing the resection. If multiple points of bleeding are observed, the operator should reaffirm that fibroid—and not myometrium—is being resected. Although endometrial polyps can often be transected at their base because they are soft and can be delivered intact through the cervix, large intact myomas often cannot be extracted easily through the cervical os. In these cases, the fibroids can be resected into small chips before being removed by suction aspiration or blind grasping.

When current is applied, the resectoscope cuts easily through a leiomyoma to produce a shaving of the tissue. The tumor is progressively shaved down to the level of the endometrium. In general, this step should be performed by pulling the loop electrode toward the operator rather than pushing, thereby decreasing the chance of perforation. Vascular involvement, if present, is usually minor. The hemostasis of cut vessels is performed, one by one, with coagulating current. Once hemostasis is achieved, the cavity is drained, the fragments of fibroid are removed, and the cavity is inspected for bleeding and adequacy of resection. Some reports have indicated that

vasopressin may be a useful adjunct to prevent excessive bleeding. Theoretically, this agent will reduce uterine blood flow and cause myometrial contraction. Corson *et al.* recommended that 5 mL be injected on each side of the cervix, into the stroma, and at the junction with the vaginal mucosa, using a solution of 20 units diluted in 30 to 50 mL of saline (16). As bleeding is usually minimal, however, routine use of vasopressin does not seem warranted.

An alternative to the hysteroscopic resectoscope is use of laser to remove submucosal fibroids. The argon and neodymium:yttrium-aluminum-garnet (Nd:YAG) lasers can effectively perform this task, while the carbon dioxide laser has not proved as effective. In a series of abdominal myomectomies, conventional surgery was associated with a 71% higher blood loss than microlaser surgery (17). A similar finding has not been demonstrated in hysteroscopic resection of fibroids, however, and there appears to be little clinical difference in hemostatic properties between the resectoscope and laser techniques. Other alternatives to traditional myomectomy, including cryomyolysis, are under investigation (18).

Hemorrhagic complications

Hemorrhagic complications of hysteroscopic surgery can result from perforation of the uterine corpus. While superior or inferior perforations can cause bladder or bowel damage, lateral damage to broad ligament vessels often produces significant bleeding. These injuries can sometimes be prevented by concomitant laparoscopy. Certainly the novice should perform all operative hysteroscopies under laparoscopic visualization. Laparoscopy adds only minimally to the morbidity of the procedure as the patient is already under general anesthesia. In the event of uterine perforation, an assessment of damage should be made either by laparoscopy or exploratory laparotomy. Simple uterine perforations may be simply observed, while more extensive damage may require laparotomy and repair.

Published series of hysteroscopic myomectomies reveal a low rate of the postoperative bleeding. Clearly, many such series are performed by skilled surgeons with a great deal of operative experience. In one series of 61 submucous leiomyomas removed using the resectoscope, none was complicated by hemorrhage. The authors reported that all interventions were performed completely and final hemostasis was always obtained, with no blood transfusions required. With the exception of one perforation (recognized immediately and repaired by laparotomy), all patients were treated successfully (19). Corson and Brooks also reported good results on 92 patients undergoing resectoscopic myomectomy (16). Only one patient experienced heavy bleeding, and she was admitted and treated successfully with one unit of autologous blood and mechanical intrauterine balloon tamponade. Corson and Brooks' series also included three uterine perforations and one case of endometritis.

When bleeding is encountered, efforts should initially be made to coagulate the bleeding site. If this strategy is not successful, a 24-French, 30-mL Foley catheter can be inserted and partially inflated with up to 10 cc of fluid to tamponade the bleeding. In one series of 55 procedures, Loffer reports the need for Foley catheter to control excessive postoperative bleeding in three patients (20). If the cervix is widely dilated, a cerclage of absorbable suture may be necessary to hold the Foley catheter in place. In some early attempts at hysteroscopic myomectomy, postoperative oozing or delayed bleeding was treated by placing a silicon rubber uterine balloon stent to tamponade the raw surfaces. The conical balloon was inflated with air or sterile saline to a 20 mL volume—considerably higher than the average uterine volume (21).

After the bleeding is controlled, the patient should be brought to the recovery room with the Foley catheter in place. If she complains of significant discomfort from uterine distention, some of the fluid can be released. The catheter should remain in place for several hours, although occasionally achievement of hemostasis may require that it be left in for as long as 24 hours. When the balloon is deflated, it should be left inside the uterine cavity for at least one hour, allowing the operator to reinflate the balloon quickly in the event that brisk bleeding mandates continued tamponade.

Other authors have reported good results with use of a vasopressin pack for control of bleeding (22). In one series, 17 patients were treated successfully with a 1-in. new gauze pack soaked in dilute vasopressin (20 units in 30 mL normal saline solution). By leaving the pack in place for just one hour, hemostasis was achieved and maintained in all cases.

In the event that coagulation and tamponade do not control bleeding, the surgeon is faced with several options. The anesthesia team should have cross-matched blood available for possible transfusion, and coagulation studies should be drawn. Ultimately, exploratory laparotomy and either uterine artery or hypogastric artery ligation may be required. Transcatheter arterial embolization of the hypogastric artery and its distal branches may occasionally represent an option for persistent hemorrhage (23, 24). Ultimately, hysterectomy may be the definitive treatment.

Conclusion

Although submucous tumors constitute only 5% of all leiomyomata (25), their presence may have profound clinical significance, as they have been implicated in menometrorrhagia, infertility, and recurrent spontaneous abortions. A safe procedure for their removal has allowed for the preservation and possibly the improve-

ment of reproductive potential in many women (26). While there are potential risks of intraoperative or postoperative bleeding, bowel damage from perforation or electrical injury, and fluid overload and electrolyte imbalance from transtubal or intravascular flow of the distention medium, these events are rare in the hands of experienced and cautious endoscopists (27). When bleeding does occur, prompt recognition and treatment should prevent serious sequelae from this procedure.

REFERENCES

1. Neuwirth RS, Amin HK. Excision of submucous fibroids with hysteroscopic control. Am J Obstet Gynecol 1976;126:95–99.
2. Romano F, Cicinelli E, Anastasio PS, Epifani S, Fanelli F, Galantino P. Sonohysterography versus hysteroscopy for diagnosing endouterine abnormalities in fertile women. Int J Gynaecol Obstet 1994;45:253–260.
3. Fedele L, Vercellini P, Bianchi S, Brioschi D, Dorta M. Treatment with GnRH agonists before myomectomy and the risk of short-term myoma recurrence. Br J Obstet Gynecol 1990;97:393–396.
4. Coddington CC, Brzyski R, Hansen KA, Corley DR, McIntyre-Seltman K. Short term treatment with leuprolide acetate is a successful adjunct to surgical therapy of leiomyomas of the uterus. Surg Gynecol Obstet 1992;175:57–63.
5. Mukherjee T, Abadi M, Copperman AB, et al. The effect of extended gonadotropin releasing hormone agonist administration on uterine leiomyomata histopathology. J Gyn Surg 1996 (in press).
6. Bonney V. The technique and results of myomectomy. Lancet 1931;220:171–175.
7. Buttram VC, Reiter RC. Uterine leiomyomata: etiology, symptomatology, and management. Fertil Steril 1981;36:433–445.
8. Berkeley AS, DeCherney AH, Polan ML. Abdominal myomectomy and subsequent fertility. Surg Gynaecol Obstet 1983;156:319–322.
9. Lamorte AI, Lalwani S, Diamond MP. Morbidity associated wih abdominal myomectomy. Obstet Gynecol 1993;82:897–900.
10. Ginsberg ES, Benson CB, Garfield JM, Gleason RE, Friedman AJ. The effect of operative technique and uterine size on blood loss during myomectomy: a prospective randomized study. Fertil Steril 1993;60:956–962.
11. Goldrath MH. Vaginal removal of the pedunculated submucous myoma: the use of laminaria. Obstet Gynecol 1987;70:670–672.
12. Ravina JH, Bouret JM, Fried D, et al. Interet de l'embolisation preoperatoire des fibromes uterins: a propos d'une serie multicentrique de 31 cas. [Value of preoperative embolization of uterine fibroma: report of a multicenter series of 31 cases]. Contracept Fertil Sex 1995;23:45–49.
13. Haning RV, Harkins PG, Uehling DT. Preservation of fertility by transcervical resection of a benign mesodermal uterine tumor with a resectoscope and glycine distending medium. Fertil Steril 1980;33:209–210.
14. Witz CA, Silverberg KM, Burns WN, Schenken RS, Oliver DL. Complications associated with the absorption of hysteroscopic fluid media. Fertil Steril 1993;60:745–756.
15. Mangar D. Anaesthetic implications of 32% dextran-70 (Hyskon) during hysteroscopy: hysteroscopy syndrome. Can J Anaesth 1992;39:975–979.
16. Corson S, Brooks P. Resectoscopic myomectomy. Fertil Steril 1991;55:1041–1044.
17. McLaughlin DS. Metroplasty and myomectomy with the CO_2 laser for maximizing the preservation of normal tissue and minimizing blood loss. J Reprod Med 1985;30:1–9.
18. Jourdain O, Descamps P, Abusada N, et al. Treatment of fibromas. Eur J Obstet Gynecol Reprod Biol 1996;66:99–107.
19. Hallez JP, Netter A, Cartier R. Methodolgical intrauterine resection. Am J Obstet Gynecol 1987;156:1080–1084.

20. Loffer FD. Removal of large symptomatic interuterine growths by the hysteroscopic resectoscope. Obstet Gynecol 1990;76:836–840.
21. Neuwirth RS. A new technique for an additional experience with hysteroscopic resection of submucous fibroids. Am J Obstet Gynecol 1978;131:91–94.
22. Townsend DE. Vasopressin pack for treatment of bleeding after myoma resection. Am J Obstet Gynecol 1991;165:1405–1407.
23. Yamashita Y, Harada M, Yamamoto H, et al. Transcatheter arterial embolization of obstetric and gynaecological bleeding: efficacy and clinical outcome. Br J Radiol 1994;67:530–534.
24. Sproule MW, Bendomir AM, Grant KA, Reid AW. Embolisation of massive bleeding following hysterectomy, despite internal iliac artery ligation. Br J Obstet Gynaecol 1994;101:908–909.
25. Novak ER, Woodruff JD. Myoma and other benign tumors of the uterus. In: Gynecologic and obstetrics pathology, 8th ed. Philadelphia, London, Toronto: W.B. Saunders, 1979.
26. Neuwirth RS. Hysteroscopic management of symptomatic submucous fibroids. Obstet Gynecol 1983;62:509–511.
27. Brooks PG, Loffer FD, Serden SP. Resectoscopic removal of symptomatic intrauterine lesions. J Reprod Med 1989;34:435–437.

Uterine Fibroids: Difficulties with Tissue Removal | 49

Charles M. March

The hysteroscopic removal of submucosal leiomyomata was first shown to be feasible by Norment in 1956 (1). Following the introduction of a high-viscosity dextran medium, Hyskon hysteroscopy fluid, as a uterine-distending medium and the application of the urological resectoscope to intrauterine surgery as demonstrated by Neuwirth, this operation gained even more popularity (2). Further modification of the urological resectoscope by the addition of an outer sheath that facilitates continuous flow of low-viscosity media (e.g., G-5-W, 3.3% sorbitol, or 1.5% glycine) made the operation even more attractive because the volume of medium utilized could be monitored more accurately and conveniently.

Two types of submucosal myomas are accessible to removal by transcervical endoscopy: the pedunculated and the sessile. The approaches to resection and extraction of these tumors differ, however, and each poses its own type of challenge.

Removal of pedunculated myomas

In the case of a small pedunculated myoma with a readily identifiable stalk, the stalk may be transected by scissors or an Nd:YAG laser. The mass is then grasped with alligator jaw forceps and extracted together with the hysteroscope. If the mass is larger than 1 cm in diameter, it should be morcellated to facilitate removal and reduce the amount of trauma to the cervix. If morcellation of the tumor is impossible, the mass may be left in situ; it is then permitted to undergo degeneration and liquefaction and aborted spontaneously. If this approach is taken, the tumor should be biopsied to verify that it is benign and the patient should be advised that she will abort a piece of tissue 7 to 14 days after the procedure.

To obviate this type of problem, Goldrath has dilated the cervix as much as 3 cm to remove large tumors (3). This approach may lead to cervical incompetence and is not advised for patients who wish to conceive in the future. If the stalk of the myoma is not accessible, as in the case of pedunculated tumors that are on the most superior aspect of the fundus, the approach to resection and removal is the same as for sessile tumors.

Removal of sessile myomas

Although sessile myomas can be resected with scissors, this method is very tedious except for the smallest tumors. A hysteroscope through which a 600-nm quartz fiber delivering Nd:YAG laser energy can be passed or a continuous-flow resectoscope is the instrument of choice for resection of sessile myomas. As the resection progresses, the fragments of tumor should be pushed cephalad to the tumor mass so that a clear view is maintained. When a large amount of resected tissue is accumulated, the telescope and sheath are withdrawn and the fragments removed with polyp forceps (Fig. 49.1). This approach is continued until the resection is complete.

If the sessile tumor occupies the most superior portion of the fundus, gaining access to it may prove difficult, as can judging the proper depth of resection. In these instances, a straight loop electrode (or a 90° loop straightened) that remains in line with the rest of the electrode or is offset only minimally should be used. The removal is accomplished by passing the loop to and fro across the tumor. Extraction of the fragments is carried out as described above.

More recently, a disposable resectoscope sheath has been introduced. This device contains a suction-morcellator which aspirates and fragments the tumor masses as they are resected. It may prove to be the ultimate solution to this problem.

Other issues in myoma removal

Special consideration must be given to tumors that are larger than 5 cm, those that have a significant (more than 25%) intramural component, and those that are attached to opposing walls. Large tumors may require a long

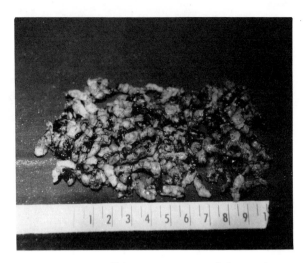

Fig. 49.1 Fragments of leiomyoma removed via resectoscope.

operating time with consequent absorption of a large amount of medium. If a significant portion of the myoma lies within the uterine wall, complete excision is not possible because the myometrial bed will bleed profusely. In such a case, the dissection is continued until the myoma has been "shaved down" to a level even with the adjacent normal myometrium (or perhaps a little below that point). Over the next few months, uterine contractions will likely force the residual tumor mass into the cavity where it will be readily accessible or may even be aborted spontaneously (4). An alternative approach was reported by Hallez, who exerted manual pressure transabdominally on the uterine wall to express the intramural portion of a submucosal myoma into the cavity (5). This technique permitted the entire myoma to be removed in one procedure.

A myoma on the opposing wall is a relative contraindication to hysteroscopic removal because of the risk that the two adjacent raw surfaces will adhere to one another. Although postoperative estrogen therapy has been used by some investigators, adhesions have devel-oped even after removal of solitary tumors (6). Although data are not available to address the relative risk of adhesion formation after resection of myomas on one or both walls, the author prefers to remove opposing wall myomas in two separate procedures.

The final approach to facilitate tissue removal is to shrink the myoma prior to excision, thereby presenting a smaller tumor mass. GnRH agonists such as leuprolide acetate or nafarelin used for two months prior to myomectomy are very effective in diminishing the size of myomas, especially those that are cellular and/or vascular. Concerns about reducing the tumor so much that it will "vanish" are probably more theoretical than real. The marked estrogen deficiency caused by a GnRH agonist will, however, lead to endometrial atrophy and perhaps predispose the patient to adhesion formation. More data are needed to establish the level of this risk.

A thorough preoperative investigation prior to hysteroscopic myomectomy is necessary to anticipate potential problems with removal of tissue. Hysterosalpingography, office hysteroscopy, ultrasound (preferably after saline infusion), and even magnetic resonance imaging may be needed to ensure that appropriate preoperative treatment is prescribed (if needed), that a one- or two-stage procedure is planned prior to surgery, that cervical trauma is minimized, and that steps are taken to reduce adhesion formation if child-bearing capacity is to be retained.

REFERENCES

1. Norment WB. The hysteroscope. Am J Obstet Gynecol 1956;71:426.
2. Neuwirth RS, Amin HF. Excision of submucous fibroids with hysteroscopic control. Am J Obstet Gynecol 1976;131:95.
3. Goldrath MH. Vaginal removal of the pedunculated submucous myoma. J Reprod Med 1990;35:921.
4. Donnez J, Gillerot S, Bourgonjon D, et al. Neodymium:YAG laser hysteroscopy in large submucous fibroids. Fertil Steril 1990;54:999.
5. Hallez JP. Single-stage total hysteroscopic myomectomies: indications, techniques, and results. Fertil Steril 1995;63:703.
6. Hallez JP, Netter A, Cartier R. Methodical intrauterine resection. Am J Obstet Gynecol 1987;156:1080.

Müllerian Fusion Defects: Complications with Resectoscopic and Laser Resection of Uterine Septums

50

Jeffrey B. Russell

Introduction

The proper diagnosis of the exact Müllerian deformity must be fully appreciated before any operative procedure can be undertaken. Historically, these abnormalities have been identified by physical examination and hysterosalpingography. Recently, however, ultrasound studies and magnetic resonance imaging (MRI) have aided in the diagnosis of Müllerian fusion defects (1). Specifically, transvaginal ultrasound has increased our ability to differentiate between septate and bicornuate uteruses (Figs. 50.1 and 50.2). Final diagnosis should be confirmed laparoscopically with external visualization of the uterus to identify one or two uterine corpuses. The fusion between the Müllerian ducts begins low in the uterine corpus, before it metamorphosizes completely from the dual system. To correct the defects that occur during the unification process, an understanding of the embryologic structures involved and their development is essential.

Hysteroscopic metroplasty is performed to alleviate problems with poor pregnancy outcome and recurrent pregnancy loss. Patients with a septate uterus are two to three times more likely to abort than those with a bicornuate uterus, and a complete septum is associated with an even higher pregnancy loss than in women with a partial or incomplete uterine septum. Buttram and Gibbons reported a 70% fetal loss in patients who had a partial septate uterus versus 80% of pregnancies in patients with a complete septate uterus (2). In a study of 240 pregnancies in 57 women before the uterine unification procedure was performed, 212 pregnancies resulted in miscarriage during the first or second trimester (3). Only 7 pregnancies subsequently went to term, with 21 pregnancies resulting in premature deliveries and only 12 of those premature infants surviving.

The etiology of recurrent pregnancy loss in patients having a uterine septum may be related to the poor blood supply, which could impair adequate implantation, or the septum's inability to expand as the fetus develops.

Perioperative

All patients should undergo a complete evaluation to eliminate all other causes of pregnancy loss before undergoing any metroplasty procedure. Patients presenting with a septate uterus prior to any documented loss of a pregnancy must be handled very carefully. They must be informed when a septum is discovered prior to any loss, as no controlled prospective information has been developed about the association between infertility and a septate uterus.

The objective of hysteroscopic metroplasty is to reduce the septum and provide one unique cavity without a division or interruption between the two halves of the uterine corpus. A preoperative evaluation of every patient must be performed similar to that conducted before any outpatient gynecologic endoscopic procedure. It involves an assessment of the patient's general health, including a thorough history and physical examination and an evaluation of current medications, previous surgical procedures, and any other medical problems. Discovery of medical problems that need further investigation may prompt a consultation with the appropriate physician. Patients with previous history of pelvic inflammatory disease, undiagnosed uterine bleeding, or pregnancy do not represent candidates for the procedure until these conditions are addressed. In addition, women with major medical or cardiovascular problems are not optimal surgical candidates. Thus, most patients undergoing hysteroscopic metroplasty are in excellent health without significant medical problems.

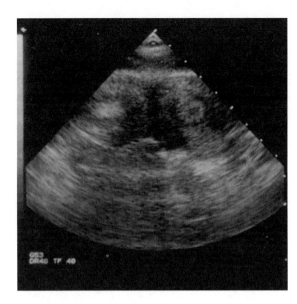

Fig. 50.1 Transvaginal ultrasound revealing two uterine cavities and two uterine corpuses (bicornuate uterus).

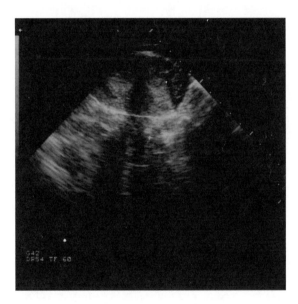

Fig. 50.2 Transvaginal ultrasound revealing one uterine corpus and two uterine cavities.

The procedure is usually undertaken in the follicular phase when pregnancy is unlikely and the endometrial lining is thin. Once the endometrial lining has been exposed to estrogen and proliferation of the endometrium has occurred, the procedure becomes slightly more difficult and carries an increased risk of infection and annoying bleeding. In addition, tubal osteums may be obscured with a thick, lush endometrial lining, making uterine landmarks more difficult to visualize. Patients with oligo-ovulation should have a negative pregnancy test, followed by a withdrawal bleed, before the procedure is approved.

Hysteroscopic metroplasty

Hysteroscopic metroplasty is performed with greater assurance of safety when combined with laparoscopy. The patient is placed under general endotracheal intubation due to the deep Trendelenburg position, which allows the laparoscopist to maneuver the uterine corpus away from the bowel during the resection of the uterine septum. The use of carbon dioxide infusion into the peritoneal cavity also facilitates examination of the uterus and surrounding structures and can help to eliminate the potential complications.

Media for distention of the uterine cavity include dextran-70 (Hyskon; Pharmacia Laboratories, New Jersey), carbon dioxide, normal saline, and glycine. Glycine is commonly used during urological procedures to avoid the high-viscosity problem frequently encountered during the infusion of Hyskon. Glycine, which does not conduct electricity, has not been associated with the sequelae of extravasation that can occur with the high amounts of pressure required for distention of the uterine cavity during the operative procedure. Although Hyskon produces bubbles during coagulation of the septum during the procedure, all liquid media have an advantage over the gaseous media because they provide a cooling effect on the uterine cavity and surrounding structures.

Several types of instruments are employed to perform the hysteroscopic metroplasty, including scissors (semi or rigid), urological resectoscopes, electric knives, rollerballs, and KTP 532, argon, or ND:YAG lasers. The ND:YAG laser has emerged as the best-suited laser for the intrauterine surgical procedure. Its power and depth of penetration produce an excellent coagulation effect while removing the septum.

Clinical outcomes

The classic Tompkins and Jones laparotomy procedure was initially performed for those patients with recurrent pregnancy loss who were identified as having a septated uterus (4, 5). It demonstrated excellent results, including a dramatic increase in the delivery of term infants. Hysteroscopic metroplasty was originally introduced by Edström in 1974 (6). Several years later Fayez compared the classic Tompkins procedure with the hysteroscopic metroplasty in two groups of patients with recurrent pregnancy loss; the study revealed a 71.4% pregnancy rate in the laparotomy group versus an 84% rate after the hysteroscopic procedure (7). Seventy-eight percent of those patients having transvaginal hysteroscopic metroplasty were delivered vaginally compared with 80% who had abdominal metroplasty performed. A small percentage (9%) of those patients who had undergone hysteroscopic metroplasty in the series of Fayez experienced a subsequent pregnancy loss.

The advantages of hysteroscopic metroplasty relate to the fact that the procedure can be performed on an outpatient basis without abdominal or uterine scarring and with minimal postoperative morbidity. In addition, little to no reduction in uterine volume is noted, pregnancy may be attempted soon after the operative procedure, and vaginal delivery is the typical mode of delivery. Studies have clearly identified transcervical hysteroscopic metroplasty as the treatment of choice for management of the uterine septums in those patients with repetitive reproductive loss (8, 9).

Complications of metroplasty

In 1986, DeCherney et al. reported resection of Müllerian fusion defects or uterine septums in 72 patients (9). They described the ability of the procedure to be performed with a septum less than 1 cm in width. As our experience with this technique has increased, so has our ability to resect larger and more vascular septums. However, the growth in the number of hysteroscopic metroplasty procedures performed has also been accompanied by more complications. These problems can arise from the actual introduction of the hysteroscope, the distending medium, the dissection itself, or the postoperative period. The actual frequency of hysteroscopic complications is difficult to estimate, as most reports come from case histories.

Complications related to introduction of the hysteroscope

The most common complication of hysteroscopic metroplasty occurs during introduction of the hysteroscope. In cervixes that have not been adequately dilated or have any amount of cervical stenosis, this instrument can penetrate the cervix and subsequently perforate the uterine corpus. Cervical stenosis clearly increases the resistance and contributes to uterine perforations. The appropriate way to relieve this problem is by slow, gentle dilatation of the cervical os with deliberate controlled insertion of the hysteroscope inside the uterine cavity. If excessive resistance is encountered with the insertion of the hysteroscope, it must be removed and further dilation performed.

If perforation has occurred, immediate identification and location of the perforation must be sought. Adequate visualization of the perforation to rule out any other organ damage must be immediately undertaken. Bleeding from the perforated area and any internal organ damage must be thoroughly evaluated before continuing with the metroplasty. If the bleeding is negligible and the patient is stable, resection of the septum may be attempted. If poor visualization is encountered because of the rapid exit of the distending medium through the uterine perforation, the procedure must be abandoned and should not be attempted for another three to six months. If the perforation reveals excessive bleeding, steps must be taken to arrest the active flow of blood from the area. These measures include initial observation, pressure, tamponade of the supporting blood vessels, and suture ligature of the perforation or the blood vessels supplying the area. Observation followed by pressure is usually sufficient to control most perforation bleeding caused by introduction of the hysteroscope. Serial hematological evaluations postoperatively will confirm cardiovascular stability.

Another complication with the introduction of the hysteroscope involves cervical laceration. Again, the area injured must be thoroughly evaluated. Any bleeding must be controlled and observation, pressure, or suture ligatures must be applied, if necessary.

Complications related to distention media

Distention media can cause several types of complications during hysteroscopic metroplasty. Several authors have reported that an air embolus to the heart with venous carbon dioxide infusion is a complication for hysteroscopic procedures (10, 11). A simple way to avoid this problem involves stethoscopic surveillance during the carbon dioxide infusion with the auscultation for characteristic metallic heart sound caused by the intracardiac presence of free carbon dioxide during the contractile phase. These typical metallic heart sounds appearing during hysteroscopy should immediately prompt an interruption of the procedure and withdrawal of the hysteroscope. The complication of carbon dioxide embolism during hysteroscopic procedures has been treated by McGraff et al. with hyperbaric oxygen therapy (12). Complications with air embolus to the cardiovascular system may be devastating. Immediate recognition of the problem and supportive measures are imperative for saving the patient's life.

Distending media can also lead to bleeding coagulopathies or anaphylaxis followed by acute respiratory insufficiency and pulmonary edema (13). Jedeikin et al. reported a bleeding coagulopathy with Hyskon with subsequent pulmonary complications (14). The infusion of glycine has been associated with metabolic risks as well. Boublai found significant fluctuations in blood levels of protein, hematocrit, glucose, and sodium in patients undergoing hysteroscopic surgery (15). Goland et al. reported high left ventricular output failure caused by extravasation of Hyskon to the systemic circulation (16). This extensive extravasation of dextran to the systemic circulation can also cause a significant shift of fluids from the third space during prolonged hysteroscopic procedures.

Other complications from distending media include vulvar and lower extremity swelling. These usually minor complications can easily be managed with bed rest and time.

The surgeon must keep track of the amount of

Hyskon used, and this fluid should be aspirated by the laparoscopist during the procedure. To minimize complications related to distention media, hysteroscopic metroplasties should be kept to less than 45 minutes. Recently, hysteroscopic pumps with constant irrigation and aspiration have been shown to alleviate fluid overload problems.

Dissection complications

When performing resection of the septum using rigid or semi-rigid scissors, electrocautery, or laser application, the division must be directed toward the center of the septum. Deviation anteriorly or posteriorly may destroy the endometrial cavity and cause thinning of the myometrial wall and subsequent perforation of the uterine corpus. Perforation of the uterine corpus is handled much like a perforation caused by introduction of the hysteroscope. Evaluation of the damaged area, observation, control of blood loss, and visualization of surrounding structures to assess damage must be immediately undertaken in the event of such an injury.

The most significant complication for the patient following perforation of the uterine corpus involves damage to the surrounding visceral contents (Fig. 50.3) The extent of the damage reflects the instrument used during the perforation. If the scissors perforate the uterine corpus, identification and visualization of the area injured is usually minimal. When damage is caused by electrocautery or laser, the depth or extent of injury may not be readily apparent because of intrinsic thermal damage.

To minimize damage to the pelvic contents, the laparoscopist should keep the peritoneal contents away from the uterine cavity. The pelvic contents may also be bathed in a Ringer's lactate solution to keep surfaces moist, thereby providing an additional level of safety.

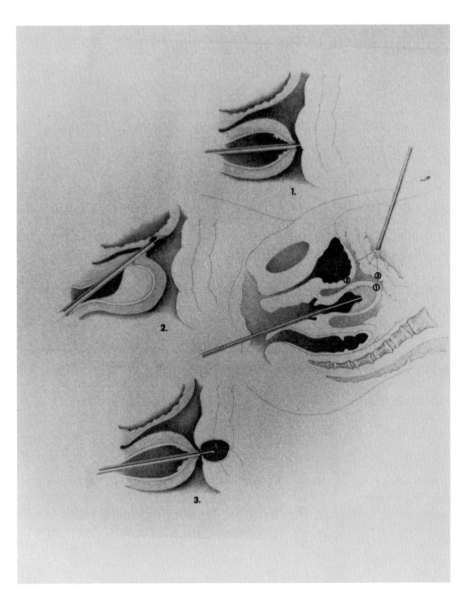

Fig. 50.3 Complications with hysteroscopic metroplasty: (1) uterine perforation; (2) uterine perforation with bladder injury; and (3) uterine perforation with bowel injury.

The assistant performing the laparoscopy can hold the bowel surface off the uterus to assure the surgeon that the bladder is completely empty. In addition, the operator can bring the uterine corpus up into the anterior pelvic cul-de-sac area to ensure an even greater margin of safety. Visualization of the hysteroscopic light by the laparoscopist may warn the operator of the thinness of the area being resected.

Occasionally electrocautery or the laser beam may enter into the abdominal cavity and injure the peritoneal contents, such as the bladder, bowel, or ureters. If this situation arises, the resection of the septum should cease and the extent of the injury should be evaluated immediately. Because the first concern is bleeding, hemostasis must be obtained as soon as possible. Landmarks of the area injured and surrounding organs must be identified before concluding the laparoscopy portion of the procedure if the operation is to be converted to an exploratory laparotomy. Locating the area of the burn or perforation at a later time may prove somewhat difficult once the orientation of the pelvic cavity changes and the area is approached abdominally. Hemostasis may be obtained with electrocautery or laser vaporization of the vessels, pressure, or suture ligature. Brisk, active bleeding should alert the surgeon to have the patient typed and crossed immediately for four units of blood. The anesthesiologist must be informed about possible volume depletion. Intraoperative consultation should be requested for areas unfamiliar to the surgeon prior to the appropriate reconstruction of the injured structure. Because hysteroscopic pelvic injury to the bowel or bladder occurs only infrequently, the assistance or consultation of the appropriate individual should be obtained without hesitation. The required resection of the injured area should be complete. The patient should be admitted to the hospital under the appropriate observation or drainage of the structure reconstructed.

Another complication encountered with transcervical hysteroscopic metroplasty is intrauterine bleeding. Because septums are avascular without adequate blood supply, bleeding is infrequently encountered. Occasionally, if the dissection is performed off midline and drifts posteriorly to the myometrial portion of the uterine corpus, venous or arterial bleeding may occur. Patience and observation will usually control most uterine bleeding. If this strategy proves unsuccessful, electrocauterizing the area with a resectoscope or using the defocused laser beam (or "nontouch" technique) to the area may coagulate the vessels. If this technique also is unsuccessful, pressure or tamponading the area manually represents an option. A pediatric Foley may be placed inside the intrauterine cavity to tamponade the walls of the uterus to inhibit further bleeding. Cessation of bleeding must be observed both internally and externally to ensure that the patient is stable and that bleeding has been controlled.

Hysteroscopic laser surgery carries a risk for the doctor as well as for the patient. The surgeon is at risk for eye injury from back scatter following tissue impact. Mandatory safety filters will eliminate this risk.

Postoperative complications

Late hemorrhage after resection of a uterine septum has been reported by Kazer et al. (17). They describe two women who presented with hemorrhage approximately seven days postoperatively. The area where the septum had been resected was identified hysteroscopically to be bleeding profusely. The patients were returned to surgery and the bleeding area was coagulated.

A long-term complication of transcervical division of a uterine septum is uterine rupture during the third trimester of a pregnancy. Women with a perforation during the hysteroscopic resection should be counseled about the possibility of a chronic defect and its potential complications. Several reports describe a uterine rupture during the third trimester incidentally with neonatal mortality and maternal morbidity (18, 19).

Conclusion

In summary, transcervical hysteroscopic metroplasty is an important procedure to perform in patients identified with a uterine septum and recurrent pregnancy loss unrelated to other physiological causes. The procedure can be performed with a high ratio of success and subsequent pregnancy outcome in the appropriately selected patients. It can be carried out in an outpatient setting without extensive abdominal or uterine resection, permitting the patient to achieve a quick and easy recovery.

Complications from the surgery may be encountered during any part of the procedure, from introduction of the hysteroscope, to final dissection of the septum (causing uterine or peritoneal organ damage), to postoperative recovery. Obeying the rules of power density and completely understanding laser physics should allow a safety factor for the hysteroscopist. Inexperience may also contribute to complications. All surgeons should be trained with hands-on courses and supervised during the early stages of the learning curve to treat Müllerian fusion defects. Although these complications are infrequent, they must be recognized immediately and treated appropriately. A consultation with the appropriate individual may be requested to assist with the reconstruction or repair of any damaged organs.

The successful completion of the transcervical hysteroscopic metroplasty procedure depends on the ability to handle any complications that may arise during the operation. This knowledge provides the surgeon with the confidence and the assurance to improve the patient's obstetrical outcome.

REFERENCES

1. Golan A, Langer, Bukovsky I, Caspi E. Congenital anomalies of the Müllerian system. Fertil Steril 1989;51:747.
2. Buttram VC, Gibbons WB. Müllerian anomalies: a proposed classification (an analysis of 144 cases). Fertil Steril 1979;32:40.
3. March CM, Israel R. Hysteroscopic management of recurrent abortion caused by septate uterus. Am J Obstet Gynecol 1987;156:834.
4. Rock JA, Jones HW Jr. The clinical management of the double uterus. Fertil Steril 1977;28:798.
5. Jones HW Jr. Reproductive impairment and the malformed uterus. Fertil Steril 1981;36:137.
6. Edström K. Intrauterine surgical procedures during hysteroscopy. Endoscopy 1974;6:175.
7. Fayez JA. Comparison between abdominal and hysteroscopic metroplasty. Obstet Gynecol 1986;68:399.
8. Daly DC, Tohan N, Walters C, Riddick DH, *et al.* Hysteroscopic resection of the uterine septum in the presence of a septate cervix. Fertil Steril 1983;39:560.
9. DeCherney AH, Russell JB, Graebe RA, Polan ML. Resectoscopic management of Müllerian fusion defects. Fertil Steril 1986;45:726.
10. Brundin J, Thomasson K. Cardiac gas embolism during carbon dioxide hysteroscopy: risk and management. Eur J Obstet Gynecol Reprod Biol 1989;33:241.
11. Obenhaus T, Maurer W. CO_2 embolism during hysteroscopy. Anesthesiologist 1990;39:243.
12. McGrath BJ, Zimmerman JE, Williams JF, Parnet J. Carbon dioxide embolism treated with hyperbaric oxygen. Can J Anaesthesia 1989;36:586.
13. McLucas B. Hyskon Complications in hysteroscopic surgery. Obstet Gynecol Surv 1991;46:196.
14. Jedeikin R, Olsfanger D, Kessler I. Disseminated intravascular coagulopathy and adult respiratory distress syndrome: life-threatening complications of hysteroscopy. Am J Obstet Gynecol 1990;162:44.
15. Boublai L, Blanc B, Bautrand E, Achilli Cornesse ME, Houvenaeghel M, Manelli JC, Aquaron R. Metabolic risks in surgical hysteroscopy. J Gynecol Obstet Biol Reprod 1990;19:217.
16. Golan A, Seidner M, Bahar M, Ron-El R, Herman A, Caspi E. High-output left ventricular failure after dextran use in an operative hysteroscopy. Fertil Steril 1990;54:939.
17. Kazer RR, Meyer K, Valle RF. Late hemorrhage after transcervical division of a uterine septum: a report of two cases. Fertil Steril 1992;57:930–932.
18. Howe RS. Third-trimester uterine rupture following hysteroscopic uterine perforation. Obstet Gynecol 1993;81:827–829.
19. Lobaugh ML, Bammel BM, Duke D, Webster BW. Uterine rupture during pregnancy in a patient with a history of hysteroscopic metroplasty. Obstet Gynecol 1994;83:838–840.

Acute Urinary Retention After Laparoscopy | 51

Samuel S. Thatcher and Piyush N. Joshi

The inability to urinate after laparoscopy has an unknown incidence with multiple etiologies possible. Undoubtedly, most laparoscopists have encountered this problem sporadically, either at the time of discharge from the ambulatory surgery center or that evening after an urgent call from the patient. As with most complications, awareness and defensive planning can significantly reduce the incidence of postsurgical urinary retention. When it occurs, this condition is easily treated with little long-term impact.

Risk factors

A careful urological and voiding history should not be initiated in an attempt to avoid complications, but rather as a component in the evaluation of all preoperative gynecological patients. Patients presenting with pelvic pain often have urological complaints. Depending on the nature of these findings, the proposed procedure may need to be altered to include preoperative or intraoperative urological evaluation and therapy.

A history including previous spinal, back, abdominal, or pelvic surgery could be responsible for compromise of the efferent or afferent nerve supply of the bladder. Nerve damage at any level may impact on bladder function. In particular, attention should be given to patients with a history of urinary retention after previous surgeries. Their past medical histories may reveal multiple sclerosis or diabetic neuropathy, which would place them at higher risk for detrusor dysfunction. Particularly prone to retention may be mentally retarded patients or patients with underlying central nervous system damage. A drug history may reveal β-adrenergic blockers or central-acting depressants used either as urological drugs or as therapy for other medical problems (Table 51.1). Preoperative ingestion of cold remedies (e.g., pseudoephedrine or cough suppressants containing parasympatholytics) can cause retention by increasing bladder neck and urethral closing pressure.

During the preoperative interview, questioning about the patient's typical voiding pattern may elicit important information. Nurses, teachers, waitresses, and others who void only when absolutely necessary may be at higher risk for retention but are easily overlooked. These "habitual holders" with large-volume bladders are characterized by early detrusor failure and "myogenic bladders." Preoperative urodynamic testing may aid in both diagnosis and management of the higher-risk patient.

Postanesthesia management

As surgeons become more aggressive and the array and complexity of procedures and patients broaden, the risk of major complications will increase. The once young, healthy, uncomplicated, "poststerilization" patients will become a minority. They will be replaced by older, more medically and surgically complex cases, requiring longer and more intensive postanesthetic recovery management.

As after laparotomy, anuria after obstruction of both ureters is possible but unlikely. It is also unlikely that the patient becomes anuric because of hypovolemia or renal compromise. While more common after open abdominal or vaginal procedures, the presence of packs or pessaries should be excluded as a cause of mechanical obstruction. Much more common is urinary retention; hence, catheterization should be performed on all patients before fluid boluses, or diuretics, are given. The surgeon should be notified whenever a catheterization is deemed necessary.

Reflex urethral spasm may follow any form of pelvic surgery. Furthermore, in a rush toward early discharge, a combination of anxiety and normal postoperative pain can inhibit urination. To counter this effect, patients should be handled in an unhurried atmosphere. Many experts do not consider urethral spasm to be due to smooth muscle activity, but rather overactivity of skeletal muscle. As such, it can be more reasonably treated with analgesics or relaxants, such as diazepam.

Table 51.1. Preoperative risk factors for urinary retention.

Constitutional
Previous episode
Large-capacity bladder

Medical
Diabetes mellitus
Multiple sclerosis
Mental retardation
Recurrent infections

Pharmacological
Cough and cold remedies
Pseudoephedrine
Propanthelein sodium
Oxybutynin chloride
Methenamine
Phenothiazines

Surgical
Spinal cord injury/surgery
Pelvic neurectomy

little detrusor tone. Probably the most common cause of retention is related to postoperative pain and/or the trauma to the pelvic structures. Almost any disturbance of pelvic viscera produces an increased urethral tone. Placement of a trocar near the dome of the bladder, ablation of endometrial implants, or transection of the uterosacral ligaments may contribute to urinary retention.

The bladder is primarily under cholinergic control with contributing ß-adrenergic action, while the urethra is an alpha-adrenergic control. Alpha-adrenergic stimulation will prompt contraction of the urethra but not the bladder, while beta-adrenergic component has the opposite effect. Consequently, it is easy to see why beta blockers can cause hypotonia of the bladder. Furthermore, the bladder is stimulated by a cholinergic activity and relaxed by anticholinergic activity (Fig. 51.1).

After laser laparoscopic surgery, two types of transient effects on the bladder may be noted. First, the detrusor may be paralyzed by direct manipulation of the bladder or laser fulguration of the bladder surface. Second, a

Patient management should be individualized after the initial catheterization. Few patients will require hospitalization, but discharge with an indwelling Foley catheter with leg bag may be advisable in some cases. It is probably better to send the patient home with a catheter than to have her return to the emergency room later that evening with symptoms of acute retention. The patient can be instructed to remove the catheter after 12 to 48 hours with a return to the physician's office only if voiding is impossible. One should heed the old adage that the drains should be withdrawn in the morning. Telephone follow-up is important and may be all the reassurance that is necessary.

All patients at risk for retention and patients who have experienced voiding difficulty in the recovery period should be encouraged not to wait for the urge to void. These patients are better managed on a "timed voiding" schedule. Sufficient analgesia should be given during the postoperative period to make voiding as comfortable as possible.

Neurological mechanism of retention

Urinary retention is a fairly common sequela of regional anesthesia and is often encountered in obstetric patients. Because virtually all laparoscopy is performed under general anesthesia, it is less likely that this anesthesia will have such an effect. The two major reasons for inability to void are either too much urethral tone or too

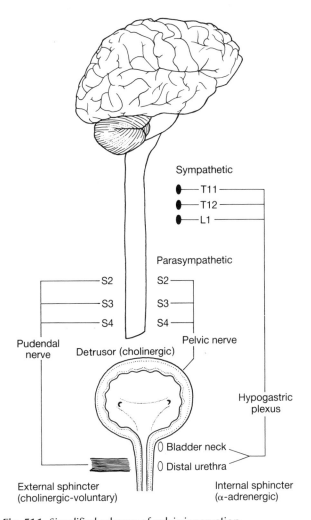

Fig. 51.1 Simplified scheme of pelvic innervation.

direct injury may affect the pelvic nerves of the bladder sulcus coursing between the bladder and broad ligament.

Pharmacology

Great care should be taken in prescribing urological medications unless a clear indication has been identified. For example, Ditropan is indicated for relief of reflex neurogenic bladder with frequency and urgency, but actually may exacerbate urinary retention. Uresid, which has an indication for inflammation and post-procedure pain, contains the parasympatholytic agents atropine and hysocyamine, which relax smooth muscle and may contribute to retention. In effect, these agents may inhibit initiation of micturation and exacerbate, rather than treat, retention.

While phenothiazines may inhibit urination, Phenergan and Vistaril, which have similarities to the phenothiazines, have not been associated with retention. Several drugs may have limited application, however. Urecholine increases detrusor tone when given at 25–50 mg three times daily. Hytrin and Cardene are alpha$_1$-receptor blockers that will decrease urethral tone and help diminish hesitancy from detrusor/internal sphincter dyssynergia. These potent drugs may cause significant hypotension and complicate the postoperative period. In general, attempts at pharmacological management of retention should be avoided in favor of analgesia and catheterization.

52 | Postoperative Nausea and Vomiting

Benjamin R. Jacobs and David G. Silverman

Seemingly identical patients undergoing identical surgeries in the care of the same physicians can experience varying postoperative courses with respect to nausea and vomiting. Thus, prevention of these symptoms is difficult. For several decades, the incidence of postoperative nausea and vomiting (PONV) following routine surgical procedures without prophylactic antiemetic therapy has remained at 15% to 40%, and is markedly higher after laparoscopic surgery (1–6).

Etiology and mechanisms

The etiology of nausea and vomiting is multifactorial and often difficult to identify. Four major neurotransmitter systems (dopamine, histamine, cholinergic, and serotonin) mediate emesis. Hence, a combination of drugs may have more antiemetic efficacy than single-drug therapy. Factors appear to interact at the vomiting center and the chemoreceptor trigger zone in the medullary region of the brain, with dopamine being a critical mediator. Physical and physiological factors (i.e., gastric distention, oral intake, movement, pain, and hemodynamic instability) affect these medullary centers as well.

Opioids are analgesic agents that induce nausea and vomiting. Their role may arise from the fact that they partially activate dopamine receptors at the chemoreceptor trigger zone. This explanation is consistent with the fact that dopamine antagonists (e.g., droperidol) are often effective in counteracting nausea and vomiting.

Adverse consequences

In 1899, Blumfield (7) wrote, "It matters little to the average patient how skillfully his anesthetic was administered, but how pleasant or unpleasant his experiences are once he returns to consciousness." Nausea and vomiting both significantly affect such experiences. A recent study involving patients undergoing outpatient laparoscopy noted that, when nausea was present, the post-anesthesia care unit (PACU) stay was prolonged by 19 minutes, as was the inability to take oral fluids; for patients experiencing both nausea and vomiting, these periods were extended by 47 minutes (8). Protracted postoperative vomiting is the leading reason for non-scheduled hospital admission from the PACU after outpatient surgery.

Vomiting is not only unpleasant, but also may lead to volume depletion, electrolyte imbalance, aspiration of gastric contents, wound dehiscence, and esophageal rupture. Fortunately, however, the incidence of such severe sequelae is low.

In most situations, treatment is indicated if a patient is vomiting. The hazards associated with a single dose of most antiemetics are small compared with the consequences and inconvenience of vomiting.

Prophylaxis and treatment

During the preoperative interview, the physician should attempt to determine whether the patient is susceptible to PONV (Table 52.1). This susceptibility may be indicated by a history of motion sickness or nausea and vomiting following previous surgeries. When a patient at increased "risk" presents, one must carefully organize the perioperative use of antiemetics (see Tables 52.2 and 52.3 for recommended doses), gastric emptying techniques, narcotics and other anesthetic agents, local or regional block supplementation, and regional anesthesia.

The most effective prophylaxis involves minimizing risk factors. The patient should receive the following care:

1. Receive positive reassurance by the physicians to help allay anxiety.

2. Be moved slowly at all times to avoid motion sickness.
3. Have a warm blanket to enhance the sense of security.
4. Have minimal pharyngeal suction at the conclusion of surgery to avoid stimulation of the gag reflex.
5. Be allowed to awaken slowly in the PACU.

Table 52.1. "Risk factors" for postoperative nausea and vomiting.

Age: young > old (peak incidence 11–14 year age group)
Ambulatory surgery
Anesthetic gases (e.g., enflurane, isoflurane, halothane)
Anxiety
Duration of surgery/anesthesia (longer surgery → ↑ PONV)
Gastric distention
Hemodynamic instability
History of postoperative nausea and/or vomiting
History of motion sickness
Movement: transport from operating room to PACU
Narcotic administration
Nitrous oxide (?)
Obesity
Pain
Pharyngeal stimulation
Position: sitting > supine
Postoperative oral intake
Preexistent medical problems (e.g., uremia)
Proximity to vomiting patient
Sex: females > males, especially during weeks 3 and 4 of menstrual cycle
Site of surgery: intraperitoneal > extraperitoneal

PACU, postanesthesia care unit.

Routine antiemetic prophylaxis for patients undergoing elective surgery is not currently justified due to the cost involved and possible side effects (e.g., sedation, dysphoria, extrapyramidal symptoms). Prophylaxis is justified, however, in patients at markedly increased risk for PONV. Minor procedures, such as emptying the stomach via an orogastric tube after the induction of anesthesia, have been shown to reduce the incidence of nausea in patients undergoing laparoscopic surgery (9).

When practical, regional anesthesia is preferable to general anesthesia for ambulatory surgical patients because it has a lower incidence of PONV than does general anesthesia, and consequently earlier discharge from the facility. Epidural anesthesia was administered to 50% of laparoscopy cases in a study at the Virginia Mason Hospital (Seattle, Washington). Following laparoscopy, nausea and vomiting were present in 38% of general anesthesia patients, compared with only 4% of those who received epidural anesthesia (1). PONV associated with epidural anesthesia is often a result of a rapid decline in arterial blood pressure. In addition to administration of 100% oxygen and use of the Trendelenburg position, atropine may prove beneficial, suggesting that nausea and vomiting may have a vagal component.

Total intravenous anesthesia (TIVA) is another method of administering anesthesia that may decrease the incidence of PONV. Propofol is a relatively new intravenous anesthetic structurally unrelated to the other sedative-hypnotics (e.g., sodium pentothal). It has been shown to have a lower incidence of postoperative emesis (1%–3%) compared with other intravenous agents (11%–15%) (10). Propofol is extremely popular in outpatient anesthesia because of its favorable recovery characteristics, including rapid emergence and low incidence of postoperative side effects. TIVA can safely be given with a benzodiazepine, propofol, narcotic, oxygen, and nitrous oxide. For patients at increased risk for PONV, narcotics and nitrous oxide can be omitted.

Table 52.2. Pharmacological prophylaxis of postoperative nausea and vomiting.

Drug	Dose (mg)	Route	Time of Administration
Droperidol (Inapsine)	0.625–1.25	IV	15–30 minutes prior to conclusion of surgery
Ephedrine	25	IM	15–30 minutes prior to conclusion of surgery
Hyoscine (Scopolamine)	1.5	Transdermal patch	3–12 hours prior to surgery
Metoclopramide (Reglan)	10	IV	15–30 minutes prior to conclusion of surgery
Ondansetron (Zofran)	8	PO	1 hour prior to surgery
Ondansetron (Zofran)	4–8	IV	Induction of anesthesia
Prochlorperazine (Compazine)	5–10	IM	Induction of anesthesia
Thiethylperazine (Norzine, Torecan)	10	IM	Induction of anesthesia

IM, intramuscular; IV, intravenous; PO, orally.

Table 52.3. Pharmacological treatment of postoperative nausea and vomiting.

Drug	Dose (mg)	Route of Administration
Droperidol (Inapsine)	0.625–1.25	IV
Ephedrine	5–25	IV, IM
Metoclopramide (Reglan)	10	IV, IM
Ondansetron (Zofran)	4–8	IV
Prochlorperazine (Compazine)	5–10	IV, IM, PR
Thiethylperazine (Norzine, Torecan)	10	IM, PR

IM, intramuscular; IV, intravenous; PR, per rectum.

Once a patient has begun to vomit, many physicians tend to rely primarily upon antiemetic drugs and to withhold narcotics. Pain itself can cause nausea and vomiting, however, and active retching may produce more pain from subsequent stress on the incision site. Effective analgesia may be achieved with local and regional analgesic techniques and nonnarcotic analgesics. Potent nonopioid analgesics (e.g., ketorolac) can be used for pain control while avoiding opioid-related side effects. If pain persists, narcotics may be necessary even though they can induce nausea and vomiting.

Several practical measures can be taken to reduce the patient's discomfort. The vomiting patient should be given more intravenous fluids—enough to offset hypotension caused by fluid loss and antiemetic drugs. Assuming adequate oxygenation, the patient should not be made to keep the oxygen mask in place while nauseated, as it often exacerbates the unpleasant stuffiness experienced by some patients. The nursing staff frequently encourages patients to take deep breaths when they feel nauseated. Although not clearly understood, this tactic is well recognized as an effective way to decrease nausea. Monitoring of the severely nauseated or vomiting patient should be continued for an hour or more in the PACU. While such monitoring does not guarantee a reduction in symptoms, it does enable observation of the patient's progress.

Although many drugs have been evaluated, no single drug has emerged as an effective prophylactic antiemetic or therapy. Because antiemetics are not entirely innocuous, and newer agents can be quite costly, aggressive prophylaxis is not routine and is typically reserved for the patients at highest risk.

Anticholinergics

Scopolamine (hyoscine) crosses the blood–brain barrier and blocks cholinergic stimulation of the vomiting center from both the gastrointestinal tract and the vestibular center. Although scopolamine is an effective antiemetic, its perioperative use has been limited by the fact that its intramuscular or intravenous administration produces relatively high plasma concentrations and is associated with a high incidence of undesirable side effects. The principal side effects are dry mouth, sedation, mydriasis, and disorientation. In addition, its antiemetic efficacy is limited with parenteral administration because of its short (1 hour) elimination half-life. This limitation has prompted development of a 0.2-mm-thick patch containing 1.5 mg of scopolamine, which delivers 5 µg/hour at a constant rate over 72 hours (total absorbed dose <0.5 mg). The patch requires three hours before providing a steady blood concentration.

Bailey *et al.* demonstrated that the transdermal scopolamine patch significantly decreased the incidence of postoperative nausea and vomiting versus placebo after outpatient laparoscopy (4). A significantly higher incidence of side effects (dry mouth, sedation, amblyopia, mydriasis, and dizziness) was noted with scopolamine than with placebo. In this study, incidence of nausea and vomiting was 62% in the placebo group and 37% in the scopolamine group. Patients treated with scopolamine also required significantly less additional antiemetic therapy and were subsequently discharged from the hospital 30 minutes earlier than the placebo patients—a statistically significant difference. The authors concluded that transdermal scopolamine is a safe and effective antiemetic for outpatients undergoing laparoscopy.

Only a small number of studies have compared atropine with placebo for the prevention of PONV. Most investigations failed to show atropine as being significantly better than placebo. Thus, this agent is not commonly used as an antiemetic preoperatively (11). Atropine (0.2–0.6 mg IV) is occasionally used in the PACU for the treatment of PONV believed to be vagally mediated, although one must be aware of its cardiovascular effects.

Antidopaminergics

Metoclopramide (Reglan) is a specific antidopaminergic drug (but not a phenothiazine) that does not possess antihistaminic properties. It increases lower esophageal sphincter tone and the rate of gastric emptying, with minimal sedation. Metoclopramide has a short half-life and should be administered at the conclusion of surgery or immediately postoperatively to have a lasting antiemetic effect postoperatively.

When compared with 10 mg of prochlorperazine (Compazine) in a 600-patient study, 20 mg of metoclopramide proved significantly more effective and lacked side effects; peak effects occurred in three hours (12).

Rao *et al.* evaluated ambulatory laparoscopy patients who had taken metoclopramide 10 mg orally either alone or in combination with cimetidine 300 mg orally at home on the morning of surgery. These patients had a significant decrease in PONV compared with either control or cimetidine-only groups (13). Rao *et al.* also noted that 10 mg of metoclopramide relieves PONV within 5 to 10 minutes of its intravenous administration and does not prolong PACU stay.

A combination of droperidol (0.5–1.0 mg IV administered 3–6 minutes prior to induction of anesthesia) and metoclopramide (10–20 mg IV administered 15–30 minutes prior to droperidol) was reportedly more effective in preventing nausea and vomiting than droperidol alone, and considerably shortened PACU stay (14).

In contrast, other studies employing doses of metoclopramide ranging from 0.3 to 3.0 mg/kg failed to show metoclopramide's value as an effective antiemetic. Kortilla *et al.* (15) observed that metoclopramide was no better than placebo for either prophylaxis or treatment of postoperative vomiting. In addition, metoclopramide may elicit a dystonic reaction, especially when given via the intravenous route.

Antihistamines

Antihistamines are excellent agents to counter motion sickness, acting mainly at the vomiting center and on vestibular pathways; they can, however, cause excessive sedation. Hydroxyzine hydrochloride (Vistaril) 25–100 mg IM is commonly administered as an adjunct to intramuscular narcotic injections. It lasts for four to six hours, during which time it also potentiates the central nervous system depressant actions of narcotics and barbiturates (and their doses may need to be reduced).

Butyrophenones

Droperidol (Inapsine) and haloperidol (Haldol) are powerful antidopaminergic agents with neuroleptic properties.

Droperidol has received much attention as an antiemetic, and studies confirm its effectiveness as such in doses of 0.625–5 mg either IV or IM (15–18). Droperidol 5 mg IM has an onset of approximately two hours; 0.625–1.25 mg IV works within 30 minutes.

Wetchler and co-workers (18) reported that droperidol 0.625–1.25 mg IV given immediately after intubation was an effective prophylactic antiemetic for outpatients undergoing laparoscopic tubal surgery. Patients who received droperidol during anesthesia had a lower incidence of nausea and vomiting in the PACU, significantly less severe emetic symptoms, and a shorter length of stay than the control group.

Intravenous droperidol is the authors' prophylactic drug of choice for two reasons: its long duration of activity (12–24 hours) and its efficacy. In the PACU, we administer droperidol 0.625–1.25 mg IV to patients who are at significant risk for postoperative symptoms or who experience persistent nausea or vomiting.

Although effective, droperidol may produce extrapyramidal symptoms, hypotension, and sedation. These side effects are generally less severe than those seen with phenothiazines.

Droperidol potentiates central nervous system depressants and, if administered during the final phases of recovery care, may prolong the time to discharge. In an outpatient setting, the maximum antiemetic dose of droperidol should not exceed 2.5 mg; with doses above 1.25 mg, drowsiness becomes more noticeable.

There have been two case reports of extrapyramidal reaction, including dystonia and motor restlessness, occurring approximately three hours after outpatients received prophylactic low-dose (0.625 mg IV) droperidol. Intravenous diphenhydramine (Benadryl) 25–50 mg is an effective treatment for extrapyramidal reactions. It may be necessary to repeat this treatment over the next 24 hours.

Haloperidol is a potent prophylactic antiemetic with a 12-hour duration of action after intramuscular injection. Tornetta (19) demonstrated that haloperidol in doses of 0.5–4.0 mg IM was effective in women undergoing minor gynecological operations without significantly prolonging emergence from anesthesia. A 2-mg dose of IM haloperidol was effective in treating vomiting. Onset occurred within 30 minutes, and duration was roughly three hours. Currently, this agent is rarely used for antiemetic purposes.

Phenothiazines

The phenothiazines are predominantly antidopaminergic agents with antiemetic, antihistaminic, and anticholinergic activity. In the past, they were often used as premedicants. Their usefulness as antiemetics is limited by extrapyramidal side effects, which may be noted as long as 24 hours after a single dose. Presently, prochlorperazine (Compazine) is the only phenothiazine that is routinely administered for both prophylaxis and treatment of anesthesia-related nausea and vomiting. Compazine also increases lower esophageal sphincter tone despite its minimal anticholinergic activity. It is effective treatment for vomiting; 5–10 mg IM takes effect in 30 to 60 minutes and remains effective for four hours. Onset of action may be hastened with intravenous injection or rectal suppository.

Thiethylperazine (Norzine, Torecan) is a phenothiazine that lacks antipsychotic activity. It is indicated only for the treatment of nausea and vomiting, and is used primarily for chemotherapy-induced nausea and vomiting. Recent reports indicate that thiethylperazine is as effective as droperidol for the prophylaxis of PONV following outpatient laparoscopy (20). Thiethylperazine 10 mg IM compared favorably with droperidol 1.25 mg IV in a placebo-controlled, 45-patient trial. No adverse reactions were reported in the group treated with thiethylperazine, and sedation was no greater than with placebo. In the droperidol group, one patient exhibited extrapyramidal side effects, and sedation scores were significantly higher than in the placebo group.

Chlorpromazine (Thorazine) 25 mg IM possesses significant prophylactic antiemetic properties. This dose is often accompanied by undue sedation and hypotension, however.

Although an effective prophylactic antiemetic, promethazine (Phenergan) causes significant sedation and delays emergence from anesthesia. It has also been effective at reducing opioid-induced nausea and vomiting when added in low concentration to the syringe providing morphine patient-controlled analgesia (PCA). When administered for the treatment of active vomiting, promethazine 12.5 mg IV has proved effective with minimal hemodynamic changes, but with varying levels of sedation.

Serotonin antagonists

Serotonin antagonists have been the most-studied antiemetics since 1990. These drugs competitively antagonize the effect of serotonin at 5-hydroxytryptamine subtype 3 (5-HT3) receptors centrally in the CTZ and peripherally in the gastrointestinal tract, and appear to lack the unwanted side-effect profiles of the other classes of antiemetics. Ondansetron (Zofran), which is structurally related to serotonin, possesses specific 5-HT3 receptor antagonism. Although a single dose of ondansetron costs roughly $16.00, many recent studies have demonstrated its efficacy in decreasing PONV with resulting earlier discharge from the PACU. Ondansetron may be administered either orally or over two to five minutes intravenously. Its major site of metabolism is the liver; for patients with moderate or severe hepatic impairment, the dose should be limited to 8 mg in 24 hours.

Khalil et al. (21) compared the prophylactic administration of IV ondansetron with placebo in 589 women undergoing elective outpatient surgery. In the PACU, 1-, 4-, and 8-mg doses of ondansetron proved significantly better than placebo in controlling emesis. Only the 4- and 8-mg doses maintained effectiveness over a 24-hour period, however. No differences were noted in awakening times or adverse events among the three doses, or compared with placebo. The most common adverse events were headache, dizziness, and shivering. The researchers concluded that either 4- or 8-mg doses of IV ondansetron are effective prophylaxis for controlling postoperative emesis, and patients with risk factors for PONV may benefit more from the 8-mg dose.

In a multicenter study (22) (580 ASA I and II female outpatients undergoing ambulatory surgery), those patients who received either 1-, 4-, or 8-mg ondansetron just before the induction of anesthesia had significantly less PONV than did the placebo patients over a 24-hour period. Ondansetron 4 mg IV was found to be the optimal prophylactic dose.

Grond et al. (23) found droperidol 2.5 mg IV more efficacious than ondansetron 8 mg IV for the prophylaxis of PONV in minor gynecological inpatient surgery. Their results agreed with those of other trials that showed droperidol to be significantly more effective than ondansetron in preventing postoperative nausea, but not postoperative vomiting. Grond et al. found a 58-minute-longer time period for arousal and a 23% greater incidence of undesirable central nervous system symptoms in the droperidol-treated group. Thus, droperidol's efficacy with respect to PONV must also take into account its propensity for side effects at this dosage.

Bodner and White (24) completed one of many studies documenting the efficacy of ondansetron in treating PONV. They studied 71 healthy females with PONV following laparoscopy. They found ondansetron 8 mg IV resolved PONV in 49% of patients, versus placebo's 8% success in resolving PONV. Cardiorespiratory variables and sedation scores did not differ significantly between ondansetron and placebo groups.

With respect to postoperative psychomotor recovery performance, several studies (25–27) have been unable to show a statistically significant difference in time to awakening or cognitive function in patients randomly receiving up to 8 mg ondansetron or placebo in outpatient surgery.

Only one case report (28) has been published associating ondansetron with an extrapyramidal reaction. The patient was a 58-year-old male cancer patient who was described as twice having "opisthotonos and difficulty moving because of stiffness and mild shortness of breath" following 10- and 7.5-mg doses of IV ondansetron; the symptoms resolved within 10 minutes. Of interest was that the same patient subsequently received ondansetron 5-mg doses every four hours (following diphenhydramine prophylaxis) for chemotherapy-induced nausea without neurologic side effects.

Sympathomimetics

The prophylactic use of ephedrine to decrease PONV is controversial. Rothenberg et al. found ephedrine 0.5 mg/kg IM prior to conclusion of anesthesia as effective as droperidol 0.04 mg/kg IM and significantly more effective than placebo in reducing PONV (29). On the other hand, Poler and White found that patients treated with ephedrine 25 mg IM before the conclusion of the procedure did not experience any reduction in emetic sequelae (30). Use of this agent generally is limited to the treatment of hypotension.

Conclusion

An important aspect of the preoperative interview is to identify the patient susceptible to PONV. Attention to controllable factors (preanesthetic medication, anesthetic drugs and techniques, and postoperative pain management) and familiarity with antiemetic agents may potentially reduce postoperative nausea and/or emesis. In the event that the first-choice drug is ineffective, we suggest that either the dose be repeated or a second agent be given, preferably one with a different mechanism of action. Aggressive IV hydration and pain management are important components of the therapeutic regimen as well.

For surgical patients without significant risk factors for PONV, we do not administer prophylactic antiemetics. In the PACU, droperidol 0.625 mg IV is the drug of choice for such patients who complain of nausea or who are actively vomiting or retching. For patients who are drowsy or for whom droperidol proves ineffective, prochlorperazine 5–10 mg IV/IM or metoclopramide 0.15 mg/kg IV is administered. Often the prochlorperazine dose is divided such that the patient receives 2.5–5 mg IV and 2.5–5 mg IM, allowing for faster onset, longer duration, and less incidence of extrapyramidal reactions.

For surgical patients with known significant risk factors for PONV, prophylactic antiemetics are administered; droperidol 0.625–1.25 mg IV (near the conclusion of surgery) or ondansetron 4–8 mg IV (immediately preoperatively) is the initial medication administered. In the PACU, initial antiemetic drug therapy for these patients who complain of nausea or who are actively vomiting or retching is either droperidol 0.625–1.25 mg IV or ondansetron 4–8 mg IV; the patient typically receives the antiemetic that he or she did not receive prophylactically. Patients who become nauseated when sitting upright or attempting to ambulate are treated with bed rest, IV hydration, and/or ephedrine 5–25 mg IV.

If PONV persists, the situation should be explained to both the patient and family, and the patient should consider spending the night in the hospital.

Many patients prefer to recover at home, and are given a compazine suppository to take with them. These patients should be instructed to call their physician, the facility, or the emergency room if their symptoms persist or worsen after leaving the hospital. The patient may then need to return to the hospital for further evaluation and possible readmission.

REFERENCES

1. Bridenbaugh LD, Soderstrom RM. Lumbar epidural block anesthesia for outpatient laparoscopy. J Reprod Med 1979;12:85–86.
2. Dent SJ, Ramachandra V, Stephen CR. Postoperative vomiting: incidence, analysis, and therapeutic measures in 3000 patients. Anesthesiology 1955;16:564–572.
3. Smessaert A, Schehr CA, Artusio JF Jr. Nausea and vomiting in immediate post-anesthetic period. JAMA 1959;170:118–122.
4. Bailey PL, Streisand JB, Pace NL, et al. Transdermal scopolamine reduces nausea and vomiting after outpatient laparoscopy. Anesthesiology 1990;72:977–980.
5. Palazzo MGA, Strunin L. Anaesthesia and emesis. 1. Etiology. Can Anaesth Soc J 1984;31:178–187.
6. Palazzo MGA, Strunin L. Anaesthesia and emesis. 2. Prevention and management. Can J Anaesth Soc J 1984;31:407–415.
7. Blumfeld J. Prevention of sickness after anaesthetics. Lancet 1899;ii:833–834.
8. Meeter SE, Kitz DS, Young ML, et al. Nausea and vomiting after outpatient laparoscopy: incidence, impact on recovery stay and cost. Anesth Analg 1987;66:S116.
9. McCarroll SM, Mori S, Bras PJ, et al. The effectiveness of gastric intubation and removal of gastric contents on the incidence of postoperative nausea and vomiting. Anesth Analg 1990;70:S262.
10. Stark RD, Binks SM, Dutka VN, O'Connor KM, Arustein MJA, Glen JB. A review of the safety and tolerance of propofol ("Diprivan"). Postgrad Med J 1985;61(suppl. 3):152–156.
11. Rowbatham DJ. Current management of postoperative nausea and vomiting. Br J Anaesth 1992;69(suppl 1):46S–59S.
12. Tornetta FJ. Studies with the new antiemetic metoclopramide. Anesth Analg 1969;48:198–204.
13. Rao TLK, Madhavareddy S, Chinthagada M, et al. Metoclopramide and cimetidine to reduce gastric fluid pH and volume. Anesth Analg 1984;63:1014–1016.
14. Doze VA, Shafer A, White PF. Nausea and vomiting after outpatient anesthesia: effectiveness of droperidol alone and in combination with metoclopramide. Anesth Analg 1987;66:S41.
15. Kortilla K, Kauste A, Auvinen J. Comparison of domperidone and metoclopramide in the prevention and treatment of nausea and vomiting after balanced general anesthesia. Anesth Analg 1979;58:396–400.
16. Patton CM, Moon MR, Dannemiller FJ. The prophylactic antiemetic effect of droperidol. Anesth Analg 1974;53:361–364.
17. Rita L, Goodarzi M, Seleny F. Effect of low dose droperidol on postoperative vomiting in children. Can Anaesth Soc J 1981;28:259–262.
18. Wetchler BV, Collins IS, Jacob I. The antiemetic effects of droperidol on the ambulatory surgery patient. Anesth Rev 1982;9:23–26.
19. Tornetta FJ. Double blind evaluation of haloperidol for antiemetic activity. Anesth Analg 1972;51:964–967.
20. Jacobs BR, O'Connor TZ. Controlled comparison of the antiemetic efficacy of thiethylperazine and droperidol in outpatient surgery. Anesth Analg 1991;72:S122.
21. Khalil NK, Kataria B, Pearson K, et al. Ondansetron prevents postoperative nausea and vomiting in women outpatients. Anesth Analg 1994;79:845–851.
22. Kovac A, McKenzie R, O'Connor T, et al. Prophylactic intravenous ondansetron in female outpatients undergoing gynecologic surgery: a multicenter dose-comparison study. Eur J Anesth 1992;9(suppl 6):39–50.
23. Grond S, Lynch J, Diefenbach C, Altrock K, Lehmann KA. Comparison of ondansetron and droperidol in the prevention of nausea and vomiting after inpatient minor gynecologic surgery. Anesth Analg 1995;81:603–607.
24. Bodner M, White PF. Antiemetic efficacy of ondansetron after outpatient laparoscopy. Anesth Analg 1991;73:250–254.

25. Kovac A, Steer P, Hutchinson M, Calkins J, Joslyn A. Effect of ondansetron in recovery time, sedation level and discharge from ambulatory surgery. Anesthesiology 1991;75:A7.

26. Lessin JB, Azad SS, Rosenblum F, Bartowski RR, Marr A. Does antiemetic prophylaxis with ondansetron prolong recovery time? Anesth Analg 1991;72:S162.

27. Pearson KS, From RP, Ostman LP, et al. Psychomotor effects of IV ondansetron in female outpatients. Anesthesiology 1991;75:A8.

28. Halperin JR, Murphy B. Extrapyramidal reaction to ondansetron. Cancer 1992;69:1275.

29. Rothenberg D, Parnass S, Newman K, et al. Ephedrine minimizes postoperative nausea and vomiting in outpatients. Anesthesiology 1989;71:A322.

30. Poler SM, White PF. Does ephedrine decrease nausea and vomiting after outpatient anesthesia? Anesthesiology 1989;71: A995.

Index